PHYSICAL ACTIVITY AND CHILDREN: NEW RESEARCH

PHYSICAL ACTIVITY AND CHILDREN: NEW RESEARCH

NOEMIE P. BEAULIEU
EDITOR

Nova Science Publishers, Inc.
New York

NOTICE TO THE READER

The Publisher has taken reasonable care in the preparation of this book, but makes no expressed or implied warranty of any kind and assumes no responsibility for any errors or omissions. No liability is assumed for incidental or consequential damages in connection with or arising out of information contained in this book. The Publisher shall not be liable for any special, consequential, or exemplary damages resulting, in whole or in part, from the readers' use of, or reliance upon, this material.

Independent verification should be sought for any data, advice or recommendations contained in this book. In addition, no responsibility is assumed by the publisher for any injury and/or damage to persons or property arising from any methods, products, instructions, ideas or otherwise contained in this publication.

This publication is designed to provide accurate and authoritative information with regard to the subject matter covered herein. It is sold with the clear understanding that the Publisher is not engaged in rendering legal or any other professional services. If legal or any other expert assistance is required, the services of a competent person should be sought. FROM A DECLARATION OF PARTICIPANTS JOINTLY ADOPTED BY A COMMITTEE OF THE AMERICAN BAR ASSOCIATION AND A COMMITTEE OF PUBLISHERS.

LIBRARY OF CONGRESS CATALOGING-IN-PUBLICATION DATA

Physical activity and children : new research / Noemie P. Beaulieu (editor)
        p. cm.
ISBN 978-1-60456-306-1 (hardcover)
    1.   Exercise for children—Case Studies. 2. Physical fitness for children—Case studies. I
       Beaulieu, Noemie P. GV443.P425 2008
       613.7'042—dc22

Published by Nova Science Publishers, Inc. New York

CONTENTS

PREFACE

Physical inactivity is a major risk factor for developing coronary artery disease. It also increases the risk of stroke and such other major cardiovascular risk factors as obesity, high blood pressure, low HDL ("good") cholesterol and diabetes. The American Heart Association recommends that children and adolescents participate in at least 60 minutes of moderate to vigorous physical activity every day. Increased physical activity has been associated with an increased life expectancy and decreased risk of cardiovascular disease. Physical activity produces overall physical, psychological and social benefits. Inactive children are likely to become inactive adults. This book presents new research in the field from around the world.

Chapter 1 - Children and young people are now recommended to take part in at least 60 minutes of moderate to vigorous physical activity daily to promote and protect healthy heart function, increase bone and muscle strength, improve mood and lower the risk of depression, and reduce the risks of obesity, osteoporosis and diabetes. Yet how easy is it for young people to achieve these required 60 minutes in modern cities that are dominated by traffic and busy roads with miles of low density urban sprawl promoting high car dependence, with young people living in increasingly larger homes built on smaller blocks with busy parents concerned about personal and traffic safety? What role does the built environment play in young people's physical activity; the neighbourhoods and homes where children live, go to school, and play? How important is it to provide communities with safe walking routes to school and with a variety of local destinations within walking or cycling distance? How important is the home, including the size of, and equipment in, the back yard? In this chapter, the authors examine the literature that explores why physical activity is so crucial to healthy physical development and why physical activity is required to enhance positive social development and psychological well-being. The authors turn their attention to studies exploring how different aspects of the built environment appear to influence the physical activity of younger children, of adolescents and the differences between males and females. Finally the authors consider whether the current norms of "good parenting" prevent or facilitate young people's physical activity.

Chapter 2 - In an island nation with easy access to water, opportunity for young New Zealanders to recreationally engage in aquatic activity abounds. While participation in aquatic activity is generally perceived as a positive indicator of a healthy lifestyle, it does have attendant negative consequences. Drowning as a consequence of aquatic activity is a significant cause of unintentional death among young New Zealanders. In spite of some evidence of the popularity of aquatic recreation, little is known about the nature of that recreation and its associated risk of drowning. It is the purpose of this chapter to ascertain what youth do in the aquatic environment and how their behaviour might exacerbate the risk of drowning inherent in water-based activities.

A 25-item questionnaire was designed to survey a nationwide sample of 15–19-year-old New Zealand high school students (N = 2,202). Students from 41 schools who were in their final year of compulsory schooling (Year 11) completed the self-complete, written questionnaire during school time to assess the nature and extent of their participation in aquatic recreation and their associated water safety knowledge and behaviour.

Almost all the youth surveyed had taken part in some swimming (98%) or other aquatic activity (94%) in the previous year. Most students had swum at public/school pools (89%) and patrolled surf beaches (76%). Two thirds of the participants reported having taken part in paddling (67%) and surfing (65%) activities. Risk of drowning was exacerbated among many students because, in addition to high levels of exposure to risk, they often reported at-risk behaviours during their activities. For example, many had swum outside patrol flags (61%) or had swum when cold or tired (56%). One half (50%) of youth reported having swum in a prohibited place or having swum alone (47%). One fifth had never worn a lifejacket (19%) or had consumed alcohol (21%) during aquatic recreation.

Even though youth that took part in this study generally reported higher levels of aquatic recreation than that previously reported for other age groups, this increased participation has attendant increased risks to health and wellbeing for youth because of the high levels of at-risk behaviour reported by some youth. When behaviour was analysed by gender, socio-economic status and ethnicity, the prevalence of risky behaviours among males was consistent and pronounced, the effect of socio-economic status and ethnicity less so. Taken separately, any of the risky behaviours is capable of heightening drowning risk; taken collectively they offer strong explanation as to why some youth, especially males, are at greater risk of drowning than others. Consequently, while encouraging youth to participate in aquatic activity, emphasis on doing so safely by educating youth about the inherent risks of drowning and their role in drowning prevention appear to be warranted.

Chapter 3 - This review presents a new approach to assessing swimming skill through the analysis of the inter-limb coordination: inter-arm coordination in the alternate strokes (front crawl and backstroke) and arm-leg coordination in the simultaneous strokes (breaststroke and butterfly). Based on Newell's concept of constraints [27], for whom constraints may be viewed as features that reduce the degree of freedom of the human motor organisation, the authors aimed to identify the three types of constraint (organismic, environmental and task), all of which can serve as control parameters in experiments designed to determine how and why inter-limb coordination in swimming changes. The lag time between the propulsion of one limb and the other, or one set of limbs and the other, has often been considered a mistake, but this type of experiment has shown that lag time can be an adaptation to a relative constraint. Scientists, coaches and instructors are invited to revisit the theoretical knowledge of biomechanics and motor control in the contexts of competitive swimming, swim training programs and instructions to beginners. Practical applications are proposed to improve inter-limb coordination in children and/or unskilled swimmers.

Chapter 4 - The purpose of this chapter is to describe the exercise capacity of children with cyanotic congenital heart disease (Fontan circulation and Tetralogy of Fallot) and secondly to summarize the available evidence on exercise training in these patients. Eleven patients with a Fontan circulation (5 males and 6 females) with a mean age of 9.5 ± 3.5 years (range 6.4-16.5) and 12 patients with Tetralogy of Fallot (7 males and 5 females) with a mean age of 12.6 ± 3.7 years (range 6.7-18.8) underwent a maximal exercise test. The results were compared to reference values for Dutch children matched for age and sex. Data were expressed as Z-scores. Moreover, based on current literature, best evidence guidelines on physical activity and exercise training will be provided.

Z-score of $\dot{V}_{O2peak}$/kg in Fontan patients was -3.17 ± 1.22 (p<0.001) and in Tetralogy of Fallot patients -1.22 ± 0.94 (p<0.01). Z-score of peak heart rate was -5.90 ± 3.28 in Fontan patients and -2.10 ± 1.98 in patients with Tetralogy of Fallot. Peak work load (p=0.009), duration of test (p=0.008), $\dot{V}_{O2peak}$/kg (p<0.001), peak heart rate (p=0.002), oxygen pulse (p=0.008), ventilation (p=0.002) and oxygen saturation (p=0.003) were all significant lower in the Fontan group compared to the Tetralogy of Fallot patients.

Conclusion: A reduced exercise capacity in patients with a Fontan circulation and patients with Tetralogy of Fallot is observed compared to reference values. Exercise capacity in Fontan patients was significantly lower compared to Tetralogy of Fallot patients. Best-evidence guidelines for physical activity and exercise training are provided.

Chapter 5 - The development of musculoskeletal system is one of the major features of childhood and adolescence. Although growth and maturation of the cardiovascular and skeletal systems have been the focus of important research activities in recent years, the muscle system has received relatively little attention and the results were somewhat controversial. This lack of information on the musculoskeletal system during growth is mainly attributable to ethical and methodological constraints associated with paediatric testing. Besides the limited use of muscle biopsies, 31-phosphorus magnetic resonance spectroscopy (^{31}P-MRS) and Magnetic Resonance Imaging (MRI) are potent tools to investigate the musculoskeletal system. In adults, MRI and ^{31}P-MRS have been used for the non-invasive estimation of muscle fibre type composition. It has been shown that MRI-derived longitudinal and transversal relaxation times were positively correlated to the relative percentage of slow-twitch muscle fibres. Also, it has been shown that the resting phosphocreatine-inorganic phosphate ratio (PCr/Pi) measured by ^{31}P-MRS could be considered as a good indicator of muscle fibre type composition. For instance, the PCr/Pi ratio in the type I muscle was shown to be clearly lower than in the type II muscle. In addition, mapping of muscles activated during exercise is another interesting issue which can be addressed using MRI. Exercise-induced transversal relaxation time changes have been used in order to locate activated muscles and also as a quantitative index of exercise intensity. This approach, along with surface electromyography, provides an interesting avenue of investigation into the changes of muscle recruitment pattern during growth. In conclusion, the advent of technologies which are non-invasive, ethical for use on children and allow muscle bioenergetics to be measured during exercise will significantly enhance scientists understanding of children's physical activity.

Chapter 6 - Gage (1991) defined energy conservation as one of the five major determinants of normal gait. The mechanical cost of walking is dependent on the amount of positive work that must be performed by the muscles to move the whole body, to accelerate body segments and to overcome energy absorption at other joints and because of antagonistic co-contractions. Positive mechanical work production requires muscular (metabolic) work. Adults prefer walking at the speed when the energetic cost is minimal (Winter, 1990). The energetics of walking is quite different in young children as the kinematics, kinetics and muscle activation patterns during gait are still maturing (Cavagna et al., 1983; Hallemans et al., 2004; Ivanenko et al., 2004; Schepens et al., 2004). Also changes in size and morphology during childhood affect the mechanical en metabolic costs of locomotion (De Jaeger et al., 2001). Mechanical work necessary to lift the body against gravity is large at the onset of independent walking, since the energy saving inverted pendulum mechanism is not yet fully mastered (Hallemans et al., 2004; Ivanenko et al., 2004). Also the work necessary to move the limbs relative to the centre of mass is greater in children than in adults (Cavagna et al., 1983; Hallemans et al., 2004; Schepens et al., 2004). Furthermore, standing energy expenditure rate is large in 3 to 4 year old children and decreases with age (De Jaeger et al., 2001). The age related decrease in metabolic energy expenditure is larger than the observed decrease in normalised mechanical work. This suggests that young children have a lower muscular efficiency of (positive) work production than adults (Schepens et al., 2004). Differences in mechanical work, metabolic energy cost and muscular efficiency between children and adults disappear by the age of 10 (Cavagna et al., 1983; De Jaeger et al., 2001; Schepens et al., 2004).

Chapter 7 - While children are among the most active segments of our society, their physical activity amounts decrease with age during school years, and a considerable portion of children are physically inactive. Physically inactive children are more likely to remain sedentary in their adulthood years, which will result in a higher rate of prevalence and premature death of lifestyle diseases. Thus, early identification of sedentary children and "untracking" of sedentary living are critical to public health promotion and disease prevention. Accumulative research results, plus the most recent findings, have documented that field-dependent children may be a less athletically skilled and physically inactive subpopulation that needs immediate attention and intervention.

Field-dependent children, which constitute one-quarter of total children and adolescents population, are consistently and constantly documented to be less competent in sport-related settings. Compared with their field-independent counterpart, field-dependent children and adolescents are less athletically skilled, less involved in school varsity sports, and slower or less effective in motor skill acquisition. In addition, in a series of studies comparing field-independent and field-dependent children's learning behaviors in physical education classes, field-dependent children are found to have more problems to understand and remember directions, have more off-task behaviors, and tend to reduce complex tasks to simpler and easier ones when performing them. As a result, field-dependent children experience much less success academically.

Given the consistent findings regarding field dependence-independence in sport-related settings and the importance of regular physical activity participation to health promotion and disease prevention, the research has recently been extended by investigating the relationship between field dependence-independence and children's physical activity participation. It has been found that, compared with field-independent children, field-dependent children are less likely to participate in organized sports, tend to choose physical activities with less energy expenditure, and have significantly smaller daily physical activity amounts. In addition, new research findings also suggest that African-American children who are less physically active than Caucasian children are significantlly more field-dependent than the latter.

This chapter will introduce the concept and assessment of field dependence-independence first, and then report the accumulated findings regarding the impact of field dependence-independence on sports levels, novel motor skill aquization, and behaviros in phsycial education. Finally, the latest research results with respect to field dependence-independence and children's physical activity participation will be reported. The possible strategies enhancing field-dependent children's sports skill and physical activity level will also be discussed.

Chapter 8 - Regular participation in physical activity is considered critical for healthy and active lifestyles among children and adults in the United States. Accordingly, many schools have incorporated running programs into their physical education curricula to maintain and enhance physical activity levels of children. Regular running has been shown to reduce the risk of coronary heart disease, obesity and enhance perceived competence and self-esteem. However, little is known about children's motivation in such programs. Even less is known about how their motivation in such programs might change over time. Inquiry into this area represents a valuable endeavor in the journey to our understanding of how motivational processes might change in children involved in physical activity. Therefore, this longitudinal study examined how children's motivation and performance changed in required running programs conducted during regularly scheduled physical education classes. Specifically, guided by the expectancy-value model of achievement choices, this study examined whether mean levels of children's expectancy beliefs, task values (importance, interest, and usefulness), intention for future running participation, and their running performance changed across grade levels and by gender. Participants (N = 90; 53 boys; 37 girls) completed a timed 1 mile run and questionnaires four times over a three-year period: twice in the fourth grade (September and May) and again at the end of the fifth and sixth grades respectively. During the study, students made the transition from elementary to intermediate school at the beginning of the fifth grade. A 13-item, 5-point Likert scale questionnaire, adapted from previous work with elementary children, assessed children's expectancy beliefs, task values, and intention for future running participation. The 1 mile run assessed the children's running performance. Results revealed no declines in children's expectancy beliefs in running across grades 4-6. But children's task values of running and intention for future running participation decreased as they advanced from elementary to intermediate school. Additionally, children's 1 mile run times consistently improved across all three grades. Lastly, there were no significant gender differences across all variables from fourth to sixth grade. Overall, this study's results are consistent with those of longitudinal classroom research that children's task values of schooling decline over the school years. They also provided empirical evidence that negative effects of school transition on children's motivation observed in the classroom also existed in the physical activity context. Research efforts should be made to help students maintain their motivation for running during the middle school years.

Chapter 9 - The purpose of the study was to determine the rate of development of motor error detection capability in elementary school children. Fifty-five children aged 6 - 11 yrs and 9 adults (mean age 26 yrs) tossed 2 oz and 4 oz beanbags with eyes closed to a floor target located 198 cm away. Participants performed 16 acquisition trials using an underhand toss, 8 trials for each weight bag using both dominant and non-dominant hands. Following each trial, the participant was asked to estimate where the tossed bag landed by placing a second beanbag at the predicted landing point. The actual landing point was then revealed to the participant. Following the acquisition trials, 8 trials were performed without feedback of the actual landing point. The mean absolute difference in distance between the actual landing point and the estimated landing point was the measure of error detection capability. Throwing accuracy was also determined by measuring the absolute distance between the landing point of the toss and the center of the target board. Acquisition accuracy improved significantly with age, from 58 cm error for the 6 yr olds to 21 cm for the adults. Error detection capability also improved significantly with age with estimation errors decreasing from 51 cm in the 6 yrs olds to 20 cm in the adults. Accuracy and estimation errors were reduced on the no feedback trials compared to acquisition. Trial-to-trial variability also improved with age for both accuracy and estimation scores. The results suggest that accuracy in force production and the ability to detect errors based on proprioceptive feedback improves markedly with age. The results imply that teachers, coaches, and clinicians can expect reliable estimations from children about their movements, particularly as they approach 11 and 12 years of age.

Chapter 10 - The regression line equation obtained through the relationship between swimming distances and respective time durations has been used to provide the estimation of the critical velocity value. This value is considered a good indirect indicator of the anaerobic threshold and, consequently, a measure of the functional aerobic capacity of swimmers. However, even in young swimmers, the majority of swimming events last less than 2.30 minutes, which reflects the importance of the anaerobic energy production as a major contributor during competition.

The purpose of this study was to assess, in young swimmers, an "anaerobic" critical velocity (AnCV), assessed with shorter test distances that could allow scientists and coaches to possess a new tool for anaerobic training control. The existence of a relationship between the AnCV and the performance during a 100 m front crawl event (first and second 50 m splits, and total time), being accepted as a good example of an anaerobic swimming effort, was tested.

A group of 32 competitive swimmers of the North of Portugal regional swimming team, 15 girls (12.3±0.7 years old, 160.5±4.7 cm, 45.6±6.6 kg and 6.3±0.5 training sessions/week) and 17 boys (13.2±0.7 years old, 169.8±9.0 cm, 54.5±7.6 kg and 6.6±0.9 training sessions/week) were included in the study. To obtain the AnCV values through the distance/duration regression line, the swimmers swam three distances in front crawl (12.5, 25 and 50 m) at maximum velocity, separated by a 30-minute rest interval. This methodology is a mode-specific non-invasive method, hypothesised to estimate parameters normally obtained from blood lactate analysis. The 100 m front crawl performance values were obtained in real competition events. Mean plus SD values for AnCV and 100 m front crawl were 1.48 ± 0.06 m/s and 68.3 ± 2.0 s, and 1.62 ± 0.06 m/s and 62.4 ± 2.6 s, respectively for female and male swimmers (differences between genders were observed for both parameters for a $p < 0.001$). It was found a strong inverse relationship between the AnCV and the 100 m front crawl time ($r = -0.84$), the first 50 m partial ($r = -0.87$) and the second 50 m partial ($r = -0.79$), all for a $p < 0.001$ ($n = 32$). The value of the AnCV converted in 100 m time was not different from the 100 m front crawl event duration for each gender group ($p > 0.05$).

To the authors knowledge, it was the first time that the anaerobic critical velocity concept was presented for front crawl, suggesting that AnCV can be used as a control parameter for the training development of anaerobic capacities.

Chapter 11 - Children's fitness, once taken for granted, is now the centerpiece of a national effort to improve the health of all Americans (e.g., Healthy People 2010). A critical focus of this effort is the role of school physical education (PE). Recently, concern has shifted to time/space/budgetary constraints and the efficacy of PE to meaningfully impact children's fitness. The purpose of this study was to examine growth rates (i.e., change) in fitness performance by children in grades 4-8 during two consecutive school years (i.e., yr.1 =grades

4-7; yr. 2=grades 5-8). The study's design was multi-cohort sequential (i.e., grades 4-8) with eight repeated measures over 21 months. The authors used the FITNESSGRAM to test each child's aerobic capacity, muscular endurance, and flexibility. Hierarchical linear modeling (HLM) analyzed the data. HLM is a multi-level form of regression that models intercept and slope for each participant and permits hypothesis testing about rate of change over time, and factors associated with change. In addition to overall growth-rates on selected fitness subtests, the authors examined the association of age, sex, body mass index (BMI) and participation in organized sports. The authors results varied considerably across the three areas of fitness, but four principal findings emerged: a) Very substantial gains occurred in aerobic performance (i.e., PACER score), ($p< .001$); b) the authors found small but significant gains in muscular endurance (pushups & curl ups) and flexibility; c) high levels of BMI (+1.5 SD) exerted a negative pull on aerobic performance, pushups and curl-ups ($p<.05$); and d) participation in after school sports was positively associated ($p< .05$) with better performance, especially PACER score. These results suggest that PE—especially in combination with sports—might foster physical fitness.

Chapter 12 - Children with moderate and severe traumatic brain injuries often have associated physical impairments such as muscle weakness, incoordination, and spasticity as long term sequelae of their injury. The current practice is to provide an individualised therapy program consisting of retraining of motor tasks, specific muscle strengthening and coordination exercises, and fitness and balance activities. However the use of an aerobic exercise program specifically prescribed to the needs of patients as part of the therapy regimen has not been used consistently or evaluated formally. This proposed randomised controlled trial aims to evaluate the benefits of including prescribed aerobic exercises as part of the therapy program in this patient population. Eligible subjects for this study will include children and adolescents aged between 6 and 16 years who have sustained moderate and severe traumatic head injuries as determined by their initial Glasgow Coma Scores (GCS) at least 12 months prior to enrolment. Patients who suffer head injuries with a GCS of 13 or higher are classified as a having mild brain injury, 9 to 12 a moderate injury and 8 or less a severe brain injury. Patients satisfying the selection criteria will be randomly allocated to the control or the intervention groups. Patients in the control group will receive standard rehabilitation therapy as per their conditions. Patients in the intervention group will receive the standard rehabilitation treatment deemed appropriate to their needs, with an extra treatment of a prescribed aerobic exercise program specified by a specialist in sports medicine. The program will last for 12 weeks with 2 sessions per week according to the requirement for significant effects which have been reported in the literature. The primary outcomes of the study are cognition/attention, functional status, mobility, general quality of life, and parental evaluation of the program. Outcome measures have been selected to assess impairment, activity and participation according to the WHO international classification of Functioning, Disability and Health. Data will be collected on each subject at baseline, and 3 months after the intervention. All outcome assessments are measured using standardised and validated clinical assessment tools, or by using calibrated electronic instruments. A standard data analytical approach for randomised controlled trails will be employed for analysing data, taking into consideration multiple outcomes and repeated measurements.

In: Physical Activity and Children: New Research
Editor: N. P. Beaulieu, pp. 1-5

ISBN: 978-1-60456-306-1
© 2008 Nova Science Publishers, Inc.

Expert Commentary

THE RELATIONSHIP BETWEEN PHYSICAL ACTIVITY AND SOCIOECONOMIC STATUS: THE ITALIAN EXPERIENCE ON CHILDREN AND ADOLESCENTS

Giuseppe La Torre[1], Elisabetta De Vito[2], Nicola Nicolotti[1] and Antonietta Monteduro[1]

[1]Institute of Hygiene, Catholic University of the Sacred Heart, Rome, Italy
[2]Chair of Hygiene, University of Cassino, Cassino, Italy

BACKGROUND

Several studies show an association between active lifestyles and a better health status and quality of life, but less evidences are available about socio-economic status (SES) and physical activity (Robert 2000; Ford 1991; La Torre 2006).

METHODS

This chapter will be divided into three parts. The first one will concern data from the Health Survey conducted by the Italian National Statistics Institute (ISTAT). The second and the third ones are cross-sectional studies concerning children and adolescents, respectively. In these studies the association between type of extra-curricular physical activity and socioeconomic status is studied.

The way in considering the SES will be different in the three studies. In ISTAT study the SES of participants was assessed by the educational level, while in the other two we used a SES index derived from parents' job activity.

The statistical analysis was conducted using parametric and non parametric tests. Moreover, multiple logistic regression models were built in order to adjust for possible confounders. The results are expressed as odds ratio (OR) and 95% Confidence intervals (95% CI).

RESULTS

ISTAT Study

Physical activity (PA) at the national level, regular, continuous or light activity, has been reported by 63,5% of Italians. As far as concerns age group, PA is performed by 80,3% of children of 6-17 of age, by 67,1% in those of 18-40 of age and 48,7% in the age group of more than 41 years.

In table 1, the results of the logistic regression are shown.

Cassino Study on Children

In this survey 264 schoolchildren entered the study, 114 males and 150 females. The study sample was formed by 59 children (22.3%) belonging to the age group ≤ 5 years, 82 (31.1%) to the age group 6-8 years and 123 (46.6%) to the older ones (≥ 9 years).

225 children (85.2%) had a normal weight, while 39 some weight problem (at risk of obesity or obesity).

Table 1. Factors associated to Physical activity

	Italy		
	OR	I.C. 95%	p
Gender			
Males	1		
Females	0,80	0,80 - 0,81	< 0,001
Smoking			
Never smokers	1		
Ever smokers	0,91	0,90 - 0,92	< 0,001
Age			
6-17 years	1		
18-40 years	1,11	1,09 - 1,12	< 0,001
≥ 41 years	0,82	0,81 - 0,83	< 0,001
Educational level			
Elementary school	1		
Junior high school	1,45	1,44 - 1,46	< 0,001
Senior high school	2,07	2,06 - 2,08	< 0,001
Degree	2,37	2,36 - 2,38	< 0,001

Concerning BMI, a statistically significant difference emerged according to age group, with older children that showed weight problems (79.5%; $\chi^2 = 20.408$, p<.0.001), while no difference did exist between genders ($\chi^2 = 0.445$; p = 0.505).

The preventive role of PA is often neglected. In fact, only 45.7% of children declared to participate in some extra-curricular PA, and factors that can influence this behaviour are parents' educational level and father's work activity.

PHASES Study on Adolescents

The survey was carried out by submitting an anonymous questionnaire to the students, randomly selected, of the high school coming from the following Italian regions: Lazio, Abruzzo, Molise, Campania, Puglia.

The submitted questionnaire permitted to collect information about the following areas:

- scholastic physical activity
- extra-curricular physical activity
- physical activity attitudes
- lifestyle habits
- parents' physical activity, education and work activity
- students' socio-demographic data.

Concerning extra-curricular physical activity, the students answered that possible types are: football, Dancing/aerobics/gymnastics, Swimming, Volleyball, Basketball, Fitness/body-building, Martial arts, cyclism, other sports (target-shooting, tennis, skiing, fencing and skating). Participants were 1121 males (46.5%) and 1290 females (53.5%), aged between 11 and 17 years (median age 12 years). 33.7% of the students attended the first class, 38.5% the second and 27.8% the third one.

Table 2. Extra-curricular physical activity

	Frequency	Percent
None	523	21,7
Football	613	25,4
Dancing/aerobic/gymnastics	361	15,0
Swimming	303	12,6
Volleyball	232	9,6
Basketball	106	4,4
Fitness/body-building	102	4,2
Martial arts	62	2,6
Cyclism	32	1,3
Other	77	3,2
Total	2411	100,0

Table 3. Type of extra-curricular physical activity and SES in Italian adolescents

	Very high	High	Medium	Medium-low	Low
None	12.2%	14.2%	21.7%	30.1%	30.3%
Football	21.6%	23.7%	24.3%	30.4%	21.2%
Dancing/aerobics/gymnastics	18.5%	15.1%	14.5%	13.1%	12.1%
Swimming	17.0%	16.6%	13.6%	7.0%	12.1%
Volleyball	10.2%	12.4%	10.2%	7.2%	6.1%
Basketball	5.8%	6.8%	3.9%	3.1%	9.1%
Fitness/body-building	6.6%	3.3%	4.3%	3.7%	3.0%
Martial arts	2.8%	3.3%	2.6%	2.0%	3.0%
Cyclism	1.8%	0.3%	1.6%	1.1%	3.0%
Other	3.6%	4.4%	3.3%	2.3%	0.0%
Tot	100.0%	100.0%	100.0%	100.0%	100.0%

Concerning extra-curricular physical activity: 21.7% declared to make no sport, while 25.4% of the students played football, 15.0% performed Dancing/aerobics/gymnastics, 12.6% did swim, 9.6% Volleyball, 4.4% basketball, 4.2% Fitness/body-building, 2.6% Martial arts, 1.3% cycled and 3.2% did other sports (Table 2).

In particular, stratifying every single extra-curricular physical activity for each of five classes of socioeconomic status (Table 3), percentage of student that didn't play any sport had gone from 12.2% in Very high, to 14.2% in High, 21.7% in Medium, 30.1% in Medium-low to 30.3% in Low class.

Football was played with highest percentage especially by students of medium-low class (30.4%). The percentage of students that played football decreased in the other classes: 24.3% in Medium, 23.7% in High, 21.6% in Very high and 21.2% in Low class.

Dancing/aerobics/gymnastics decreased from Very high class (18.5%) to low class (12.1%). Variables like Swan, Volleyball, Fitness/body-building and Martial arts decreased from higher to lower SES classes too.

"Other sport" showed a similar trend: they passed from 3.6% in the Very high class to 2.3% in Medium-low class, but no student of Low SES class played this type of activities.

We can suppose that the trend of these sport depends from the cost of the activities: to play football can be less expense than play swimming, dance, martial arts, target-shooting, tennis, skiing, fencing or skating.

REFERENCES

De Vito E., Arzano I., Berardi D., Capelli G., Gentile A., Langiano E., La Torre G. Prevenzione dell'obesita' infantile: risultati di uno studio pilota in Italia Centrale. *Igiene Moderna* 2004; 121: 301-13.

Ford ES, Merritt RK, Heath GW, Powell KE, Washburn RA, Kriska A, Haile G. Physical activity behaviors in lower and higher socioeconomic status populations. *Am J Epidemiol* 1991; 133 (12): 1246-1256.

ISTAT – *Indagine campionaria sulle condizioni di salute e sul ricorso ai servizi sanitari* 1999-2000.

La Torre G, Iarocci G, Quaranta G, Mannocci A, Ricciardi G. Determinanti dell'attività fisica in Italia. *Igiene e Sanità Pubblica* 2006; 62: 271-82.

La Torre G, Masala D, De Vito E, Langiano E, Capelli G, Ricciardi G, & PHASES collaborative group. Extra-curricular physical activity and socioeconomic status in Italian adolescents. *BMC Public Health* 2006; 6(1):22.

Robert G, Harell S, Bradley B: The influence of physical activity, socioeconomic status, and ethnicity on the weight status of adolescents. *Obesit Research* 2000; 8: 130-39.

In: Physical Activity and Children: New Research
Editor: N. P. Beaulieu, pp. 7-33

ISBN: 978-1-60456-306-1
© 2008 Nova Science Publishers, Inc.

Chapter 1

PHYSICAL ACTIVITY AND YOUNG PEOPLE: THE IMPACT OF THE BUILT ENVIRONMENT IN ENCOURAGING PLAY, FUN AND BEING ACTIVE

Sally F. Kelty[*][†], *Billie Giles-Corti*[†], *Stephen R. Zubrick*[‡]

*Centre for the Built Environment and Health. School of Population Health, M707, University of Western Australia, 35 Stirling Highway, Crawley, 6009, Western Australia

[†]Centre for the Built Environment and Health.
School of Population Health, M707, University of Western Australia, 35 Stirling Highway, Crawley, 6009, Western Australia

[‡]Centre for Developmental Health, Curtin University of Technology and Telethon Institute for Child Health Research. PO Box 855, West Perth, 6872, Western Australia

ABSTRACT

Children and young people are now recommended to take part in at least 60 minutes of moderate to vigorous physical activity daily to promote and protect healthy heart function, increase bone and muscle strength, improve mood and lower the risk of depression, and reduce the risks of obesity, osteoporosis and diabetes. Yet how easy is it for young people to achieve these required 60 minutes in modern cities that are dominated by traffic and busy roads with miles of low density urban sprawl promoting high car dependence, with young people living in increasingly larger homes built on smaller blocks with busy parents concerned about personal and traffic safety? What role does the built environment play in young people's physical activity; the neighbourhoods and homes where children live, go to school, and play? How important is it to provide

[*] Corresponding author: Sally Kelty (Ph.D., BA (Hons)., Bcom). Email: sally.kelty@uwa.edu.au; Tel: 061 8 64887371; Fax: 061 8 64881199.
[†] Email: Billie.Giles-Corti@uwa.edu.au
[‡] Email: S.Zubrick@curtin.edu.au
[†] Email: Billie.Giles-Corti@uwa.edu.au
[‡] Email: S.Zubrick@curtin.edu.au

communities with safe walking routes to school and with a variety of local destinations within walking or cycling distance? How important is the home, including the size of, and equipment in, the back yard? In this chapter, we examine the literature that explores why physical activity is so crucial to healthy physical development and why physical activity is required to enhance positive social development and psychological well-being. We then turn our attention to studies exploring how different aspects of the built environment appear to influence the physical activity of younger children, of adolescents and the differences between males and females. Finally we consider whether the current norms of "good parenting" prevent or facilitate young people's physical activity.

INTRODUCTION

Why do we Need to Discuss Children's Physical Activity at all?

A century ago it would have been unnecessary to write a chapter examining how the built environment could be shaped to encourage youth to be more physically active. People were habitually active: they walked for miles each day. Children were more active before, after, at and en route to school and there were few labour saving devices in homes. Social norms and expectations of the times also resulted in children being engaged in more physically demanding work. However, over the past 50 years there has been a huge societal shift from a lifestyle that was by definition physically active to one that is predominantly sedentary (WHO, 2004). In contemporary lifestyles, the advancement in technology has removed many opportunities for incidental physical activity (PA). Most adults now have sedentary jobs and travel longer distances to work in cars. Most households have many labour saving devices that minimise energy expenditure and maximise convenience, from washing machines, TV remote controls to motorised lawnmowers (Booth, 2000; National Health Forum (NHF), 2007). Moreover, many adults now experience more sedentary working conditions (desk-bound) yet have longer working hours than their parents did during the 1970s (Campbell, 2005). Children in many western nations, like their parents, also lead more sedentary lives with many children doing less than 30 minutes of daily PA (Booth, 2000; Janssen et al., 2005)

Along with more sedentary lives there have also been dramatic changes in the types of foods we eat from fresh unprocessed raw foods to the more convenient packaged highly processed and calorie dense foods (Sallis & Glanz, 2006; Wells et al., 2007). In the US, it is estimated that many children regularly consume over 200 calories in excess of their daily requirements to maintain a healthy weight based on the amount of physical activity in which they engage (Saris & Blair, 2003). A recent Western Australia study showed that since the 1980s, both children and adolescents had increased their consumption of confectionary and snack foods, and decreased their consumption of fruit and vegetables (Hands, Parker, Glasson, Brinkman, & Read, 2004). A recent Federal Australian government report (Australian Institute of Health and Welfare (AIHW), 2006) argued that the imbalance between calorie intake and energy expenditure derived from physical activity is a primary factor influencing the global obesity epidemic. Currently in Australia approximately 18% of boys and 22% of girls aged 15 or under are overweight or obese (AIHW, 2005). With childhood obesity currently rising by 1% annually it is estimated that if this trend is not curbed, by 2025 over one half of young Australians will be overweight and close to one quarter of youth will be obese (Australian Society for the Study of Obesity (ASSO), 2004).

The upward trend in sedentary lifestyles among young people is not just an Australian social phenomenon but is observed worldwide. A recent systematic review of research involving 137,593 child participants across 34 nations found childhood obesity was strongly associated with lower levels of daily physical activity and increased hours spent watching TV (Janssen et al., 2005). People who are obese during adolescence are more likely to remain obese as adults (ASSO, 2004). Adolescents and adults who are severely obese (Body Mass Index (BMI) > 35) are more likely to reduce their life expectancy by 3 to 7 years (AIHW, O'Brien, & Webbie, 2004; Centres for Disease Control and Prevention (CDC), 2007).

Nevertheless, encouraging PA is not just about preventing obesity. There is a substantial body of literature suggesting that physically active youths are both physically and psychologically healthier. Increasing levels of PA in young people is an international priority (WHO, 2004). In order to do so, it is now recognised that programs designed to encourage people to change their diets and be more active may be insufficient to reduce obesity and sedentary lifestyles (Giles-Corti, 2006). Rather, researchers, policy makers and practitioners now recognise that multi-level interventions are required that also consider the role played by the built environment in increasing the PA of both adults and young people (NHF, 2007).

The built environment (BE) is defined as *"the neighbourhoods, roads, buildings, food sources, and recreational facilities in which people live, work, are educated, eat and play"* (Sallis & Glanz, 2006, p.90). It has been suggested that by examining how buildings, neighbourhoods, town and cities are planned and developed we will be able to see how urban and rural environments in the 21st century afford people the opportunity to be more active, especially incidental opportunities encountered in our everyday lives (NHF, 2007). For example, climbing a few flights of stairs rather than riding an escalator or taking the lift.

Fit as a Fiddle: Why Being Active is so Critical for Healthy Physical Development

Apart from obesity, physical inactivity is a leading contributor to the burden of many preventable diseases (Stephenson & Bauman, 2000). There is now strong evidence for the association between physical inactivity and health and that by increasing physical activity, especially during childhood, coronary heart disease, high blood pressure, high cholesterol, sleep apnoea and endometrial, and breast and colon cancers can be prevented or the symptoms better managed (CDC, 2007; WHO, 2004).

Of growing concern is that Type 2 diabetes and fatty liver disease, commonly diagnosed in middle aged adults, is increasingly being diagnosed in adolescents as young as 15 (Baur, 2002; Booth et al., 1997). In 2003, one of the most comprehensive Australian studies of physical activity, obesity and health was carried in New South Wales with a sample of 5500 males and females children aged 5 to 16 years. The findings highlighted growing concerns in that almost 20% of the 15 and 16 year olds sampled had high blood pressure, low concentrations of HDL and high concentrations of LDL cholesterol (all disease markers for the development of Type 2 diabetes and cardiovascular disease). Furthermore, 40% of the obese 15 year old boys had elevated alanine aminotransferase (ALT) levels, an indicator of fatty liver disease. These biomarkers were more prevalent in the physically inactive and obese children. For example, 70% of obese adolescent boys had very high insulin and high ALT levels (Booth et al, 2006). However, it is noteworthy that even children who have developed chronic diseases function better if they are physically active (Goldberg, 1995).

Being physically active as a child is vital for optimal skeletal, joint and muscle growth. Developing a stronger skeletal frame through moderate to vigorous intensity PA (MVPA) creates higher bone density and bone mineral content; both vital for protecting against osteoporosis in later life (Matthews et al., 2006). Bass et al., (1998) observed that MVPA engaged in during the pre-pubertal years, especially for females, represented the optimal time to develop high bone density. As bone density developed before puberty is maintained into adulthood this represents one way that women can help protect themselves from osteoporosis onset after menopause (Bass et al., 1998; Matthews et al., 2006). Paediatric researchers over the past 20 years have found that stronger bones, joints and muscles are developed through moderate to vigorous weight bearing exercise, such as football, ballet, dancing, athletics, rounders/softball and basketball. To accrue this benefit young people require only three hours each week of weight bearing PA (Vicente-Rodr´iguez, 2006).

Thus, encouraging physical activity in childhood makes sense. It is vital for the development of physically healthy adults and insignificantly reduces the risk of developing debilitating chronic diseases.

Healthy Body Healthy Mind: Creating Psychological and Social Well-being through PA

As noted above, children who do not meet the 60 minutes per day of MVPA are more likely to be overweight or obese and hence at greater risk of developing incapacitating chronic diseases in adulthood (Booth et al., 2006). Overweight and obese children have poorer mental health outcomes which can lead to debilitating and prolonged clinical conditions. For example, many overweight and obese children have a negative self body image, have very low self-esteem, experience recurrent suicidal ideation, demonstrate obsessive-compulsive behaviour, and report generalised social anxiety (Chess & Thomas, 1984). Research with obese young people has found strong correlations between more severe clinical depression and high levels of peer rejection, social isolation, and higher levels of on-going ridicule from siblings and parents (Petersen, 2004). Ridicule and social ostracism occurring across a range of social domains (at school, in the community and at home) creates or exacerbates the psychological distress that overweight young people experience (Wodarski & Wodarski, 2004).

Social psychologists have found two prominent factors underpinning "social rejection" for obese children and adults. First, people perceived as obese/overweight are considered to have breached the accepted norm of beauty in most western nations, for women this equates to a toned and slim form, for men a lean and muscular form. Second, because the norm is perceived as "breached", overweight people are then widely stereotyped as lazy, unmotivated to care about their appearance and less intelligent (Rapp-Paglicci, Dulmus, & Wodarski, 2004). Finally, adolescents and adults who are obese are significantly less likely to form lasting relationships and marry, and are more likely to experience entry discrimination into higher education and discrimination in the workplace (Wodarski & Wodarski, 2004).

In contrast, young people who are within a healthy weight range and are physically active, especially those who participate in sports and clubs at and after school, have been found to be more popular among peers, to have higher self-esteem, a more positive body image, have higher self-confidence in their ability to perform across a range of social skills and settings, and overall appear to have more positive mental health and optimism for the future (Rapp-Paglicci et al., 2004; Singer, 1992; WHO, 2004). Young people who are members of sporting teams or have active hobbies (such as dancing or martial arts) are less likely to become regular and heavy smokers, less likely to become acquainted with and then mix with delinquent peers, or take illicit drugs (Akers, 1997). They also self-report feeling a stronger bond to their community, are more likely to feel connected with their school and tend to achieve higher academic marks overall (Chappell & Wilson, 2005; Peterson, 2004).

Young people who participate in team sports or are club members are provided with a rich environment in which specific social skills can be enhanced. For example, young people at clubs learn about teamwork and group co-operation, sharing resources, reading the body language of others, self-discipline, learn to accept loss and defeat, to have improved communication skills, learn sportsmanship, leadership and conflict resolution (Petersen, 2004). Although these skills are not acquired through physical activity directly they are learned in specific social environments. Within sporting clubs young people are exposed to the places and times where certain behaviours are encouraged and rewarded (such as teamwork and gracious losing) while other behaviours are discouraged (bullying or vocal outbursts) (Akers, 1997). According to Petersen (2004) as the skills leant through club memberships are usually generic they are readily transferable to other settings such as in school. It is possible that these generic skills (such as gracious losing, teamwork and co-operation) acquired through sports clubs account in part for why members are more popular with their peers (Petersen, 2004).

In addition to exposure to behavioural rules in sporting clubs, vital skills can also be gained by being active in the neighbourhood (Cornell & Hill, 2006; Rissotto & Giuliani, 2006) that. For example by cycling or walking around local areas young people increase their spatial and local knowledge (where streets connect, location of shops), increase road safety (knowing where they are and how to operate pedestrian crossings), enhance problem solving (mentally retracing and reversing a route taken for the return trip) and develop environmental awareness of fauna and flora and (Cornell & Hill, 2006; Joshi, MacLean & Carter, 1999; Rissotto & Giuliani, 2006).

Activity outside of the home provides young people with the opportunity to increase the social capital of their neighbourhood. For example, active young people are more likely to become acquainted with their neighbours, to learn the unspoken rules of etiquette in road and cycle path user behaviour, and meet store owners and operators of local services (Putnam, 1995). Increasing local area knowledge and becoming acquainted with people in the community enhances the social capital of neighbourhoods by creating communities where people feel they have a bond. This provides young people with a sense of belonging and a sense of place in the world. It is likely that where children experience good interactions with places and people in their neighbourhoods, these positive interactions can lead to an increased engagement in their community and active civic engagement throughout adulthood (Stone, 2001). In practical terms cohesive communities provide young people with safer places to play and be active in two ways. First, more cohesive communities (for example where neighbours monitor each others properties and intervene when faced with suspicious behaviour) are associated with having lower crime rates and less delinquent behaviour (Andrews & Bonta, 1998). Second, as more people socialise and become involved in their communities there is more natural surveillance present simply because a wide range of people are out and about in the neighbourhood (Putnam, 1995; Stone, 2001).

Encouraging PA makes sense from a psychological perspective. Young people who are physically active appear on average to be happier, have more positive thoughts about themselves and their abilities, are more optimistic about their future. Young people who keep physically active by exploring their communities appear to gain the additional benefits of richer and more detailed environmental knowledge and potentially a stronger sense of place and belonging in their local community.

Full of Zip or Quiescent: How Active Are Australian Young People?

Recently endorsed Australian PA guidelines recommend that young people aged 5 to 12 years engage in at least 60 minutes of MVPA each day and limit television viewing and electronic media usage to below two hours a day (Commonwealth Department of Health and Aging, 2006). A sizeable minority of young Australians do not meet these guidelines.

A survey of 5-12 year old children from Brisbane, Queensland found that approximately 20% of the sample were overweight or obese, 14.7% did not meet the recommended 60 minutes of daily MVPA, and 31% of the sample spent more than 2 hours daily watching TV or playing computer games (Spinks, Macpherson, Bain, & McClure, 2007). Of the children who did not engage in 60 minutes of MVPA they were 28% more likely than their peers to be overweight. Of the children who spent more than 2 hours per day watching TV or using computers they were 63% more likely to be overweight (Spinks et al., 2007). Similar results were observed in New South Wales (NSW) with approximately 25% of the 5500 boys and girls surveyed not meeting the 60 minutes of daily MVPA (Booth et al., 2006). The study also observed that obese and overweight boys and girls spent between one to 10 hours more per week in sedentary activates (TV watching, church, crafts, music practice) than their peers with a healthy weight. This study did however find some encouraging results. Compared with an earlier child and adolescent dataset collected by the same research team five years earlier in 1997, of the 75% of healthy weight children and adolescents from the 2003 study who met or exceeded 60 minutes of daily MVPA they had significantly higher levels of cardio-respiratory fitness as recorded by a standard 20-meter shuttle run test (Booth et al., 1997; Booth et al., 2006).

Children's physical activity can take various forms including organised sports during and after school and active recreations such as cycling round the neighbourhood with friends. One means of increasing physical activity in young people is through active transport, especially walking or cycling to and from school. However, there have been marked decreases in the number of Australian children engaging in active transport (Salmon, Timperio, Cleland, & Venn, 2005) Recently, Harten & Olds (2004) estimated that active transport is decreasing in Australia by approximately 1.5% per year. They noted that in Adelaide in 1985 approximately 56% of children used active transport to and from school. By 1998, the number of children using active transport had fallen to 25% (Harten & Olds, 2004). Similar decreases in incidental physical activity provided by walking to school have been observed in the UK (Hillman, Adams, & Whitelegg, 1990), in Italy (Rissotto & Giuliani, 2006) and in the US

(McDonald, 2007). In Britain, the US and in Australia the incidental form of physical activity of walking and cycling to school has been replaced for most children by passive transport: being driven to and from school by car.

HOW THE BUILT ENVIORONMENT INFLUENCES THE PA OF YOUNG PEOPLE

It has become apparent that the way we design our environments can facilitate an active lifestyle (Sallis & Glanz, 2006). People may be more likely to cycle if there are cycle paths present rather than riding on roads (Pikora, Giles-Corti, Bull, Jamrozik, & Donovan, 2003). People may be more likely to walk to local shops, if there are footpaths/sidewalks present rather than having to walk on the road or garden verges (Frank et al., 2006).

Most of the research on PA and built environments (BE) has focused on adults with a relative lack of evidence about how the BE influences the PA of young people. Furthermore, although research shows that the BE can have an influence on physical activity and young people, it appears this influence is not uniform across all ages or genders. In the section that follows, the available evidence is reviewed. Where gender and age differences are observed these will be highlighted.

The literature review is presented in five themes. Four of these themes reflect the framework developed by Pikora et al., (2003) based on their analysis of the public health, transport and urban planning literature. The SPACES framework (see Figure 1), identified four constructs representing distinct aspects of the BE that correlated with higher levels of walking and cycling: functional aspects (i.e. physical aspects, direct routes, footpaths); safety features (i.e. street lighting, surveillance); aesthetics (green space, urban decay); and destinations (distances to and types of places in the neighbourhood, land zoning). For this review, a fifth theme was added to represent an expansion of the SPACES framework and covers the physical aspects of the home environment associated with higher levels of PA in young people, such as the size of the back garden/yard and presence of play equipment.

Which Functional Aspects of the BE Influence the Physical Activity of Youth

Functional aspects of the BE are a group of variables that facilitate the ease with which people can engage in physical activities like walking or cycling, such as footpaths, amount of cars, or gradient of the walking route. Research examining functional aspects with child and/or adolescent samples has mainly focused on the provision and type of footpaths, street connectivity, intersections, traffic speed and urban density.

Five construct themes of how the BE can influence physical activity levels				
External environment				Internal environment
Functional	Safety	Aesthetic	Destination	The home
Direct route **Gradient** **Intersection distance** **Kerb type** **Path location** **Path maintenance** **Street type** **Street width** **Traffic control devices** **Traffic speed** **Traffic volume** **Type of path** **Density/Sprawl** **Street connectivity**	**Crossing aids** **Crossing Lighting** **Verge width** **Surveillance**	**Cleanliness** **Sights** **Garden maintenance** **Parks** **Pollution** **Trees** **Architecture** **Street maintenance**	**Local facilities** **Parks** **Public transport** **Services** **Shops** **Vehicle parking** **Bike parking** **Land mix**	**Play equipment** **Garden** **Home gym** **Exercise DVDs** **Exercise area**

Figure 1. The expanded Pikora et al., (2003) SPACES framework to include the original four constructs together with the inclusion of the home physical environment.

Several studies have found that higher levels of walking for both children and adolescents are associated with the presence of footpaths en route from home to school and home to recreational venues (Boarnet, Anderson, Day, McMillan & Alfonzo, 2005; Evenson, Scott, Cohen, & Voorhees, 2007; Ewing, Schroeer & Green, 2004; and McMillan, 2007. A few researchers explored further whether certain features of footpaths increased levels of walking. In a US sample of male adolescents higher levels of brisk walking was recorded (by accelerometers) when footpaths were free of physical obstructions and where trees had been planted along the paths (Jago, Baranowski, Zakeri, & Harris, 2005). In contrast, Copperman & Bhat (2007) and Mota, Delgado, Almeida, Ribeiro, and Santos (2006) found no relationship between walking levels and condition of footpaths. Furthermore, Ziviani, Kopeshke & Wadley (2006) found that in an Australian sample of primary school children there was no association between the physical condition of footpaths and whether paths were sheltered or covered and the number of children walking to and from school.

The above findings appear to support the hypothesis that regardless of age and gender providing footpaths can increase PA levels. Clearly the presence of a footpath is at least necessary in prompting greater PA. However, the evidence about the provision of shade (and quality of the footpaths) is mixed. As only two studies were identified that have explored the presence of trees on paths further replication is essential. For example, given the risk of skin cancer through sun exposure, especially in Australia and in the US (Edlich et al., 2004), it would be premature to assume that shade trees are not necessary on paths. Moreover, as discussed below, little is known about how the aesthetics of neighbourhoods influences young people's physical activity or the decisions made by parents to allow their children to walk locally. Thus, the presence of attractive streetscapes may have an indirect (rather than direct) influence on young people's PA and this warrants further investigation.

Another aspect of enquiry has been on whether the general walkability of neighbourhoods influences PA. Walkable neighbourhoods, according to Sallis and Glanz (2006) are those which are designed for ease of pedestrian travel, characterised by streets based on the traditional grid system with high levels of connectivity between them offering direct routes; moderate to high urban density; and mixed land use with residential dwellings, shops, utilities, services and parks all within walking distance. In contrast, low walkable neighbourhoods are those where land use is zoned either residential or industrial, with poor access to shops and services and with disconnected street networks based on cul-de-sacs that eventually feed into high speed arterial roads creating a traffic hazard barrier for walkers and cyclists (Sallis & Glanz, 2006). The visible differences between traditional and conventional urban designs can be seen in Figures 2 and 3 below[1].

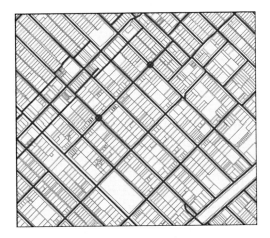

Figure 2. High walkable traditional neighbourhood.[2]

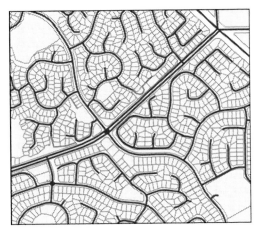

Figure 3. Low walkable conventional neighbourhood.[3]

---

[1] Road and cadastre/lot parcel data provided by Department of Planning and Infrastructure, Perth, Western Australia, 2006.

[2] Figure.2. Traditional grid system of a high walkable inner city suburb in Perth, Western Australia. Suburb is mixed residential (detached Edwardian houses, semi-detached cottages, modern blocks of flats) with mixed retail (shops, pubs, cafés, cinema, hardware, supermarkets) within walking distance.

A few studies have focused on how walkability is associated with higher levels of walking to school (referred to as active transport). In their sample of 9 to 11 year olds, Braza, Shoemaker and Seeley (2004) found that regardless of gender, young people walked to school more often if they lived in a neighbourhood with better street connectivity and higher population density. Similar results were observed in a sample of 11 to 15 year old adolescent girls (Norman et al., 2006), as well as in a sample of to 10 year old boys and girls (McMillian, 2007) and in small sample of older adolescent males and females (Kligerman, Sallis, Ryan, Frank, & Nader, 2007). In contrast, Timperio et al., (2006) found higher levels of walking to school to be associated with less direct routes (poorer street connectivity) for children in the 10 to 12 age range. Nevertheless, these investigators found that routes with gentler inclines were associated with more walking to school for younger children (aged 5 to 6 years).

Walkability is also associated with higher levels of PA in local neighbourhoods out of school hours (evenings and weekends). Frank, Kerr, Chapman, and Sallis (2007) using a large US sample of 3161 males and females aged 5 to 20 years, found significant between-group differences in out-of-school PA. For children aged 5 to 8 years, overall walkability (combined density, street connectivity and land mix) of neighbourhoods was not associated with out of school PA. For children aged 9 to 11, of all three walkability variables measured, only higher density predicted higher levels of PA. For 12 to 15 year olds, two variables were significant: the higher the density and better the street connectivity the higher the out-of-school PA. For older adolescents their recorded levels of PA were lowest of all the age groups. However in the older adolescents who did leave their homes, higher PA was only predicted by better street connectivity. Another study found similar results. Using a sample of Dutch 6 to 12 year olds, de Vries, Bakker, van Mechelen, & Hopman-Rock (2007) found that in 10 cities throughout the Netherlands higher levels of weekly PA was predicted by residential density (but only up to a limit of six stories per building), better street connectivity and more manned zebra crossings. Conversely, Copperman & Bhat, (2007) found that in their US sample of younger children (aged 12 and under) higher levels of out of school PA was associated with low density single zoned land use (urban sprawl).

When the results are combined, it appears that different types of land use and density are associated with different types of PA for children of different ages. Several prominent issues are apparent. First, because most young people are required to attend school this aspect of their lives becomes a prompt for incidental daily PA. The research tells us that the higher the overall walkability of routes to local schools the more children will walk or ride their bikes to school. Second, for out-of-school hours the results are more variable suggesting that a developmental interaction exists between age, density and land use. For younger children some researchers observed that higher density encourages PA (de Vries et al., 2007) while other researchers found that lower density encourages PA (Copperman & Bhat, 2007). In contrast, higher density neighbourhoods with mixed land use is associated with more activity for older children, especially boys (aged 11 and above). The results discussed above highlight the complexities depending upon the age of children and the types of behaviours predicted (either playing at the weekends or walking to school) and suggests that complex developmental interactions exists between age, gender, density and land mix. Given the dearth of research to date and the inconsistency of findings, more detailed studies are

---

[3] Figure 3 is a suburb established in the 1990s on the urban fringe, 14km from Perth, Western Australia. The suburb is primarily detached dwellings with few retail services and no shops within walking distance of most homes.

essential before firm recommendations can be offered related to the impact of neighbourhood density on the PA of young people, particularly with young children and out-of-school hours.

In summary, the literature on the functional aspects appears to provide empirical support for an association between higher levels of PA in young people when certain environmental conditions are present, such as the provision of footpaths and higher density neighbourhoods for older children and adolescents. These appear to interact with developmental age and PA behaviours (i.e. attending school). However, based on the existing research, two questions warrant further investigation. First, do the quality aspects of walking routes (i.e. condition of footpaths, physical geography, available shade) independently contribute to the likelihood of increased PA? Second, what is the nature of the function that links neighbourhood density and land mix to PA for children of differing ages and differing developmental requirements (after school, during school holidays and over weekends)?

Which Safety Aspects of the BE Influence the PA of Children and Adolescents?

Safety aspects of the BE include both objective and subjectively measured variables assessing how safe people actually are, or believe they are, while being active in their neighbourhood. Safety variables include presence of street lighting, level of crime, safe places to cross roads and community surveillance. Objective measures of safety are usually obtained from a Geographic Information System (GIS) or from observer checklists (McMillian, 2007; (Timperio et al., 2006), for example, the number of manned traffic crossings within a kilometre radius around a school. Subjective variables involve self-reported perceptions, either from parents or young people, about how safe they perceive their neighbourhood. Australian research has shown that parental concerns about safety in neighbourhoods is significantly associated with children engaging in lower levels of out of school PA (Timperio, Crawford, Telford, & Salmon, 2004) and with the less active children being significantly more likely to be overweight or obese (Salmon et al., 2005; Timperio, Crawford, Telford, & Salmon, 2005).

The main safety concern for parents in both Australia (Timperio et al., 2004) and in the US (McMillan, 2007) appears to be exposure to traffic, especially on busy roads with fast travelling vehicles. Children are less likely to walk to and from school if they have to cross busy roads (Timperio et al., 2006). As Sallis and Glanz (2006) point out, parental concern about traffic exposure is highly understandable given the high rates of childhood injury and death following vehicle accidents. In Australia, motor vehicle accident is the leading cause of death of children aged one to 14 years (Cross & Hall, 2005). In 1995, a Western Australian case control study of child pedestrian behaviour identified three environmental factors that predicted the likelihood of child pedestrian injury (Stevenson, Jamrozik, & Spittle, 1995). Two factors related to safety, namely: personal exposure to high traffic volume and the presence of visual obstructions, such as parked cars creating unsafe places to cross roads (Stevenson et al., 1995).

Parents, especially those with younger children, report being concerned about encounters with strangers who may harm their child (Valentine & McKendrick, 1997). An Australian qualitative study found that "stranger danger" was cited as one of the main reasons for parents restricting their children's ability to go out into the neighbourhood and be independently mobile (Veitch, Bagley, Ball, & Salmon, 2006). Of interest, research has found that children are also concerned about stranger danger (Joshi, MacLean, & Carter, 1999), although their concerns about stranger danger are not at the same level expressed by their parents (Timperio et al., 2004, 2005).

Where parents and children's concerns are similar is regarding the risk posed by unsafe destinations, especially public spaces and parks. Both parents and children have raised concerns about the risk of bullying and antisocial behaviour from delinquent teenagers, as well as the risk associated with used syringes found in public places (Trayers et al., 2006; Veitch et al., 2006). As most of this research has been based on subjective report we have limited knowledge about the level of risk posed by these concerns.

Other prominent safety concerns are surveillance and street lighting. Evenson et al., (2007) found that adolescent girls who had a healthy weight and who were more physically active, compared with their inactive and overweight/obese peers, were more likely to believe their neighbourhoods were safe places in which to be active. These teenagers perceived that there was good surveillance because other walkers and joggers were visible in the area. They were also less concerned than their inactive peers with antisocial behaviour and more likely to judge their neighbourhood as having a low crime rate. McMillian (2007) also found that the surveillance was an important community feature and that younger children were more likely to walk to school if at least 50% of the homes they passed en route had windows facing the street. Evenson et al., (2007) also observed that adolescent girls were more physically active in neighbourhoods where the streets were well lit and when traffic volume was higher on the routes they walked. The association between higher PA and higher traffic volume appears to be counter-intuitive finding given that the main concern of parents and children is traffic risk and given the very real risk of pedestrian injury being high. As this was not a qualitative study the participants were not asked to elaborate about why the presence of more cars influenced more walking. It is possible that the presence of more cars along popular walking routes may provide adolescent girls with additional surveillance simply because more people are around. In addition, it is also possible that the routes used by adolescent girls are to reach destinations and that cars are also using the same route to get to the same destination. Future research using better developmental methods (both quantitative and qualitative) that probe motives for walking, destination, and tasks undertaken would help elucidate this seemingly counterintuitive finding.

Overall the literature supports the hypothesis that safety concerns - whether subjectively or objectively measured - impacts upon the PA levels of young people. The literature suggests that traffic safety, stranger danger, presence of antisocial behaviour in public spaces (gangs or drugs), and lack of street lighting impacts upon whether children are allowed by their parents to be physically active in their neighbourhoods. Furthermore, despite traffic being a major risk for most children it appears to be associated with increased PA for some – notably, adolescent girls. The evidence suggests that as children and young people are to be encouraged to undertake more PA, then it is encumbent upon society to provide safe places to cross roads, well lit streets that make users feel safe in the evenings and a reduction in the levels of antisocial behaviour and drug use in public spaces.

What Aesthetic Aspects of the BE Influence the PA of Children and Adolescents?

The aesthetic aspects of the natural or built environment make being physically active more pleasurable and interesting. Just for a moment, imagine a beautifully maintained garden or park. Now imagine a run down inner city ghetto. It is not difficult to envisage how the aesthetics of an environment may impact on a decision to walk for 30 minutes rather than drive.

The idea that aesthetics is important is not new. For example, the sound of trickling water and its ability to induce mental calmness has been noted in Japanese literature since the 14th Century (Young & Young, 2005). Due to the association between water and tranquillity, streams and water features are essential elements in the Japanese garden (Young & Young, 2005). Other examples of aesthetic variables include the absence or presence of litter or urban decay, the maintenance of private and public gardens and parks and presence or absence of interesting architecture. Several researchers have explored the association between aesthetically pleasing environments (such as parks) with mental health. For example, Kuo and Taylor (2004) found a significant reduction in ADHD symptoms for both boys and girls who were exposed on a weekly basis to green space. Given the calming and pleasing ambiance of some public places it is surprising that more systematic research has not been carried out into how this aspect of the BE can influence the PA of young people.

In a sample of 422 primary school children, de Vries et al., (2007) found that higher levels of PA was associated with the aesthetic features, namely: higher ratings of overall local neighbourhood attractiveness; more green space (parks and gardens); less visible litter; less urban decay; less concrete covered playgrounds. In a Scottish study of 352 adolescent girls, Whitehead, Biddle, O'Donovan and Nevill (2006) found that the aesthetic qualities of local neighbourhoods and sports facilities were important to their female sample. Furthermore they found that one of the main factors associated with whether girls aged 14 and above were physically active at the weekends was whether they rated their overall neighbourhood as attractive with enjoyable scenery. The older girls in the Whitehead et al sample also reported they used sports centres (such as swimming pools) more when the facilities themselves were aesthetically pleasant places to visit. Similar results were found in a sample of Portuguese adolescent girls in that higher levels of PA were reported by the girls who rated their neighbourhoods as more aesthetically pleasuring places to wander around and which offered them interesting things to look at (Mota et al., 2006).

Based on the aesthetic literature to date three issues are prominent. First, although there have been very few studies the findings suggest that young people are more likely to be physically active in neighbourhoods that offer interesting scenery and places to visit. Second, although only tentative evidence is available, it appears that neighbourhood aesthetics may encourage more PA as children age. However, it is not clear how strong the correlation is between aesthetics, age and higher levels of PA. Third, the small number of studies to date are limited to mostly Europe and the US. The extent to which these results can be generalised to Australian and other children and adolescents is not clear.

What Destination Factors Influence the PA of Children and Adolescents?

Destination variables refer to the variety of places and the type of land mix found in neighbourhoods. For example, the mix and number of homes, parks, sports centres, shops, cinemas or public services contained in a geographical area. Recent research with Western Australian adults found that people were more likely to walk if they had a variety of destinations within approximately 400 meters walking distance from their home (McCormack, Giles-Corti, & Bulsara, 2007). The research on young people appears to mirror the finding for adults, namely that the presence and proximity of destinations matters.

Public spaces, especially parks with sports pitches, and sports centres (i.e., recreation centres) are significantly associated with higher MVPA in young people. Research from Australia, Europe and the US suggests that regardless of age (5 to 17 years old) or gender the closer parks and sports centres are to young people's home the more likely they are to use them and the higher their weekly PA. These results have been observed regardless of whether PA is measured through self-report, such as an exercise or PA journal (Brodersen, Steptoe, Williamson, & Wardle, 2005; Carver et al., 2005; de Vries et al., 2007; Frank et al., 2007; Gordon-Larsen, Nelson, Page, & Popkin, 2006; Timperio et al., 2004) or objectively, such as with pedometers or accelerometers (Cohen et al., 2006; Epstein et al., 2006; Evenson et al., 2007).

With respect to proximity when parks and sports centres are within 800 meters of the homes of both children and adolescents (aged 8 to 16) it appears that young people are more likely to use the facility as well as more likely to walk or cycle to get there from their homes (Cohen et al., 2006; Epstein et al., 2006). When facilities are within 800 meters from participants' homes, objective measurement of weekly MVPA has been shown to increase from between 17.2 minutes to 38.9 minutes per week (Epstein et al., 2006). Proximity and choice of venue has also been observed to be important. Evenson et al., (2007) found that when adolescent girls had a choice of between 9 to 14 different physical activity venues close to home, on average their MVPA was higher by 84.9 minutes per week compared with girls who only had 4 venues near their home. Finally, as long as children are able to get to venues, even having one sports centre or dance club within 8kms from their homes has been shown to reduce the risk of being overweight or obese by 5% (Gordon-Larsen et al., 2007).

Certain aspects of parks also have been found to be associated with increasing weekly PA of young people. For example, parks with higher quality sporting pitches and better overall amenities like fresh drinking water were the preferred places for both boys and girls and were significantly associated with higher levels of PA (Cohen et al., 2006). These researchers also found that parks with skateboards ramps were positively associated with higher weekly PA for boys, although negatively associated with girl's PA. As this study was quantitative it is not clear why the presence of a skateboard ramp had a negative impact on the PA of girls. As it is vital that all young people be encouraged to be more active further investigation is required of negative consequences for certain sub-groups e.g., girls. Moreover, further investigation is required of aspects of parks that encourage multiple users such that they encourage boys to use skateboard ramps whilst simultaneously providing girls with an environment that encourages their PA.

Although on balance the evidence supports the claim that proximate places are important for physical activity, a number of studies found no association between PA venues and weekly levels of PA. A critique of these studies suggests they involved younger children and it may be possible that parental concerns about safety limit younger children's independent mobility including access to parks and sports centres (Adkins, Sherwood, Story, & Davis, 2004; Kligerman et al., 2007). Furthermore, Whitehead et al., (2006) found that in their female adolescent sample simply having a proximate sports centre was not sufficient to increase PA levels. In this study, it was the girls' response to the aesthetic qualities of the sports centres that made a difference in whether they went to a sports centre or not.

Higher levels of out-of-school hours PA are also significantly associated with higher levels of urban density and mixed zoned neighbourhoods. These aspects of the neighbourhood are especially significant for older children and adolescents. For example, in the US and Europe, adolescents aged 12 and older appear to be more active in neighbourhoods that have homes on smaller blocks and where there is a variety of shops, restaurants or fast food venues they can walk or cycle to (Copperman & Bhat, 2007; Frank et al., 2006; Mota et al., 2006; Norman et al., 2006). In contrast, for children aged 12 years and under in Australia and in the US, no association, or a negative association, was found between PA and the density or land zoning of neighbourhoods (Carver et al., 2005). It is possible that these results reflect the levels of independent mobility that children have rather than density or land use mix per se. It may be no coincidence that some aspects of the environment only appear to be influential after age 12 and that adolescence marks the time that many parents begin to permit their children greater independent mobility and freedom to explore their local environment (Peterson, 2004).

The research above suggests that sport centres and parks are important places and that having access to these destinations close to young people's homes can significantly increase weekly MVPA. In the last few years researchers have started to explore further what aspects of parks and sports centres young people like and subtle differences are apparent. What is lacking however from this research is why young people use certain facilities and not others. If we are to encourage young people to get more active and go outside and have fun they need to have access to places they want to use. This knowledge can only be gained if young people are asked what they need, what they would like, what they can afford financially, and what they would use and important, why. This type of research appears to be lacking in the literature. Greater developmental precision is called for in undertaking this type of research.

How Aspects of the Home Environment Can Influence the Physical Activity of Youth

A significant finding is that aspects of the BE appear more influential for male adolescents than female adolescents and younger children. It is possible that functional, safety and destination variables appear more influential for male adolescents because males usually have more independent mobility and with parents not allowing female adolescents and younger children the same level of freedom (Peterson, 2004). Due to parental restrictions, the internal home environment maybe more influential in facilitating the PA levels of some young people than external BE aspects discussed above.

Access to home PA equipment and a range of other variables that may influence PA levels was explored in a recent Australian study with 518 boys and girls aged 5 to 12 years (Spinks, Macpherson, Bain, & McClure, 2006). Insufficient daily PA (less than 60 minutes of MVPA) was predicted by four separate variables, namely: more than two hours of television or electronic entertainment; not participating in organised sport; being driven to school; and not having outdoor play equipment in the home garden (such as a swing). However when the four variables were entered into regression model outdoor play equipment became insignificant and was not associated with levels of PA. Several other studies have also found no association between levels of PA and outdoor play equipment for both pre-school children (Sallis et al., 1993) and 11 year olds (Trost, Pate, Ward, Sanders, & Riner, 1999).

In a recent study Whitehead et al (2006) found that even having access to a garden was not significantly associated with levels of PA. However, access to internal home PA equipment was associated with PA but only where certain individual social variables were present. For example, younger girls (aged 11 to 13) were more likely to be active in their homes if their mothers were also active. For the older girls (aged 14 to 16) access to home PA equipment was associated with higher weekly PA although only for the girls who had been previously identified as highly active. Similar results were found by Rushovich et al., (2006) in their sample of adolescent girls. The Rushovich et al., study explored using accelerometers whether girls home alone after school with limited access to sports centres and parks were physically active or not. They found that girls who were home alone after school spend more time being sedentary (watching TV and talking on the telephone) than girls with access to sports centres. However, of interest was that the home alone girls also danced around their homes more and were on average slightly more physically than their sports centre attending peers, but only by 7.55 minutes per week. Rushovich et al., concluded that the results suggest that being home alone is not necessarily a barrier to being active.

To date we have limited knowledge of how active young people are at home. The findings to date suggest that access to physical equipment (i.e., garden swings) or to a garden is not related to PA levels. The research also suggests that it is vital to combine environmental with individual variables when considering the home as a facilitator of PA. For example, as Rushovich et al., (2006) found, girls who are more motivated to be physically active at home may just need access to a hi-fi or the radio and they will dance for longer and more vigorously than their peers who are in organised sport or attending sports centres.

In summary further research predicting PA behaviours for young people in their homes is needed. Recent trends in the significant increases in the working hours of adults implies that the average Australian adult will spend less time at home than they do now (Campbell, 2005). If parents are working longer hours it may be possible that children (especially adolescents) are at home unsupervised in the evenings for longer periods of time. Furthermore, given an increase over the past 20 years in risk-aversive parenting (fear of letting children out of the home; (Gill, 2007) it is also possible that young people left unsupervised in the evenings or weekends may also not be permitted to leave their homes. Future research could explore several questions. For example, do Australian children need access to a garden, and if so what size is required; do young people need outdoor play equipment to be PA or not? What types of activities and games do young people like to do in their home and what conditions facilitate these? For example, is access to certain types of equipment or toys related to higher levels of fun and higher levels of MVPA? Whether children will have access to active toys and equipment or are restricted to their homes most of the week is often controlled by parents. We now turn our attention to how parents can be either a barrier or a facilitator of PA.

WHETHER YOUNG PEOPLE CAN PLAY: HOW THE NORMS OF "GOOD PARNETING" PREVENT OR FACILITATE PLAY, FUN AND PA

Parents can facilitate or constrain PA by controlling whether, when and where young people can play and be active. According to Rissotto and Giuliani (2006) over the past three decades there has been a change in parenting style from one that encourages independence in children to a style where the focus is on protection and avoidance of risk. Increasingly, this shift is now mirrored in the policies and actions of town planners and city councils concerned with safety and litigation (Gill, 2007).

Historically parents encouraged their children to go outside and play after school and for most of the weekend days. Children were also usually allowed to play outside of the fence boundaries of their home (such as in the street with neighbourhood children or in parks and natural undeveloped land) (Rissotto & Giuliani, 2006; Pyle, 2007). The freedom to move around the environment unsupervised provided children with the opportunity to connect with nature (such as catching tadpoles in streams), to have adventures and learn from experience and mistakes (e.g., which trees are safe and unsafe to climb), to play make believe games with their friends and to enjoy being active and young (Pyle, 2007). According to Marano (2006) this traditional style of parenting that allowed children to be independently mobile would now be considered verging on child neglect in the beliefs held in today's society. As Rissotto and Giuliani (2006) noted, this style of parenting has declined in most of Europe with children having their freedom restricted due to safety concerns.

The contemporary style of parenting in most western nations is not just about protecting children but rather over-protecting them. According to Gill (2007) underpinning this style is an almost zero-tolerance approach to allowing children to experience any kind of risk, however remote or small. To place this change in parenting style in perspective the shift to "parental over-protection" appears to have occurred at the same time as dramatic changes occurred in the urban landscape that include increases in the number of cars on the roads, declines in the amount of public spaces to play in and less natural bush land to explore (Pyle, 2007). According to Rissotto & Giuliani (2006) these three changes in the urban landscape have led to the dehumanising of many towns and cities, especially in northern Europe, and to reductions in people's sense of community.

In addition to safety concerns about physical hazards, another safety concern of modern parents is stranger danger. Stranger danger concerns represent a barrier to young people's ability to be active because parents do not allow their children the freedom to walk to school or explore the neighbourhood unsupervised (Veitch et al, 2006). Of interest, unlike the concern about traffic hazards which represents a high risk of harm for children, stranger danger has a fairly remote probability of occurring. For example, in the UK it has been estimated that the probability of a child being murdered by a stranger is less than 3 in a million, whereas the probability of a child being killed by a car each year is estimated at approximately 200 in a million children (Benians, 2006). In addition, although in Australia parental fears of stranger danger have risen over the past three decades, officially recorded criminal convictions for such offences over the same period do not mirror the rise in parental fear and show no significant increase in the number of sexual assaults against children or child abductions *by strangers*. What the official statistics show however is that the real risk of sexual or physical abuse for children is not from strangers but rather from members or acquaintances of their own family. It is estimated that approximately 80% of all sexual and violent crimes perpetrated against children is by people they know (e.g., fathers, mothers, uncles, family friends, babysitters) (Chappell & Wilson, 2005; Australian Institute of Criminology, 2004). Several commentators have hypothesised that this mismatch between heightened "stranger danger" and the low risk of such an event is a combination of perceived fear, often media driven (i.e., where one-off, albeit horrific, events are given worldwide prominent coverage, such as the abduction in Liverpool of Jaimie Bolger in 1993) combined with the new style of "over-protective" risk-aversive parenting style (Gill, 2007; Pyle, 2007). This new style of parenting is underpinned by a set of norms stating that a "good parent" is one who places more importance on protecting children from any harm however small the risk. These norms also provide that parents who allow their children greater independence to explore their environments, walk to school, and spend the day unsupervised with their young friends are "irresponsible, negligent and bad parents" (Rissotto & Giuliani, 2006).

One way that this protective style of parenting has provided a barrier for young people's daily PA is their walk or cycle to and from school. As mentioned earlier, active transport is one of the big reductions in young people's incidental daily PA. This decrease has occurred at the same time as cities have become more congested, with more cars on the roads, and heightened perceived "stranger danger" concern. For example, in 1970 approximately 80% of British children aged 7 or above walked to school, many of whom were unescorted by parents or adults. By 1990, this figure had reduced dramatically with only 10% of British school children walking to and from school (Hillman et al., 1990).

In summary, parents can facilitate or constrain young people's PA. It appears that the recent change in the norms of being a "good parent" has led parents to constrain their children's PA rather than facilitate it. Certainly it is society's responsibility to provide safe places for everyone, young and old alike, to be active without the worry of having to negotiate unnecessary traffic hazards. However, with regards to stranger danger, despite the real risk of abduction by strangers being remote, today's parents appear unwilling to allow even the smaller chance of this possibility eventuating.

CONCLUSION

What we Know, what we Should Do about it and what we still Need to Find out

Being physically active as a child makes sense from both a physical and psychological perspective and appears to be associated with more positive long term outcomes. Children who are active develop stronger skeletal frames, joints and supporting muscles which help prevent osteoporosis in later life (Vicente-Rodr´iguez, 2006). Being active assists children to maintain a healthy body weight which in turn reduces the risk of developing a number of debilitating chronic diseases in adulthood (Booth et al, 2006). Young people who are a healthy weight are less likely to be ridiculed or ostracised by peers (due to their physical appearance) and also self-report having higher self-esteem, a more positive self body-image and being more optimistic about their futures. They also have higher academic achievements at school and college than their overweight and obese peers (Singer, 1992).

In this chapter we examined how different aspects of the BE can act as facilitator or a barrier for young people to be active, stay healthy and have fun. The summary below presents the key points identified from the literature as well as highlights areas that warrant further exploration. Where applicable, policy implications based on findings are discussed.

Key Findings, Policy Implications and Future Research Directions

Functional Aspects of the Built Environment
The literature to date:

- Infrastructure provides opportunities for, and promotes activity. Regardless of their age, for more young people to walk/cycle to school infrastructure (footpaths, etc) is important.
- Developmental interactions occur between age, density, land mix use and type of activity. For young people regardless of age and gender, the higher the urban density the more likely they are to walk or cycle to school. For out-of-school PA, younger children are more active in low density settings (urban sprawl/cul-de-sacs). However, adolescents are more active in higher density suburbs with mixed land use (i.e., a mix of residential and retail).
- Fruitful questions for research include:
- Given the presence of infrastructure, do the quality components of it matter to the level of activity? Does the condition of paths or availability of shade influence levels of activity in young people? We know very little about whether the quality of walking and cycling routes influences levels of PA.
- Is density influential in facilitating or constraining physical activity? For whom? What are the relationships between age, gender, density and physical activity? Is there an optimal range or configuration of urban density with respect to facilitating physical activity?

Safety Aspects
The literature to date:

- Parents and young people are both concerned about having safe places to cross busy roads, and that there is surveillance in the community (people visibly around), and that streets are well-lit.
- Parental concern about stranger danger is associated with decreases in the proportion of children who walk to school.
- While car accidents are the biggest killer of children aged 14 and under, and both parents and children report concerned about traffic, evidence shows that when teenage girls walk, they are more likely to do so near traffic.
- The policy implication for known hazards, such as traffic, is that on popular walking/cycling routes young people are given the safety features they need to feel safer and be protected. For example, make sure there are enough pedestrian controlled traffic lights, ensure there is adequate street lighting on popular routes.

- Fruitful questions for research include:
- What level of street lighting is required to make young people feel safe when walking or cycling? How far are they willing to walk to use safe road crossing points?
- Where safety concerns (which limit children's PA) are based on subjective concerns about harm (perceived unsafe public spaces and stranger danger) we need to objectively investigate whether some public spaces in some areas are unsafe (such as having discarded injecting needles present)? We need to explore whether these concerns are warranted and if so how we can improve the safety levels of public spaces.

Destination Aspects

The literature to date:

- Destinations, and distances to destinations appears to matter. The implication is that if you want young people to be active in their communities they need somewhere to go.
- Young people will walk to parks and recreation/sports centres if they are within approximately 800m of their homes. Young people with access to transport will travel for several kilometres to attend more specialised clubs, such as martial arts or dance clubs.
- Directions for future research:
- What facilities are available in local communities and are they well matched with the needs of young people? What sort of walking/cycling routes are there to get to these venues (for example street lighting/footpaths – safety features)?
- Are there enough local places where young people can have adventures? What sorts of public open space do young people want and does that differ by age? For example, do today's young people like natural bushland/countryside or more manicured parks? Are children permitted to be rowdy, play, have fun and be active (or do contemporary social norms insist that children be quiet, not run, and not deface property with chalk or paint, such as hopscotch grids drawn on footpaths/roads.
- To what extent are current city and town regulations able to promote activity or are there legislative barriers or fears of litigation that reduce promotion of activity?

Aesthetics Qualities of the Neighbourhood

The literature to date:

- The meagre evidence to date suggests that aesthetics do matter with more pleasant environments appearing to facilitate PA (especially for adolescents).
- Future research questions:
- What do young people think about the aesthetic quality of their communities? If aesthetics matter, at what age does the quality and ambiance of the environment influence levels of PA and why? There is a need for both naturalistic and experimental data that test the relationship between activity and the aesthetic quality of the environment.

- Some literature suggests that it is the quality of destinations rather than just having access to destinations per se that influences PA levels of adolescents. What are the features of parks, public spaces and shopping centres that attract young people to them?

The Home Environment
The literature to date:

- A sizable minority of children now spend over 2 hours a day watching DVDs, playing computer games or pursuing other sedentary behaviours at home. However, not all young people at home alone after school and at the weekends are physically inactive. Some research suggests that the majority of children left unsupervised at home will find ways to be active at home, such as dancing to music DVDs.
- Future research questions:
- There is insufficient evidence to be able to conclude what sort of home environment facilitates higher levels of PA. What equipment and facilities at home influence levels of PA? Does having access to a garden make a difference to activity levels and what size of playing space is associated with different levels of PA? What type of garden design influences higher levels of PA? For example, the presence of mature trees for climbing, or having grass rather than paving or vice versa?
- Does access to a home gym, music or exercise DVDs influence PA levels?

In conclusion, over the past four decades the lifestyles of children in many western societies has changed dramatically. Cities and towns have become more congested with cars, pollution, and with more buildings taking up most or all of available land. This has left very little natural green space left for young people in which to play (Pyle, 2007). At the same time as the urban landscape has changed the physical activity of children reduced to such a level (often as low as 30 minutes or less per day; Janssen et al., 2005) that calorific intake now exceeds physical activity. This imbalance is said to be a prominent factor in the global obesity epidemic and why 18 to 25% of young people are overweight or obese (AIHW, 2006; WHO, 2004). With childhood obesity currently rising by 1% annually, it is estimated that by 2025 half of all Australian youth will be either obese or pre-obese (ASSO, 2004). If a serious attempt is to be made about stopping the obesity epidemic then society needs to find and use all the different ways available to encourage people to be more active. Exploring the ways in which we can ensure that the built environment provides a place where people can enjoy being active is one such way. We end this chapter with two quotes from the National Heart Foundation? (2007).

*Good-**quality** environments and healthy people are the dual keys to the 'triple bottom line' of the best possible sustainable, economic and social development.*

Some people will stay fit and be active regardless of their environments, even when there are non-existent, inappropriate or decayed facilities. However, for most of us we are physically active only when certain social and environmental conditions are in place.

For the health and wellbeing of future generations it is imperative that we better understand the social and environmental conditions that encourage and facilitate children's physical activity and provide an important prevention and treatment context for the emergent rise in population levels of obesity.

REFERENCES

Adkins, S., Sherwood, N. E., Story, M., & Davis, M. (2004). Physical activity among African-American girls: The role of parents and the home environment. *Obesity Research, 12* (Supplement), 38s-45s.

Akers, R. L. (1997). *Criminological theories: Introduction and evaluation* (2nd ed.). California, CA: Roxbury Publishing.

Andrews, D. A., & Bonta, J. (1998). *The psychology of criminal conduct* (2nd ed.). Cincinnati, OH: Anderson Publishing co.

Australian Institute of Criminology (AIC) (2004). *Australian crime: Facts and figures 2004.* Canberra; Australian Capital Territory.

Australian Institute of Health and Welfare (AIHW). (2005). *A picture of Australia's children.* Canberra, ACT, Australia: AIHW.

Australian Institute of Health and Welfare (AIHW). (2006). *Australia's Health 2006.* Canberra, ACT, Australia: AIHW.

Australian Institute of Health and Welfare (AIHW)., O'Brien, K., & Webbie, K. (2004). *Health, wellbeing and body weight: characteristics of overweight and obesity in Australia, 2001.* Canberra, ACT, Australia: AIHW.

Australian Society for the Study of Obesity (ASSIO). (2004). *Obesity in Australian children.* Retrieved August 12, 2007 from the World Wide Web: http://www.asso.org.au/ freestyler/gui/files//factsheet_children_prevalence.pdf.

Bass, S., Pearce, G., Bradney, M., Hendrich, E., Delmas, P. D., Harding, A., et al. (1998). Exercise before puberty may confer residual benefits in bone density in adulthood: studies in active prepubertal and retired female gymnasts. *Journal of Bone and Mineral Research, 13,* 500-507.

Baur, L. (2002). Child and adolescent obesity in the 21st century: An Australian perspective. *Asia Pacific Journal of Clinical Nutrition, 11,* 524-532.

Benians, C. (2006). *Kid gloves - are we over-protective of our children?* Retrieved October, 1, 2007 from the World Wide Web: http://www.familiesonline.co.uk/article/articleview/ 1735/1/37/.

Boarnet, M. G., Anderson, C. L., Day, K., McMillan, T. L., & Alfonzo, M. (2005). Evaluation of the California safe routes to school legislation. *American Journal of Preventive Medicine, 28,* 134-140.

Booth, M. (2000). What proportion of Australian children are sufficiently active? *Medical Journal of Australia 173* (Supplement 7), S6-S7.

Booth, M., Macaskill, P., McLellan, P. P., Okely, T., Patterson, J., Wright, J., et al. (1997). *NSW Schools Fitness and Physical Activity Survey.* Sydney, Australia: NSW Department of School Education.

Booth, M., Okely, A. D., Denney-Wilson, E., Hardy, L., Yang, B., & Dobbins, T. (2006). *NSW Schools Physical Activity and Nutrition Survey (SPANS) 2004: Full Report.* Sydney, Australia: NSW Department of Health.

Braza, M., Shoemaker, W., & Seeley, A. (2004). Neighborhood design and rates of walking and biking to elementary school in 34 California communities. *American Journal of Health Promotion, 19*, 128-136.

Brodersen, N. H., Steptoe, A., Williamson, S., & Wardle, J. (2005). Sociodemographic, developmental, environmental, and psychological correlates of physical activity and sedentary behavior at age 11 to 12. *Annual of Behavioral Medicine., 29*, 2-11.

Campbell, I. (2005). *Long Working Hours in Australia: Working-Time Regulation and Employer Pressures.* CASR Working Papers Number 2005-2. Centre for Applied Social Research, Canberra, ACT, Australia.

Carver, A., Salmon, J., Campbell, K., Baur, L., Garnett, S., & Crawford, D. (2005). How do perceptions of local neighborhood relate to adolescents' walking and cycling? *American Journal of Health Promotion, 20*, 139-147.

Centres for Disease Control and Prevention (CDC). (2007). *Physical activity and good nutrition: Essential elements to prevent chronic disease and obesity. At a glance 2007.* Atlanta: CDC.

Chappell, D., & Wilson, P. (2005). *Issues in Australian crime and criminal justice.* Chatsworth, NSW, Australia: LexisNexis Butterworths.

Chess, S., & Thomas, A. (1984). *Origins and evolution of behavior disorders : From infancy to early adult life.* New York: Brunner/Mazel.

Cohen, D. A., Ashwood, J. S., Scott, M. M., Overton, O., Evenson, K. R., Staten, L. K., et al., (2006). Public parks and physical activity among adolescent girls. *Pediatrics, 118*, 1381-1389.

Commonwealth Department of Health and Aging. (2006). *Australia's physical activity recommendations for children and young people.* Retrieved August 12, 2007 from the World Wide Web: http://www.health.gov.au/internet/wcms/publishing.nsf/Content/health-pubhlth-strateg-active-recommend.htm

Copperman, R. B., & Bhat, C. R. (2007). An analysis of the determinants of children's weekend physical activity participation. *Transportation 34,* 67-87.

Cornell, E. H., & Hill, K. A. (2006). The problem of lost children. In C. Spencer & M. Blades (Eds.), *Children and their environments: Learning, using and designing space* (pp. 26-41). New York: Cambridge University Press.

Cross, D. S., & Hall, M. R. (2005). Child pedestrian safety: the role of behavioural science. *Medical journal of Australia, 182,* 318-319.

de Vries, S. I., Bakker, I., van Mechelen, W., & Hopman-Rock, M. (2007). Determinants of activity-friendly neighbourhoods for children: Results from the SPACE study. *American Journal of Health Promotion, 21*, 312-659.

Edlich, R. F., Winters, K. L., Cox, M. J., Becker, D. G., Horowitz, J. H., Nichter, L. S., et al., (2004). National health strategies to reduce sun exposure in Australia and the United States. *Journal of Long-Term Effects of Medical Implants, 14.*

Epstein, L. H., Raja, S., Gold, S. S., Paluch, R. A., Pak, Y., & Roemmich, J. N. (2006). Reducing sedentary behavior: The relationship Between park area and the physical activity of youth. *Psychological Science, 17*, 654-659.

Evenson, K. R., Scott, M. M., Cohen, D. A., & Voorhees, C. C. (2007). Girls' perception of neighborhood factors on physical activity, sedentary behavior, and BMI. *Obesity, 15*, 430-445.

Ewing, R., Schroeer, W., & Green, W. (2004). School location and student travel. *Transportation Research Record, 1895*, 55-63.

Frank, L. D., Kerr, J., Chapman, J., & Sallis, J. (2007). Urban form relationships with walk trip frequency and distance among youth. *American Journal of Health Promotion, 21*, 305-311.

Frank, L. D., Sallis, J. F., Conway, T. L., Chapman, J. E., Saelens, B. E., & Bachman, W. (2006). Many pathways from land use to health. *Journal of the American Planning Association, 72*, 75-87.

Giles-Corti, B. (2006). People or places: what should be the target? *Journal of Science in Medicine and Sport, 9,* 357-366.

Gill, T. (2007). Playing it too safe, *RSA e-Journal* (Vol. April 2007). Retrieved September 14, 2007 from the World Wide Web: http://www.thersa.org/journal/article.asp?articleID=1006

Goldberg, B. (1995). *Sports and exercise for children with chronic health conditions.* Champaign, IL: Human Kinetics.

Gordon-Larsen, P., Nelson, M. C., Page, P., & Popkin, B. M. (2006). Inequality in the built environment underlies key health disparities in physical activity and obesity. *Pediatrics 117*, 417-424.

Hands, B., Parker, H., Glasson, C., Brinkman, S., & Read, H. (2004). *Physical activity and Nutrition Levels in Western Australian Children and Adolescents Report.* Perth, Western Australia: Western Australian Government.

Harten, N., & Olds, T. (2004). Patterns of active transport in 11-12 year old Australian children. *Australian and New Zealand Journal of Public Health, 28*, 167-172.

Hillman, M., Adams, J., & Whitelegg, J. (1990). *One false move...A study of children's independent mobility.* London: Policy Studies Institute.

Jago, R., Baranowski, T., Zakeri, I., & Harris, M. (2005). Observed Environmental Features and the Physical Activity of Adolescent Males. *American journal of Preventative Medicine, 29,* 98-104.

Janssen, I., Katzmarzyk, P., Boyce, W. F., Vereecken, C., Mulvihill, C., Roberts, C., Currie, C., Pickett, W., & the Health Behaviour in School-Aged Children Obesity Working Group (2005). Comparison of overweight and obesity prevalence in school-aged youth from 34 countries and their relationships with physical activity and dietary patterns. *Obesity Reviews, 6,* 123-132.

Joshi, M. S., MacLean, M., & Carter, W. (1999). Children's journey to school: Spatial skills, knowledge and perceptions of the environment. *British Journal of Developmental Psychology, 17*, 125-139.

Kligerman, M., Sallis, J. F., Ryan, S., Frank, L. D., & Nader, P. R. (2007). Association of neighbourhood design and recreation environment variables with physical activity and body mass index in adolescents. *American Journal of Health Promotion, 21*, 274-277.

Kuo, F. E., & Taylor, A. F. (2004). A Potential Natural Treatment for Attention-Deficit/Hyperactivity Disorder: Evidence From a National Study. *American Journal of Public Health 94*, 1580-1586.

Marano, H. E. (2006). A nation of wimps, *Psychology Today (Vol. Jan/Feb)*: European Journal of Social Psychology.

Matthews, B. L., Bennell, K. L., McKay, H. A., Khan, K. M., Baxter-Jones, A. D. G., Mirwald, R. L. (2006). Dancing for bone health: A 3-year longitudinal study of bone mineral accrual across puberty in female non-elite dancers and controls *Osteoporosis International, 17*, 1043-1054.

McCormack, G. R., Giles-Corti, B., & Bulsara, M. (2007). The relationship between destination proximity, destination mix and physical activity behaviors, *Preventive Medicine* (Vol. 10.1016/j.ypmed).

McDonald, N. C. (2007). Active transportation to school: Trends among U.S. schoolchildren, 1969-2001. *American journal of Preventative Medicine, 32*, 509-516.

McMillan, T. E. (2007). The relative influence of urban form on a child's travel mode to school. *Transportation Research Part A (41)*, 69-79.

Mota, J., Delgado, N., Almeida, M., Ribeiro, J. C., & Santos, M. P. (2006). Physical activity, overweight, and perceptions of neighborhood environments among Portuguese girls. *Journal of Physical Activity and Health, 3*, 314-322.

National Health Forum (NHF) (2007). *Building Health: Creating and enhancing places for healthy, active lives. What needs to be done?* London: NHF.

Norman, G. J., Nutter, S. K., Ryan, S., Sallis, J. F., Calfas, K. J., & Patrick, K. (2006). Community Design and Access to Recreational Facilities as Correlates of Adolescent Physical Activity and Body-Mass Index. *Journal of Physical Activity and Health, 3*, 118-128.

Peterson, C. (2004). *Looking forward through the Lifespan: Developmental psychology* (4th ed.). Sydney: Prentice Hall.

Pikora, T., Giles-Corti, B., Bull, F., Jamrozik, K., & Donovan, R. (2003). Developing a framework for assessment of the environmental determinants of walking and cycling. *Social Science and Medicine 53*, 1693–1703.

Putnam, R. D. (1995). 'Bowling alone: America's declining social capital'. *Journal of Democracy, 6*, 65-78.

Pyle, R. (2007). *Losers, weepers: The extinction of experience and the diminishing baseline.* Come outside and play: A mutli-disciplinary symposium. University of Western Australia, Perth, Australia.

Rapp-Paglicci, L. A., Dulmus, C. N., & Wodarski, J. S. (Eds.). (2004). *Handbook of preventative interventions for children and adolescents.* Hoboken, New Jersey: John Wiley & Sons, Inc.

Retrieved September 13, 2007 from the World Wide Web:

Rissotto, A., & Giuliani, M. V. (2006). Learning neighbourhood environments: The loss of experience in a modern world. In C. Spencer & M. Blades (Eds.), *Children and their environments: Learning, using and designing space* (pp. 75-90). New York: Cambridge University Press.

Rushovich, B. R., Voorhees, C. C., Davis, C. E., Neumark-Sztainer, D., Pfeiffer, K. A., Elder, J. P., et al. (2006). The relationship between unsupervised time after school and physical activity in adolescent girls. *International Journal of Behavioral Nutrition and Physical Activity 3*, 1-9.

Sallis, J. F., & Glanz, K. (2006). The role of the built environment in physical activity, eating, and obesity in children. *The Future of Children, 16*, 89-108.

Sallis, J. F., Nader, P. R., Broyles, S. L., Berry, C. C., Elder, J. P., & McKenzie, T. L. (1993). Correlates of physical activity at home in Mexican-American and Anglo-American preschool children. *Health Psychology, 12*, 390-398.

Salmon, J., Timperio, A., Cleland, V., & Venn, A. (2005). Trends in children's physical activity and weight status in high and low socio-economic status areas of Melbourne, Victoria, 1985-2001. *Australian and New Zealand Journal of Public Health 29*, 337- 342.

Saris, W. H. M., & Blair, S. N. (2003). How much physical activity is enough to prevent unhealthy weight gain? Outcome of the IASO 1st Stock Conference and consensus statement. *Obesity Reviews 4*, 101-114.

Singer, R. S. (1992). Physical activity and psychological benefits: A positive statement of the International Society of Sport Psychology (ISSP). *The Sports Psychologist 6,* 199-203.

Spinks, A. B, Macpherson, A., Bain, A., & McClure, R. (2006). Determinants of sufficient daily activity in Australian primary school children. *Journal of Paediatrics and Child Health 42,* 674–679.

Spinks, A. B., Macpherson, A. K., Bain, C., & McClure, R. J. (2007). Compliance with the Australian national physical activity guidelines for children: relationship to overweight status. *Journal of Science and Medicine in Sport, 10*, 156-163.

Stephenson, J., & Bauman, A. (2000). *The cost of illness attributable to physical inactivity in Australia.* Canberra: CDHAC and Australian Sports Commission.

Stevenson, M., Jamrozik, K., & Spittle, J. (1995). A case-control study of traffic risk factors and child pedestrian injuries. *International Journal of Epidemiology 24*, 957-964.

Stone, W. (2001). *Measuring social capital: Towards a theoretically informed measurement framework for researching social capital in family and community life.* Australian Institute of Family Studies, Melbourne, Victoria

Timperio, A., Ball, K., Salmon, J., Roberts, R., Giles-Corti, B., Simmons, D., et al. (2006). Personal, family, social, and environmental correlates of active commuting to school. *American Journal of Preventative Medicine, 30*, 45-51.

Timperio, A., Crawford, D., Telford, A., & Salmon, J. (2004). Perceptions about the local neighborhood and walking and cycling among children. *Preventative Medicine, 38*, 39-47.

Timperio, A., Crawford, D., Telford, A., & Salmon, J. (2005). Perceptions about the local neighborhood and their relationship to childhood overweight and obesity. *International Journal of Obesity, 29*, 170-175.

Trayers, T., Deem, R., Fox, K. R., Riddoch, C. J., R, N. A., & Lawlor, D. A. (2006). Improving health through neighbourhood environmental change: are we speaking the same language? A qualitative study of views of different stakeholders. *Journal of Public Health 28*, 49-55.

Trost, S., Pate, R., Ward, D., Sanders, R., & Riner, W. (1999). Determinants of physical activity in active and low-active, sixth grade African-American youth. *Journal of School Health, 69*, 29-34.

Valentine, G., & McKendrick, J. (1997). Children's outdoor play: exploring parental concerns about children's safety and the changing nature of childhood. *Geoforum 28*, 219-235.

Veitch, J., Bagley, S., Ball, k., & Salmon, J. (2006). Where do children usually play? A qualitative study of parents' perceptions of influences on children's active free-play. *Health & Place 12*, 383-393.

Vicente-Rodr´iguez, G. (2006). How does Exercise Affect Bone Development during Growth? *Sports Medicine 36*, 561-569.

Wells, N. M., Ashdown, S. P., Davies, E. H. S., Cowett, F. D., & Yang, Y. (2007). Environment, Design and Obesity: Opportunities for Interdisciplinary Collaborative Research. *Environment and Behavior, 39,* 6-33.

Whitehead, S. H., Biddle, S. J. H., O'Donovan, T. M., & Nevill, M. E. (2006). Social–Psychological and Physical Environmental Factors in Groups Differing by Levels of Physical Activity: A Study of Scottish Adolescent Girls. *Pediatric Exercise Science, 18,* 226-239.

WHO. (2004). *Young people: need to move for health and wellbeing.* Geneva, Switzerland: World Health Organization. Retrieved July 21, 2007 from the World Wide Web: http://www.who.int/moveforhealth/about/2004/en/print.html

Wodarski, L. A., & Wodarski, J. S. (2004). Handbook of preventative interventions for children and adolescents. In L. A. Rapp-Paglicci, C. N. Dulmus & J. S. Wodarski (Eds.), *Handbook of preventative interventions for children and adolescents* (pp. 301-320). Hoboken, New Jersey: John Wiley & Sons, Inc.

Young, D. E., & Young, M. (2005). *Art of the Japanese garden.* Singapore: Tuttle Publishing.

Ziviani, J., Kopeshke, R., & Wadley, D. (2006). Children walking to school: Parent perceptions of environmental and psychosocial influences. *Australian Occupational Therapy Journal, 53,* 27-34.

In: Physical Activity and Children: New Research
Editor: N. P. Beaulieu, pp. 35-63

ISBN: 978-1-60456-306-1
© 2008 Nova Science Publishers, Inc.

Chapter 2

YOUTH AQUATIC RECREATION: THE PLEASURES AND PITFALLS OF AN AQUATIC LIFESTYLE IN NEW ZEALAND

Kevin Moran[*]

Health and Physical Education, School of Social and Policy Studies, Faculty of
Education, The University of Auckland, Private Bag 92601, Symonds St,
Auckland 1150, New Zealand
Watersafe Auckland Inc, PO Box 8163, Symonds St, Auckland, New Zealand

ABSTRACT

In an island nation with easy access to water, opportunity for young New Zealanders to recreationally engage in aquatic activity abounds. While participation in aquatic activity is generally perceived as a positive indicator of a healthy lifestyle, it does have attendant negative consequences. Drowning as a consequence of aquatic activity is a significant cause of unintentional death among young New Zealanders. In spite of some evidence of the popularity of aquatic recreation, little is known about the nature of that recreation and its associated risk of drowning. It is the purpose of this chapter to ascertain what youth do in the aquatic environment and how their behaviour might exacerbate the risk of drowning inherent in water-based activities.

A 25-item questionnaire was designed to survey a nationwide sample of 15–19-year-old New Zealand high school students (N = 2,202). Students from 41 schools who were in their final year of compulsory schooling (Year 11) completed the self-complete, written questionnaire during school time to assess the nature and extent of their participation in aquatic recreation and their associated water safety knowledge and behaviour.

Almost all the youth surveyed had taken part in some swimming (98%) or other aquatic activity (94%) in the previous year. Most students had swum at public/school

---

[*] Telephone: +649 6238899 ext 48620; Facsimile: +649 6238836; Cellphone: 027 654 9944; Email: k.moran@auckland.ac.nz; watersafe.ak@xtra.co.nz; Website: www.auckland.ac.nz

pools (89%) and patrolled surf beaches (76%). Two thirds of the participants reported having taken part in paddling (67%) and surfing (65%) activities. Risk of drowning was exacerbated among many students because, in addition to high levels of exposure to risk, they often reported at-risk behaviours during their activities. For example, many had swum outside patrol flags (61%) or had swum when cold or tired (56%). One half (50%) of youth reported having swum in a prohibited place or having swum alone (47%). One fifth had never worn a lifejacket (19%) or had consumed alcohol (21%) during aquatic recreation.

Even though youth that took part in this study generally reported higher levels of aquatic recreation than that previously reported for other age groups, this increased participation has attendant increased risks to health and wellbeing for youth because of the high levels of at-risk behaviour reported by some youth. When behaviour was analysed by gender, socio-economic status and ethnicity, the prevalence of risky behaviours among males was consistent and pronounced, the effect of socio-economic status and ethnicity less so. Taken separately, any of the risky behaviours is capable of heightening drowning risk; taken collectively they offer strong explanation as to why some youth, especially males, are at greater risk of drowning than others. Consequently, while encouraging youth to participate in aquatic activity, emphasis on doing so safely by educating youth about the inherent risks of drowning and their role in drowning prevention appear to be warranted.

1. INTRODUCTION

1.1. A Recreation: An Overview

Aquatic recreational activities such as swimming, boating and fishing have long been identified as popular forms of leisure time pursuits in developed countries, especially where access to closed water (such as swimming pools) and open water environments (such as the sea, rivers and lakes) is plentiful. In New Zealand, an island nation with more than 15,000 kilometres of coastline extending over ten degrees of latitude, fast-flowing rivers and large tracts of inland water, opportunities for New Zealanders to engage in aquatic recreation abound. Proximity to water pervades all aspects of life in New Zealand and 95% of its population live within an hour's drive of a beach. A national survey in 2000 reported that eight out of ten adults had participated in some type of water-related activity in the previous twelve months (Water Safety New Zealand, 2000). Such is the popularity of aquatic activity, that the aquatic environment has been identified as the second most important site for public leisure and recreation (Russell & Wilson, 1992).

New Zealanders are not alone in their propensity to indulge in aquatic recreational activity. In nearest-neighbour Australia, swimming ranked second behind walking as the most popular activity among adults with over 2.2 million Australians swimming at least once in the 12 months prior to interview (Ausport, 2003). In the Active People Survey of 2006, Sport England reported that indoor swimming was the most popular recreational activity undertaken by adults during the previous year with almost one third (30.9%) of the 363,724 respondents having taken part (Sport England, 2006). A water sports survey also conducted in the UK in 2006 reported that up to 13.8 million people, just over a quarter (28%) of the UK adult population, had taken part in some aquatic-oriented activity in the previous year (British Marine Federation, 2006). A survey of sports participation in Scotland in 2000 found that swimming (23%) was the second most popular activity behind walking during the two months prior to interview (31%) (Sport Scotland, 2001). In Ireland, a study of water-based leisure activities found that 1.48 million people, almost half (49%) of the adult population, had participated in some form of water-based activity in the year preceding the survey (Marine Institute, 2004). Similarly high levels of aquatic activity have been reported in other European countries that use the COMPASS (Coordinated Monitoring of Participation in Sports) framework including Italy (Italian Statistical Institute, 2000), Switzerland (Lamprecht & Stamm, 2002), Germany and the Czech Republic (Rychtecky, 2002).

In contrast to the high levels of aquatic activity reported above, in the United States, the national Health Interview Survey (NHIS) of 1991 reported swimming for exercise ranked only ninth among common physical activities, with only 6.5% of respondents reporting that they had been swimming in the two weeks prior to interview (Centers for Disease Control and Prevention [CDC], 1996). However, caution is advised when making international comparisons because of the differing survey methodologies, differing measurement modes and definitions of what constitutes sport, physical activity and leisure pursuits (Statistics Canada, 2000).

Enthusiasm for aquatic recreation is not confined to adults; on the contrary, evidence suggests that proportionally more youth engage in aquatic activity than older age groups and that participation declines with age. For example, among Australian youth aged 15-24 years, the activities that attracted the most participants were swimming (17.7%) and aerobics/fitness (17.6%), whereas in the oldest age group (over 65 years), walking (36.4%) and golf (10.4%) attracted the most participants (Ausport, 2003). Evidence also suggests that swimming is highly popular among children less than 15 years of age. In Canada, for example, one quarter (24%) of children aged 5-14 years reported swimming regularly, making it the second most popular activity behind soccer (31%) (Statistics Canada, 2000). Evidence from the US suggests that participation rates may decline rapidly even within the youth age group. The 1992 NHIS-YRBS study found that, overall, half (55.3%) of young people aged 12-21 years had participated in running, jogging or swimming for exercise in the seven days preceding the survey (for further details, refer to Chapter 5 of *Physical Activity and Health: A report of the Surgeon General*, 1996). However, that percentage fell sharply from a peak for 13/14 year-olds (males 74.3%, females 80.5%) to a low at 21 years of age (males, 39.8%, females 30.3%), reinforcing concerns regarding physical inactivity among youth.

Some evidence suggests that popularity of aquatic activity differs between male and female youth. In New Zealand, a national survey of youth recreation identified swimming as the most popular physical activity amongst 18-24 -year-old males and the second most popular activity for females of the same age group (Hillary Commission, 1999). A study of 15-year-old New Zealanders reported that over half (54%) cited swimming as their most frequently reported form of physical activity (Reeder, Stanton, Langley & Chalmers, 1991). A survey of 750 young people in the 13-17-year-age group showed that swimming for females and surfing for males were the most popular out-of-school activities (Hillary Commission, 1998).

Among Scottish youth aged 12-18 years, swimming was the activity most females had engaged in the four weeks prior to interview (42%), for males it was the second leading activity (36%) behind soccer (77%) (Sport Scotland, 2001). In England, more than half (55%)

of 6-16-year-old females had participated in swimming out of school hours, making it their most popular activity, ahead of cycling (45%) and walking (23%) (Sport England, 2002). By comparison, the same study found swimming ranked third among males behind football (57%) and cycling (53%) with almost half (48%) of male youth reporting that they had been swimming in their own time. In the United States, swimming was also popular among 5-12th grade students, although a gender difference in participation was again evident with swimming the most frequently reported activity for girls but the fifth most frequently reported activity for boys (Ross & Gilbert, 1985).

1.2. The Pleasures of Aquatic Activity

Popularity in things aquatic is not new. In antiquity, the Greeks and Romans identified the delights of immersion in water as the lifeblood of civilised pleasures. Indulgence in swimming and bathing were well in keeping with Juvenal's famous maxim *mens sana in corpore sano* (Lenček & Bosker, 1999). The prophylactic and therapeutic values of swimming have long been used to promote participation with claims that it plays an important role in the formation of physical, mental and spiritual well-being, especially among the young. Perhaps not surprisingly then, the teaching of swimming and water safety has traditionally held a prominent position in the curriculum of schools, particularly in New Zealand and Australia. By way of example, as far back as 1919, specific mention was made of the prophylactic and practical values of swimming in the official education syllabus (Board of Education, 1919) and its inclusion is worthy of quoting at length:

> Ability to swim is a permanent possession of much practical value. It makes possible the enjoyment of a particularly invigorating and healthful form of exercise, attractive in its sporting possibilities for younger people, and capable of being indulged in with benefit until well on in life. Its importance for our seafaring population is tragically emphasised by the many lives that are lost for want of early instruction in swimming. (p. 225).

In today's climate of technological advance, reduced physical exertion in everyday living and the onset of hypokinetic diseases such as type 2 diabetes, obesity and premature cardiovascular failure, the functional value of regular aerobic activity to the maintenance of health has been well identified (for example, *Physical activity and health: A report of the Surgeon General*, 1996). A brief foray into the extensive research literature on the role that physical activity plays in health and wellbeing provides some indication of its reification as a community good. Aerobic exercise, such as swimming, has been identified as of particular value to the cardiovascular system because of its associated improvement in myocardial muscle function (Pavlik, Olexo, Osvath, Sidó, & Frenkl, 2001), improved cardiac capillarisation (McKirnan & Bloor, 1994; Tomanek, 1994) and enhanced respiratory capacity (Rumuka, Aberberga-Augskalne & Upitis, 2007; Wells, Plyley, Thomas, Goodman & Duffin, 2005). Swimming has been recommended as of particular rehabilitative value for the overweight (Murase, Haramizu, Shimitoyodome & Tokimitsu, 2005), those suffering from articular diseases and musculo-skeletal injuries because of its reduced load bearing (Biro, Fugedi & Revesz, 2007) and asthma (Welsh, Kemp & Roberts, 2005; Matsumoto, Araki, et al., 1999). In addition, swimming has been advocated as an appropriate exercise for young people because it helps build and maintain healthy muscles, bones and joints (Biro, Fugedi & Revesz, 2007). Furthermore, swimming has also been associated with psychological wellbeing with some evidence that it improves mood enhancement (Netz, 2003; Berger & Owen, 1988) and stress reduction (Berger & Owen, 1992; Oda, Matsumoto, Nakagawa & Moriya, 1999).

It would appear then that the hedonistic pleasures associated with aquatic activity of old are currently well supported by evidence of its prophylactic and therapeutic worth - values that are especially appropriate in today's developed world where the paramount belief among many in the health and education sectors is that recreational activity must not only be pleasurable, it must also be functionally good for you.

1.3. The Pitfalls of Aquatic Activity

Whilst increased participation in recreational aquatic activity is generally perceived as a positive indicator of a healthy lifestyle, it does have attendant pitfalls - negative consequences that are frequently iterated in New Zealand via high profile media coverage of drowning and rescue incidences, especially during the summer months. Death by drowning in New Zealand has been consistently among the highest per head of population recorded in developed nations, with an average of over 130 fatalities per annum over the past decade (Water Safety New Zealand, 2000). In spite of a decline in death by drowning in recent years, New Zealand compares poorly internationally with drowning rates more than double those in countries such as Australia and the USA (Langley & Smeijers, 1997; Langley, Warner, Smith, & Wright, 2002; Mackie, 1999; Water Safety New Zealand, 2000).

Drowning as a consequence of aquatic activity is a significant cause of unintentional death among young New Zealanders. Between 1980 and 1994, a total of 544 New Zealand youth and young adults in the 15-24 year age group died in unintentional drowning incidents (Langley et al., 2002). Young males in the 15-19 year age groups had one of the highest age-specific rates of drowning-related deaths (7.9 per 100,000 person years) from 1989-1998 (Injury Prevention Research Unit, University of Otago, 2003). The drowning incidence for males dramatically rises in 15-22 year olds, whereas female deaths by drowning peak in the pre-school years (Child and Youth Mortality Review Committee [CYMR], 2005). In the decade from 1992-2001, approximately one half of the New Zealand youth drowning fatalities occurred during recreational activity (Source: Water Safety New Zealand Drownbase™, 2004). Surf lifesaving rescue statistics illustrate the potential for even greater loss of young lives. In the five years from 1995-2000, young people between 10-19 years of age comprised the largest group of victims with a total of 2,363 youngsters rescued from the surf (Surf Lifesaving New Zealand, 2000).

High rates of youth drowning and rescue however, are not confined to New Zealand. Young people between the ages of 15-19 years are consistently over-represented in the drowning statistics of most developed countries and, globally, drowning is the second leading cause of injury-related death among children and youth, exceeded only by deaths from motor vehicle incidents (Brenner, 2002). Even though youth have been identified as one of the most at-risk age groups for drowning in New Zealand (Chalmers, McNoe, & Stephenson, 2004; CYMR, 2005; Langley et al., 2002) and most other developed countries (for example, Brenner, Trumble, Smith, Kessler & Overpeck, 2001, in the United States; Mackie, 1999, in

Australia; Royal Society for the Prevention of Accidents [RoSPA], 2002, in Great Britain), the underlying reasons why youth appear to be at greater risk of drowning than other groups are poorly understood. This lack of understanding of the drowning phenomenon has led to frequent demands for more research on risk factors that contribute to youth drowning from within the field of injury prevention (CDC, 2002; Harborview Injury and Prevention Research Centre, 2000). Surprisingly though, drowning is not mentioned in *Physical activity and health: A report of the Surgeon General* (CDC, 1996, refer page 143) as being among potential adverse effects of swimming activity ('swimmer's shoulder' and 'swimmer's ear' – otitis externa – however, do get a mention!).

Swimming has been identified in many studies as the activity most frequently engaged in prior to drowning (CYMR, 2005; Langley et al., 2002; Quan & Cummings, 2003; Smith & Brenner, 1995). These studies also show that drowning as a consequence of swimming also takes place in a variety of settings. In the United States, Smith and Brenner (1995) reported that youth drowning most commonly occurs in natural bodies of fresh water, whereas the most common sites in New Zealand for the 15-19 year age group between 1980-2002 were rivers, offshore, surf beaches and lakes, in descending order of frequency (CYMR, 2005). Some studies have also found that much youth swimming activity is done at remote, unsupervised sites (CDC, 1992; Smith & Brenner, 1995). Other studies have identified the prevalence of at-risk behaviours in relation to swimming alone (CDC, 1992; Smith & Brenner, 1995), boating (Howland et al., 1996), and alcohol consumption during aquatic activity (Gulliver & Begg, 2005; Orlowski, 1987; Smith et al., 2001).

In order to understand the risks associated with aquatic recreation therefore, knowledge is needed of where, how often, and with whom youth take part in aquatic recreation and what risky behaviours they may engage in that may exacerbate the risk of drowning or injury. The remainder of this chapter provides comprehensive information on what New Zealand youth do in terms of their indulgence in aquatic recreation in a country well blessed with opportunity to engage in such leisure time pursuit. Importantly, it will help explain why young New Zealanders are considered a high risk group in terms of drowning by examining firstly, the nature and extent of youth aquatic recreational activity and secondly, by ascertaining the nature and extent of risky behaviours associated with that activity.

2. NEW ZEALAND: A CASE STUDY OF YOUTH AQUATIC RECREATION

The following cross-sectional case study of New Zealand youth examines the findings of a large-scale national survey undertaken in 2003 entitled the *New Zealand Youth Water Safety Survey 2003* (Moran, 2003).

2.1. Methods

The population studied consisted of Year 11 adolescent students whose ages ranged from 15-18 years and who were enrolled in full-time study at New Zealand state and private schools. The nationwide survey of 2,202 youth that made up the sample population comprised of 4% of a target population of approximately 50,000 Year 11 students. A stratified random sampling frame based on school type and geographical region was used to select 41 schools in which to conduct the survey. The survey instrument used to gather data was a written questionnaire that took 45 minutes to complete under the direction of trained and independent survey administrators during school time.

A draft questionnaire was subjected to cognitive testing in two pilot studies and, subsequently, content validity was determined by a group of water safety experts including representatives of Water Safety New Zealand, Surf Lifesaving New Zealand, and Watersafe Auckland Incorporated. Two further pilot studies were carried out one month apart to establish reliability of the survey instrument immediately prior to the commencement of the main survey. Reliability of the questionnaire was established by comparing chi-square analyses of results from the same class of Year 11 pupils carried out one month apart immediately prior to the commencement of the main survey. A nationwide survey, entitled *New Zealand Youth Water Safety Survey 2003* (Moran, 2003), was then conducted in the selected schools during the second school term in June-July, 2003.

The questionnaire included a range of forced-response questions about student participation in aquatic activities and their water safety knowledge, attitudes and behaviours. A question on how frequently and where swimming activities took place was included in the questionnaire. The question was similar to those included in the 1992 YRBSS survey of American youth that also used a 12-month recall period, varying swim locations and an ordinal scale of frequency response (Waxweiler, Harel & O'Carroll, 1993). A question on participation in aquatic recreation other than swimming was designed in a similar way to elicit information on frequency and type of aquatic activity. For swimming and other aquatic activities, four response categories with numerical descriptors of frequency that ranged from *never, not often (1-9 times), quite often (10-19 times)* and *very often (20 times+)* were included to describe student participation in aquatic activity.

Ten at-risk behaviours associated with swimming activities and six at-risk behaviours associated with other forms of aquatic recreation were included in the survey. The forced response questions asked students how many times in the previous year they had engaged in at-risk behaviours using four frequency categories that included *never, sometimes, mostly* and *always*. However, because there were so few responses in the *always* category, the *mostly* and *always* data were combined and are reported here as an *often* category. Youth were also asked a follow-up question on the influence of friends and peer groups on water safety via a question on student observation of their friends' at-risk aquatic-related behaviours. The question was structured so as to elicit yes/no categorical responses with a third option to provide for those students who had never been with friends in the situation described. The eight at-risk behaviours included common unsafe practices such as swimming outside patrol flags, not wearing a lifejacket in a boat and mixing alcohol/drugs with aquatic activity.

Data on aquatic recreation and associated water safety behaviours were analysed using a number of socio-demographic variables including gender, socio-economic status via the decile rating of the school attended and ethnicity. For ease of interpretation, socio-economic status is reported in three categories – low-decile, mid-decile and high-decile school rating (a standard government evaluation based on a range of socio-demographic indicators such as average income per household) that correspond to low-, mid- and high-socio-economic status. While recognizing the limitations of agglomerating several peoples into one category (Rasanathan, Craig & Perkins, 2004), ethnic groupings were broadly based on Statistics New Zealand classification that included European, Maori, Pacific Islands, and Asian people.

Data from the completed questionnaires were entered into Microsoft Excel X for statistical analysis using SPSS Version 12.0 in Windows. Frequency tables were generated for all questions and, unless otherwise stated, numbers and percentages are expressed in terms of response frequency within groups of students. Chi-square tests for relatedness or independence were used to compare categorical data of one or more variables. Mann Whitney U Tests were used for analysis of significant differences between independent variables on dependent measures. The Kruskall-Wallis H Test was used for analysis of ordinal data when the independent variable had more than two levels.

In cases where Kruskall-Wallis H Tests indicated the need for multiple comparisons, Mann-Whitney U Tests were used to determine differences between groups. A Bonferroni correction was applied in these multiple comparisons by dividing the .05 level of significance by the number of comparisons made in order to reduce the likelihood of Type 1 error (Ntoumanis, 2001). To test the degree of relationship between two variables, ordinal data were initially tested for linearity using scatter plots to give a preliminary indication of relationship and, where appropriate, then analysed using Spearman Rank Correlation Tests to determine the strength of that relationship.

2.2. Results

The results of the study are presented in five sections. The first three sections present evidence of the 'pleasures' of aquatic recreation expressed in terms of:

2.2.1 Recreational swimming
2.2.2 Other aquatic recreation and
2.2.3 Ownership of, or access to, aquatic recreational equipment (such as surfboards and fishing gear)

The final two sections of results present evidence of the 'pitfalls' of aquatic recreation expressed in terms of:

2.2.4 Risky swimming behaviour and
2.2.5 Risky behaviour in other aquatic recreation

2.2.1. Recreational Swimming

Almost all youth (n = 2164; 98%) reported that they had engaged in some swimming activity in the previous year. Figure 1 shows that public swimming pools were the most frequently reported site for swimming (89%), followed by: patrolled surf beaches (76%); un-patrolled surf beaches (68%); flat-water beaches (65%) and lakes or ponds (64%). Private pools (52%) and rivers/creeks (47%) were the least frequented swimming sites.

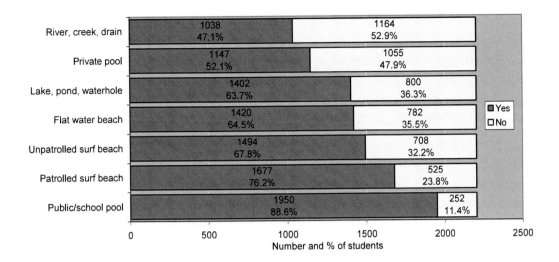

Figure 1. Youth swimming activity by location in the previous year.

In terms of frequency of participation, almost one half of youth reported swimming between 1-9 times at a public pool (n = 980; 45%), and more than one third (38%) swam there either *quite often* (n = 499; 23%) or *very often* (n = 327; 15%). Many youth reported swimming at patrolled surf beaches either *quite often* (n = 442; 20%) or *very often* (n = 471; 21%). Fewer students had swum at un-patrolled surf beaches either *quite often* (n = 342; 16%) or *very often* (n = 337; 15 %), flat water beaches either *quite often* (n = 282; 13%) or *very often* (n = 296; 13%), or in a lake either *quite often* (n = 305; 14%) or *very often* (n = 211; 10%). Rivers and creeks were the least frequented of all swimming locations with more than one half of students *never* using them for swimming (n = 1164; 53%).

Analyses of swimming frequency and location by gender, socio-economic status and ethnicity revealed some differences in patterns of swimming activity. When the frequency of swimming activity was summated and compared, the results of a Mann-Whitney *U* test (see Table 1) found no significant difference between male and female self-reported swimming activity. Table 1 also shows that no significant differences were found in the male/female use of public pools, lakes and ponds, and un-patrolled surf beaches. However, significantly more females than males reported swimming in the safe confines of home pools, at patrolled surf beaches, and at flat-water surf beaches. In contrast to this, more males swam *very often* at un-patrolled surf beaches (males 15%, females 11%) and fewer males swam *very often* at patrolled surf beaches (males 10%, females 15%).

Significant differences were also found when swimming activity was analysed against socio-economic status via the decile rating of the school attended, with youth from low-decile schools (lower socio-economic status) reporting less swimming activity than others. Inter-group analyses using Mann-Whitney *U* tests found no significant difference in swimming activity between youth attending mid-decile and high-decile schools, but significant differences between youth attending low-decile schools and those from both mid-decile (*U* = 153934.5, *p* = <.001), and high-decile schools (*U* = 237283.5, *p* = <.001). They were more likely than students from mid- or high-decile schools to report *never* having used any of the aquatic locations for swimming and less likely to report *quite often/very often* using any location for swimming activity. For example, more youth from low-decile schools *never* used public pools (15% compared with 10% respectively) or private home pools (55% compared with 47% and 44% respectively). Similar patterns of higher frequency use by youth from high-decile schools and lower frequency use by youth from low-decile schools were discernible for all other swimming locations.

Significant differences were also found when total swimming activity was analysed against ethnicity. Inter-group analysis of swimming activity found no significant differences between the amount of swimming among youth who self-identified as of European and Maori origin. European youth reported significantly more swimming activity than Pacific Islands youth ($U = 100777.0$, $p = <.001$) or Asian youth ($U = 57887.5$, $p = <.001$). Similarly, Maori youth also reported more total swimming activity than Pacific Islands youth ($U = 29993.0$, $p = <.001$) and Asian youth ($U = 116692.0$, $p = <.001$). For example, European and Maori youth were twice as likely as Pacific Islands youth and six times more likely than Asian youth to report having used patrolled surf beaches *very often* (17% and 18% compared with 9% and 3% respectively). Asian youth reported least swimming activity irrespective of location. For example, more than two thirds of Asian youth (69%) reported *never* using un-patrolled surf beaches compared with one quarter of European (26%) and Maori youth (25%).

Table 1. Differences in Location and Frequency of Swimming Activity by Gender

		% who reported swimming	Mann-Whitney U	p
Home pool	Female	56.6	550013.5	<.001*
	Male	41.9		
Public pool	Female	90.7	589719.0	.321
	Male	86.7		
Patrolled surf beach	Female	79.0	567939.0	.012*
	Male	73.6		
Un-patrolled surf beach	Female	68.0	590110.5	.338
	Male	67.7		
Flat-water beach	Female	67.6	556640.0	<.001*
	Male	61.7		
Lake, pond	Female	64.5	601608.5	.884
	Male	62.9		
River, creek	Female	45.7	578716.5	.064
	Male	48.4		
	Total Swimming Activity		577621.5	.080

* statistically significant.

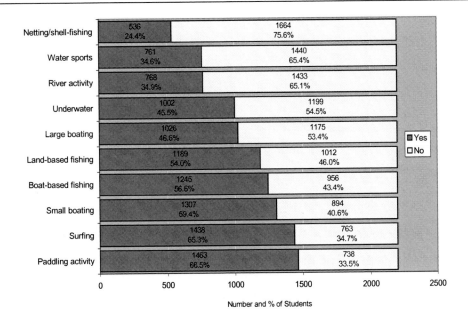

Figure 2. Youth participation in aquatic recreation other than swimming in the previous year.

2.2.2. Other Aquatic Recreation

Students were asked what aquatic recreational activity other than swimming they had participated in during the previous year. Almost all students (*n* = 2079; 94%) reported having done some water-based recreational activity other than swimming. Figure 2 shows that two thirds of youth reported taking part in paddling activities (67%) and surfing (65%) and more than half reported taking part in small craft boating (59%), boat-based fishing (57%) and land-based fishing (54%). River-based activity such as rafting/tubing (35%), other water sports such as water-skiing (35%) and netting/shell-fishing activity (24%) were the least reported activities.

In terms of frequency of activity, a majority of students reported that they participated *not often* (between 1-9 times per year) in all activities except surfing. Typically, between one half and two thirds of students reported participating less than 10 times per year in paddling activity, small boat activity, boat-based fishing, large craft activity, land-based fishing, underwater activity, and water sports. One third of students who had surfed reported participating *quite often* (n = 397; 18%) or *very often* (n = 361; 16%).

Significant differences were found when participation in aquatic recreation was summated and analysed by gender (*U* = 529123.5, *p* = <.001). Table 2 shows that significantly more males than females reported taking part in small-craft boating, fishing from a boat, land-based fishing, netting/shell-fish gathering and underwater activity. No significant differences were found in male/female self-reported participation in large craft boating, paddling, river, surfing and other water sport activities. However, fishing activity, either from a boat or land, was strongly gender-oriented, with more females than males *never* participating in boat-based fishing (females 51%, males 37%) or land-based fishing (females 57%, males 36%). More males reported participating *very often* in boat-based (males 12%, females 9%) land-based fishing (males 11%, females 3%) and surfing (males 19%, females 14%).

Table 2. Other Aquatic Recreation in the Previous Year by Gender

		% who reported taking part	Mann-Whitney U	p
Small-craft boating	Female	56.6	554223.0	<.001*
	Male	61.8		
Large-craft boating	Female	45.5	591067.0	.351
	Male	47.7		
Paddling activity	Female	66.1	602782.5	.951
	Male	66.9		
Boat-based fishing	Female	62.9	512475.5	<.001*
	Male	49.4		
Land-based fishing	Female	42.9	453693.0	<.001*
	Male	63.9		
Netting/ Shell-fishing	Female	18.5	534197.5	<.001*
	Male	29.6		
Surfing activity	Female	66.1	591034.5	.377
	Male	64.7		
River activity	Female	34.1	593308.0	.408
	Male	35.6		
Water sport activity	Female	34.5	602244.5	.911
	Male	34.7		
Underwater activity	Female	42.5	561289.0	.002*
	Male	48.2		
Total aquatic recreation (other than swimming)			529123.5	<.001*

* Statistically significant.

Significant differences were found when aquatic recreation activity was summated and analysed against socio-economic status. Significantly less participation was found among youth from low-decile schools compared with those from mid- decile ($U = 174018.5$, $p = <.001$) and high-decile schools ($U = 240280.0$, $p = <.001$), but no difference was found between youth from mid- and high-decile schools. Low-decile school students were least likely to participate in any aquatic recreational activities except for land-based fishing and underwater activity. More students from high-decile schools than from mid- or low-decile schools participated *very often* in small craft boating (14% compared with 8% and 6% respectively), large craft boating (13% compared with 7% and 4% respectively), surfing (19% compared with 16% and 12% respectively), and water sports (11% compared with 8% and 3% respectively).

When aquatic recreation was analysed by ethnicity, European youth reported higher levels of participation than all other ethnic groups in aquatic recreation that involved boat or paddling craft. More European and Maori youth than Pacific Islands and Asian youth reported taking part *very often* in surfing (20% and 19% compared with 8% and 3% respectively). More Maori and Pacific Islands youth than European and Asian youth participated in netting/shell-fish gathering activities (35% and 37% compared with 21% and 15% respectively). Asian youth had lower levels of participation in any aquatic recreational activity except for land-based fishing, where their participation was no different from that of European students, but less than that of Maori and Pacific Islands students.

2.2.3. Ownership of, or Access to, Aquatic Recreational Equipment

Most students (*n* = 1959, 89%) reported ownership of, or access to, some form of aquatic recreational equipment. The most-frequently reported items were body (boogie) boards, fishing gear and snorkelling gear. Almost three quarters of students (74%) reported the availability of body boards, more than two thirds (68%) had access to fishing gear and over one half (53%) owned, or had use of, snorkelling gear. Approximately one third of all students reported ownership of, or access to, surfboards (34%), small boating craft (33%) or paddle craft (32%). One quarter of all students (25%) reported having access to a large boat or yacht.

Table 3 shows that when ownership of, or access to, aquatic recreational equipment was analysed by gender, slightly more females reported ownership of, or access to, body boards (females 77%, males 71%) but more males reported ownership of, or access to, surfboards (males 40%, females 28%). There was also a noticeable gender difference with respect to fishing gear, with more males than females claiming ownership of, or access to, fishing gear (males 72%, females 64%). Similar proportions reported access to small boats (males 33%, females 34%), paddle craft (males and females 32%) and snorkelling gear (males 55%, females 52%).

When analysed by socio-economic status, students from high-decile schools reported greater ownership of, or access to, every type of aquatic equipment included in the survey. Not surprisingly, the difference between students from low-decile and high-decile schools was especially noticeable in the availability of high-cost equipment including surfboards (low-decile 30%, high-decile 39%), body boards (low-decile 62%, high-decile 80%), paddle craft (low-decile 22%, high-decile 38%), and large boat (low-decile 17%, high-decile 30%).

Table 3 also shows that, when analysed by ethnicity, more European and Maori than other youth reported ownership of, or access to, any aquatic recreational equipment. European students reported greater access to boating and paddle-craft than all other groups and Maori students reported greatest access to surfboards and fishing gear. Pacific Islands and Asian youth were less likely than Maori and European youth to own, or have access to, any aquatic equipment. Asian youth were the least likely of all groups to own, or have access to, any aquatic equipment, although over one third owned, or had access to, a body board (37%) and four out of ten owned, or had access to, fishing gear (43%).

Table 3. Ownership of, or Access to, Aquatic Equipment by Gender, Socio-economic Status via Decile Rating of School Attended and Ethnicity

	Surfboard n %	Body board n %	Paddle craft n %	Small boat n %	Fishing gear n %	Snorkelling gear n %
Male	470 40.1	834 71.2	368 31.5	390 33.3	838 71.6	638 54.5
Female	287 27.8	793 76.9	328 31.8	347 33.6	658 63.8	535 51.9
Low-Decile	188 29.8	392 62.2	141 22.4	174 27.6	414 65.7	303 48.1
Mid-Decile	208 32.7	484 76.0	201 31.6	211 33.1	426 66.9	341 53.5
High-Decile	361 38.6	751 80.3	355 38.0	352 37.6	656 70.2	529 56.6
European	510 38.4	1115 83.3	507 37.9	527 39.4	982 73.3	792 59.1
Maori	164 40.4	316 77.8	111 27.3	122 30.1	282 69.5	241 59.4
Pacific Islands	40 19.6	96 47.1	38 18.6	41 20.1	119 58.3	82 40.2
Asian	32 15.5	76 36.9	36 17.5	37 18.1	88 43.1	39 19.1
Other ethnicities	11 23.9	24 52.7	4 10.1	10 21.7	25 54.3	19 40.1
Total	757 34.4	1627 73.9	696 31.6	737 33.5	1496 67.9	1173 53.3

Table 4. Frequency of Self-reported Risky Swimming Behaviours in the Previous Year

Risky behaviours	Never		Sometimes		Often	
	n	%	n	%	n	%
Swum in clothing	1506	69.2	533	24.5	138	6.3
Swum alone	1151	52.9	832	38.2	194	8.9
Dived into unknown depth	1462	67.2	509	23.4	206	9.5
Swum unsupervised	574	26.4	883	40.6	720	33.1
Swum after alcohol/drugs	1665	76.5	421	19.3	91	4.2
Swum in prohibited area	1093	50.2	888	40.8	196	9.0
Swum when cold/tired	952	43.7	1026	47.1	199	9.1
Swum outside patrol area	845	38.8	930	42.7	402	18.5
Dived into shallow water	1736	79.7	352	16.2	89	4.1
Ignored safety directions	1327	61.0	711	32.7	139	6.4

2.2.4. Risky Swimming Behaviour

Students were asked whether they had engaged in ten at-risk behaviours related to swimming activity. Table 4 shows that swimming without supervision was the most frequently reported at-risk behaviour to happen *often* (33%). Diving into shallow water headfirst (4%) and using alcohol/drugs when engaged in swimming activity (4%) were the at-risk behaviours least likely to happen *often*.

When swimming behaviours were analysed by gender, significant differences were evident with males reporting higher incidence of risky behaviours in all but one of the ten at-risk swimming behaviours, the exception being swimming in everyday clothing (see Table 5). Females were more likely than males to *never* have performed any risky behaviours and males were more likely to have *often* performed risky behaviours when swimming. For example, males were twice as likely to report *often* swimming alone (males 12%, females 6%), diving headfirst into an unknown depth of water (males 13%, females 6%), swimming in a prohibited area (males 11%, females 6%), swimming when cold or tired (males 12%, females 6%), swimming outside a patrolled area at a surf beach (males 24%, females 12%) and diving headfirst into shallow water (males 6%, females 2%). In contrast to this, more females than males reported *never* swimming in prohibited areas (females 57%, males 44%); swimming outside patrol areas (females 43%, males 34%); ignoring water safety directions (females 67%, males 54%); swimming alone (females 60%, males 47%) or unsupervised (females 31%, males 22%).

Socio-economic status, as measured by the decile rating of the school attended, did not influence the incidence of risky swimming behaviour to any great extent. No significant differences were found between the risky swimming behaviours of students attending mid- and high-decile schools. However, youth from low-decile schools were more likely than those attending high-decile schools to have swum in clothes (low-decile 35%, high-decile 28%), ignored safety directions (low-decile 49%, high-decile 45%) and dived in without checking the depth (low-decile 36%, high-decile 30%).

Inter-group analysis of risky swimming behaviour by ethnicity found some differences in swim behaviours among ethnic groups. European and Asian youth were less likely than Maori and Pacific Islands youth to swim when clothed, dive in without checking the water depth, and dive headfirst knowing that the water was shallow. More Asian youth than all other ethnic groups reported *never* having engaged in any of the risky swimming practices. For example, more Asian youth than European, Maori and Pacific Islands youth reported *never* swimming unsupervised (48% compared with 25%, 19% and 25% respectively) and *never* swimming outside patrolled areas at a surf beach (70% compared with 35%, 31% and 48% respectively). Almost half of European (45%) and Maori youth (47%) reported *sometimes* swimming outside surf patrol areas and some stated that they did so *often* (21% and 23% respectively). More European and Maori youth than Asian and Pacific Islands youth reported using alcohol/drugs in conjunction with swimming activity either *sometimes* or *often* (24% and 32% compared with 11% and 19% respectively).

2.2.5. Other Aquatic Recreation Behaviour

Students were asked if they had engaged in six at-risk behaviours commonly associated with aquatic activities other than swimming (see Table 6). Almost one fifth (19%) of respondents reported that they *never* wore lifejackets during boating activity and more than one quarter (28%) *never* checked the weather or water conditions beforehand. Table 6 also shows that almost half (42%) reported having done the activity alone and one fifth (21%) reported having used alcohol/drugs in association with aquatic activities.

Table 7 shows significant differences between the reporting of risky behaviours among males and females, with the exception of checking the weather/water conditions beforehand. In terms of frequency of reporting risky behaviour, more females than males reported *never* having performed any of the risky behaviours, and more males reported *sometimes* or *often* performing any of the at-risk behaviours during aquatic recreation. For example, more than two thirds of females *never* did aquatic activity on their own compared to one half of males (females 67%, males 51%), and more females than males *never* used alcohol/drugs in conjunction with aquatic activity (females 85%, males 74%). Fewer females *never* told an adult beforehand (females 6%, males 11%), *never* wore lifejackets (females 16%, males 22%), or *never* had adult supervision (females 7%, males 14%). In addition, more females than males reported *always* telling an adult of their intentions beforehand (females 45%, males 32%), *always* wearing lifejackets (females 35%, males 28%), or *always* having adult supervision (females 22%, males 17%).

Table 5. Differences in Risky Swimming Behaviours in the Previous Year by Gender

Risky Behaviour		% who reported this behaviour	*Mann-Whitney U*	*p*
Swim on your own	Female	42.8	535332.5	<.001*
	Male	52.1		
Dive without checking	Female	24.9	500927.0	<.001*
	Male	41.2		
Swim unsupervised	Female	69.4	507742.5	<.001*
	Male	77.9		
Swim after alcohol	Female	20.6	558671.0	<.001*
	Male	27.8		
Swim in prohibited place	Female	43.5	516746.0	<.001*
	Male	56.4		
Swim when cold/tired	Female	55.4	566604.0	<.006*
	Male	58.0		
Swim outside patrol area	Female	56.6	507777.0	<.001*
	Male	66.0		
Dive into shallow water headfirst	Female	14.6	528039.0	<.001*
	Male	26.9		
Ignore safety directions	Female	32.7	513179.0	<.001*
	Male	45.9		
Swim in everyday clothing	Female	30.4	5854228.5	.134
	Male	32.7		

* statistically significant.

Table 6. Risky Behaviour during Other Aquatic Recreation in the Previous Year

Behaviour	Never n	%	Sometimes n	%	Often n	%
Told adult beforehand	184	8.9	605	29.1	1290	62.0
Had adult supervision	223	10.7	915	44.0	942	45.3
Wore a lifejacket	392	18.9	560	27.0	1124	54.2
Checked weather/water	591	28.4	670	32.2	819	39.4
Did the activity alone	1212	58.3	713	34.3	154	7.4
Used alcohol/drugs	1642	79.0	360	17.3	77	3.7

Table 7. Differences in Risky Swimming Behaviours in the Previous Year by Gender

Risky Behaviour		% who reported this behaviour	*Mann-Whitney U*	*p*
Never told adult beforehand	Female	6.4	512631.7	<.001*
	Male	11.1		
Never had adult supervision	Female	7.4	537894.5	<.001*
	Male	13.7		
Never wore a lifejacket	Female	15.9	548062.5	<.001*
	Male	21.6		
Never checked weather/water	Female	26.3	593899.0	.499
	Male	33.1		
Never doing the activity alone	Female	66.9	514564.5	<.001*
	Male	50.8		
Never used alcohol/drugs	Female	85.4	535957.5	<.001*
	Male	73.5		

* Statistically significant with Bonferroni correction.

No significant differences were found when risky behaviour during aquatic recreation was analysed by socio-economic status. When risky behaviours were analysed by ethnicity, more Maori, Pacific Islands and Asian than European youth either *never* or *sometimes* wore a lifejacket when boating (56%, 57%, 54% compared with 40% respectively). More Maori, Pacific Islands and Asian youth than European youth *never* or *sometimes* told an adult of their intentions before participating in aquatic recreation (47%, 46%, 47% compared with 33% respectively). While the differences in alcohol consumption between ethnic groups was not significant, more Asian and Pacific Islands youth than European and Maori youth reported *never* using alcohol/drugs in conjunction with aquatic recreation (91% and 83% compared with 79% and 73% respectively). In contrast to this, more European and Maori youth than Asian or Pacific Islands youth reported *sometimes* using alcohol/drugs (18% and 24% compared with 6% and 10% respectively).

2.3. Discussion

2.3.1. Exposure to Risk of Drowning

Results of the study confirm that New Zealand youth do frequently engage in a wide range of aquatic recreational activities. Most youth had engaged in swimming and other water-related activities in the previous year, which would suggest that not only are such activities relatively accessible but also that the 'pleasures' associated with aquatic recreation are widely recognised by youth. The high levels of participation found in this study would tend to reinforce previous suggestions by Langley and Smeijiers (1997) that the high drowning rates among New Zealand youth when compared to American youth are the consequence of greater exposure to water and higher exposure to risk because of youth fondness for aquatic recreation.

Yet high incidence of drowning may be more than a reflection of greater exposure to risk. In the case of youth swimming (the activity most frequently engaged in prior to drowning), much of the activity took place in relatively safe environments with almost all youth (n = 1950; 88%) having swum at public or school pools. Such sites can be considered relatively low-risk since they generally are closely regulated and supervised environments. Drowning statistics confirm that they are infrequent sites of youth drowning, accounting for only 8 deaths (7%) in the 15-19 year age group between 1992-2001 (Source: WSNZ Drownbase™, 2002). That most youth swimming in New Zealand took place in relatively safe environments is consistent with observations made in overseas studies on youth drowning incidence. For example, Brenner, Trumble, Smith, Kessler and Overpeck (2001) found that of 407 unintentional drowning incidents among 15-19 year old American youth in 1995, only 47 (12%) occurred in swimming pools compared with 280 (69%) that occurred in freshwater locations.

The frequency of New Zealand youth swimming activity at high-risk locations such as un-patrolled surf beaches and other open water locations was not great. Less than one sixth of students had swum more than 20 times in the previous year at any location other than patrolled surf beaches. In the case of rivers, less than one in ten had swum in a river or creek more than 20 times in the previous year and more than half of students (53%) had never used them. In spite of this low usage, more people drown in rivers than in any other New Zealand aquatic environment and one fifth of victims (21%) are less than 18 years of age (WSNZ, 2002). Given the relatively low exposure to high-risk environments reported by youth who took part in this study, it would appear that the reasons for increased drowning as a consequence of recreational swimming at these sites lie elsewhere than in high frequencies of exposure to risk.

Evidence of high exposure to risk also fails to adequately explain the complex nature of drowning risk when applied to other forms of aquatic recreation. Surfing and paddling activities were the most popular activities other than swimming, with approximately two thirds of youth having engaged in surfing (*n* = 1438; 65%) and paddling activities (*n* = 1463; 67%). Thus, on the basis of exposure to risk, one would expect surfing and paddling activities to be major contributors to the youth drowning statistics. However, this is not the case since these activities accounted for only 12% ($n = 7$) of youth fatalities from 1992-2001 (Source: WSNZ Drownbase™, 2004). Furthermore, surf rescue statistics from 1990-1995 show that surfing was almost six times less likely than swimming (surfing 10%, swimming 57%) to be the activity engaged in prior to rescue (Moran, 1996). Reduced drowning and rescue incidence may be attributed to the presence of buoyancy aids (lifejackets, wetsuits and the in-built flotation in surfboards, kayaks and wave skis). Alternately, another plausible explanation might lie in the relatively high frequency in which youth participated, with one third (34%) of students surfing *often* or *very often*. Such frequent exposure might have allowed opportunity to develop appropriate skills and knowledge with which to counter any increased risk associated with increased surfing participation. In other words, frequent surfing activity, rather than exacerbating risk through greater exposure to danger, might have actually reduced risk by providing opportunity to develop compensatory risk-reducing skills and abilities.

In contrast to surfing and paddling activity, fewer students participated in boating activity in small craft ($n = 1307$; 59%) or large craft ($n = 1026$; 47%). More importantly perhaps, most of those who had participated in small craft boating reported making less than 10 trips in the previous year ($n = 834$; 38%) and only one in ten students reported making more than 20 trips ($n = 222$; 10%). Yet in spite of much less exposure to risk than surfing or paddling previously discussed, boating accounted for more than one-quarter ($n = 16$; 27%) of recreational drowning fatalities in the 15-19 year age group between 1992-2001 in New Zealand (Source: WSNZ Drownbase™, 2004). Lack of experience and opportunity to develop water safety skills as a consequence of only occasional boating activity might be a more plausible explanation for high incidence of boating fatalities than high exposure to risk. Similar conclusions have been reported elsewhere with lack of experience in youth being strongly associated with increased risk of fatal boating incidents in a study on recreational boating in Ohio (Molberg, Hopkins, Paulson & Gunn, 1993). Given the high level of mortality associated with youth boating and the extent of casual boating reported in this study, interventions aimed at making youth boating practice safer through targeted boating education might help reduce boating fatalities among youth.

One frequently cited reason why more males drown than females is because males are exposed to greater risk as a consequence of their higher participation rates in aquatic recreation (Brenner, et al., 2001; Howland et al., 1996; Quan & Cummings, 2003). Howland et al. (1996) found that males in the 16-25 year age group had significantly more total annual aquatic activity days for the prior year (males 61.4 days, females 51.5 days; $p = .02$) and did more swimming in natural bodies of water. However, when swimming activity was analysed by gender in the present study, no significant difference was found in the total amount of swimming activity between males and females. Gender-based differences in frequency of risk exposure as a result of swimming activity are thus unlikely to account for the extensive differences in drowning incidence between males and females in this age group.

When the other dimension of risk exposure, the extent or magnitude of drowning risk from swimming was considered, some differences were evident between males and females in their choice of swimming location. More females than males swam at low-risk locations including private pools (females 57%, males 47%), flat-water beaches (females 68%, males 62%) or patrolled beaches (females 79%, males 68%), whereas more males swam *often/very often* at un-patrolled surf beaches, lakes and ponds, or rivers and creeks. Gulliver and Begg (2005) reported similar results with 21-year-old Dunedin females more likely to choose low-risk locations such as patrolled surf beaches (females 59%, males 55%), and males more likely to use un-patrolled beaches (males, 52%, females 41%).

However, irrespective of these gender-related differences in choice of low- and high-risk locations for swimming, it is unlikely that poor choice of location alone can adequately explain why six times more young New Zealand males than females (males 18, females 3) aged 15-19 years drowned while swimming between 1992-2001 (Source: WSNZ Drownbase™, 2004). Paradoxically, even though significantly more females than males swam at patrolled surf beaches, almost twice as many males (males 63%, females 37%) in the 16-19 year age group were involved in surf incidents necessitating rescue between 1995-2000 (Source: SLSNZ Rescue Statistics, 2004). On patrolled surf beaches at least, drowning risk from swimming for males would appear to be more about what male youth bring to the activity in terms of their practice of water safety and less about increased exposure to risk through more frequent participation.

Males did report higher levels of participation than females in aquatic activities other than swimming, especially in the traditionally male-oriented outdoor pursuits of boat- and land-based fishing, netting and shell-fish gathering, and underwater activity. For example, almost two thirds ($n = 737$; 63%) of males had engaged in boat-based fishing compared with less than one half (n = 508; 49%) of females. Gulliver and Begg (2005) have reported similar gender-oriented differences in boating activity (males 73%, females 57%) among young adult New Zealanders. However, even though statistically significant, these differences in activity level are unlikely to fully account for the seven-fold difference in boating fatalities (males 14, females 2) between 1992-2001 among youth (Source: WSNZ Drownbase™, 2004). Drowning risk for males during boating recreation, like swimming activities previously discussed, appears to again be more about differences in what male youth bring to their aquatic activity than simply a reflection of differences in risk exposure.

Some differences in levels of participation, and therefore exposure to risk of drowning were evident when aquatic recreation was analysed by ethnicity, with European and Maori youth engaging in more activity than Pacific Islands and Asian youth. On this basis, drowning risk, measured by risk exposure alone, should be greater for European and Maori students since they engaged in much greater aquatic activity than others. However, drowning and surf rescue statistics for the 16-19 year age group do not confirm this possibility. European youth, who constitute 61% of the youth population, are only slightly over-represented in drowning statistics, comprising 63% of the drowning toll from 1992-2001 (Source: WSNZ Drownbase™, 2004). In addition, the proportion of surf rescue incidents in which they were victims (62% of surf rescues from 2001-2004), closely matched their representation in the population (Source: SLSNZ Rescue Statistics 2005).

Some evidence was found among New Zealand youth to support the contention of Smith and Brenner (1995) that students from specific ethnicities, including indigenous populations, were at greater risk as a consequence of "increased exposure to dangerous bodies of water such as rivers and lakes and decreased access to protected (supervised) swimming areas" (p. 159). Maori students, like their European counterparts, took part in more aquatic activity than other minority groups and were most likely to have often used un-patrolled surf beaches, lakes or rivers. They are also over-represented in youth drowning statistics, comprising 21% of the youth population yet 32% of drowning victims from 1992-2002 (Source: WSNZ Drownbase™, 2004). In addition, more than one third of Maori compared with one fifth of European youth (35% vs. 21%) had participated in netting/shell-fish gathering. The risk of drowning for Maori youth may therefore be exacerbated by their participation in the collection of seafood via fishing and netting/shell-fish gathering activity. These findings among Maori youth may be indicative of increased incidence of drowning among the adult Maori population as postulated by Langley et al. (2002) and help explain why Maori drown at nearly twice the rate of non-Maori (WSNZ media release, 18 November, 2003).

The impact of socio-economic status on drowning risk as a consequence of differing levels of participation in aquatic recreation was not great. Students from high-decile schools took part in more swimming and other aquatic recreational activity, whereas those from low-decile schools took part in considerably less. Not surprisingly, more students from high-decile schools than those from mid- or low-decile schools participated more frequently in activities that required some capital expense including, for example, small craft boating (14% compared with 6% and 8% respectively). The only exceptions to this pattern were land-based fishing and netting/shell-fishing where no significant differences in participation were found across socio-economic groups. The reasons for this probably lie in the economic importance of fishing and shell-fish gathering among lower socio-economic groups. For example, more students from low-decile schools frequently took part in land-based fishing, a possible reflection of ease of access and low cost of participation (25% compared with 19% and 16% respectively).

2.3.2. Youth Behaviour in the Aquatic Environment

The extent of risky behaviours of youth who took part in the study suggests that the pleasures of an active aquatic recreational lifestyle potentially can turn into pitfalls when the practice of water safety is ignored. Two factors thought to heighten drowning risk in youth aquatic activity are lack of adult supervision and doing the activity alone (Howland et al., 1996; Smith & Brenner, 1995). Almost one half of the youth taking part in the study reported having swum alone ($n = 1026$; 47%) or undertaken other aquatic activity ($n = 867$; 42%) alone. Socio-economic status and ethnicity did not unduly influence this practice but gender did. Females were more likely to *never* swim alone (females 58%, males 47%) or do other aquatic activity alone (females 67%, males 51%), whereas males were twice as likely as females to *often* swim alone (males 13%, females 6%).

As well as swimming alone, a widespread lack of adult supervision was reported. Three quarters of youth (74%) had swum without adult supervision, the most frequent at-risk behaviour reported, and of these, one third (33%) reported that they *often* did so. Lack of adult supervision was somewhat less evident in respect of aquatic activity other than swimming. While a greater proportion of students reported some adult supervision during other forms of aquatic recreation, less than half (45%) reported *mostly* or *always* having adult supervision. Differences in supervision were again evident by gender with more female aquatic activity supervised, but even then, one in every four females reported that they did most of their swimming unsupervised (males 38%, females 26%). These results are similar to those reported in the 1991 Youth Risk Behaviour Survey (YRBSS) in the United States which found that almost one half of males and one third of females did most of their swimming unsupervised (CDC, 1992).

Given the extensive practice of youth aquatic activity without adult supervision reported here and in other studies (CDC, 1992; Howland et al., 1996; Smith & Brenner, 1995), it is unlikely that youth drowning risk could be reduced by appeals for greater adult supervision (through more parental involvement or increased professional life-guarding). Similarly, attempting to engage youth in more regulated, adult-assisted aquatic activity is likely to be resisted by independent-minded youth and is thus unlikely to offer any realistic diminution of drowning risk. What a continuation of youth aquatic activity without adult control does, however, is place an even greater premium on the coping skills of youth. It therefore would seem critical to invest in education by providing youth with water safety life-skills that would allow them to make informed decisions about their own safety as they move towards adulthood and independence.

The frequent reporting of risky behaviour at surf beaches is a cause of concern given that most respondents (76%) had swum at a patrolled surf beach in the previous year and youth are the age group most frequently rescued from the surf as previously reported. Four in every ten students (39%) reported having swum outside a patrolled area in the previous year and more than two thirds of students (68%) had seen their friends swim outside patrol areas at surf beaches. More males than females reported swimming outside patrolled areas (males 65%, females 56%). In addition, more males than females had observed their peers swimming outside patrolled areas (males 75%, females 61%). This greater risk-taking behaviour by young men in the surf helps explain why twice as many males were rescued by surf patrols in the five summer seasons from 2000-2004 (Source: SLSNZ Rescue Statistics, 2000-2004). Furthermore, the observation that a quarter of male youth reported *often* swimming outside patrol flags, in spite of extensive public promotion of the necessity to 'Swim between the flags', reinforces claims by Baker and Dietz (1979) that many injuries result less from lack of knowledge or skill than from failure to apply what is known. It tends also to temper claims that providing safer alternative swimming sites and lifeguard facilities may be more effective than teaching high-risk groups such as male adolescents not to swim in hazardous sites (Smith & Brenner, 1995).

Risk of drowning was exacerbated by the consumption of alcohol during aquatic recreation. Approximately one quarter of youth reported having used alcohol in association with swimming activity (24%) and during other aquatic activity (21%) in the previous year. Strong gender-based differences in behaviour were again evident, with more than one quarter of males having reported some alcohol intake during swimming activity (males 28%, females 19%) and almost twice as many males consuming alcohol during other forms of aquatic recreation (males 27%, females 15%). More males also had observed friends drinking alcohol during aquatic activity (males 33%, females 24%). The percentage of students in this study who claimed to have mixed alcohol with aquatic activity is similar to the proportion of alcohol-associated youth drowning incidents from 1992-2001 (Source: WSNZ Drownbase™, 2002). Whereas one fifth (21%) of students reported some alcohol consumption during aquatic activity in the present study, alcohol was known to be associated with approximately one sixth (17%) of recreational drowning incidents in the previous decade. The drowning statistics also reflect the strong gender bias reported in this study on the role of alcohol in aquatic recreation, with no young female victims of alcohol-related recreational drowning during that period, compared with almost one-fifth (18 %) of young male fatalities being alcohol-related.

Most males who had reported some alcohol consumption during swimming activity (28%) also reported having swum unsupervised (86%), outside the patrolled areas (77%), in a prohibited place (77%) or alone (57%). Similarly, most males who reported consuming alcohol during other aquatic activity (31%) also reported having no adult supervision (76%), not checking conditions before setting out (70%), not wearing a lifejacket (68%) and not telling an adult beforehand (66%). This clustering of unsafe behaviours among males perhaps explains the over-representation of males in drowning statistics as suggested in previous studies. Howland et al. (1996) found that the association between drinking and other risk-taking behaviours was strongly gender-oriented, with males who had consumed alcohol on their last aquatic activity day more likely to swim without lifeguard supervision (males 37%, females 26%) or to swim alone (males 15%, females 4%). Similarly, in a study of young male U.S Army soldiers, Bell, Amoroso, Yore, Senier, Williams, Smith and Theriault (2001) found that alcohol use was associated with a ten-fold increase in reckless behaviour such as violation of safety rules and swimming in an unauthorised area, particularly by those less than 21 years of age. Furthermore, a recent study in Oklahoma by Levy et al. (2004) suggests that those who consumed alcohol during the day were 3.5 times more likely to suffer a submersion injury and that the risk was especially high for underage drinkers aged 15-20 years.

In the area of boat safety, indifference among youth towards the use of buoyancy aids also was likely to exacerbate drowning risk. One fifth of students ($n = 394$; 19%) reported that they never wore lifejackets during boating activity, while two thirds ($n = 1181$; 67%) reported that they had seen their friends not wear a lifejacket. That a substantial number of students did not see the necessity to wear a lifejacket is a cause for concern especially since it is widely reported that the wearing of buoyancy aids could prevent most boating fatalities (United States Coastguard, 2003). A study of 15-19-year-olds in Washington State by Quan, Bennett and Williams (2002) found a similar lack of awareness among a focus group of 84 teenagers who rated being in a small boat without a lifejacket as the least dangerous of ten aquatic-related activities. They also reported that none of 40 young drowning victims in Washington State from 1997-1999 were wearing lifejackets and that observed lifejacket use was lowest in those older than 14 years of age.

Greater resistance to lifejacket use was evident among males with fewer females *never* wearing lifejackets (females 16%, males 22%) and more females *always* wearing them (females 35%, males 28%). Also, more males reported observing that their friends had not worn lifejackets (males 72%, females 59%). Quan, Bennett, Cummings, Trusty and Treser (1998) found similar resistance to the wearing of buoyancy aids by male youth and adults in a study of 4,000 boaters in the US Northwest. They suggested that infrequent use of lifejackets was a factor in the higher incidence of boat-related drowning among adolescent males, and that an understanding of user/non-user attitudes may help in structuring safety messages specifically targeted at this high-risk group. On the evidence of unsafe behaviours towards lifejacket use among youth reported here, similar action targeted specifically at young New Zealand males would also appear appropriate.

More European youth than Maori, Pacific Islands and Asian youth had *mostly* or *always* worn a lifejacket during boating activity in the previous year (60% compared with 44%, 43% and 47% respectively). Similar ethnic differences were reported in Canada where the Canadian Red Cross (1998) found lesser proper lifejacket use among drowning victims from indigenous groups compared with non-indigenous Canadians (6% compared with 11%). However, whether failure to use lifejackets among different ethnic groups reflects unfamiliarity with boating activity, antipathy to their use, or their cost (students attending low-decile schools also showed a less positive attitude to lifejacket use than those attending medium- or high-decile schools) requires further study.

Another area of potentially dangerous boating practice is the lack of safety preparation beforehand. Only one fifth (20%) of youth *always* checked the weather and water conditions before setting out, whereas more than a quarter (28%) *never* checked conditions. Furthermore, more than one third (38%) *never* or only *sometimes* told an adult of their intentions beforehand. Not surprisingly, males were again to the fore in this risk-taking behaviour with less than a third (32%) *always* advising an adult of their intentions compared with almost half (45%) of females. Clearly, many young New Zealanders do not comply with the fundamental preparatory advice to any boater of always checking conditions before setting out and of always informing a responsible person of your intentions. Whether such widespread unsafe practice reflects a lack of safety knowledge however, or is a deliberate decision to ignore such advice, or a combination of both, is difficult to ascertain and requires further study.

2.4. Conclusion

This study found ample evidence of frequent aquatic activity among New Zealand youth. For example, almost all (98%) had participated in some swimming activity, three quarters had swum at a surf beach and two thirds had engaged in surfing or paddling activity. On the basis of the evidence of participation reported in this study, it would appear that, like their adult counterparts, young New Zealanders enthusiastically engage in a lifestyle of aquatic recreation that maximises the opportunities available in an aquatically-blessed environment. However, the potential benefits associated with frequent physical activity for youth (and the population at large) would appear tempered by the very real dangers of drowning inherent in any human interaction with an aquatic environment and as indicated by the high rates of rescue and drowning in New Zealand. Furthermore, it would appear from the abundant evidence of risky behaviours found in this study among youth when engaged in aquatic recreation that endorsement of frequent physical activity especially in the aquatic environment needs to be strongly predicated on the need for *safe* participation.

How youth behaved around water appears to offer strong culminating evidence as to why youth have been consistently reported as one of the most at-risk groups for drowning. Moreover, this chapter has highlighted salient gender-related differences in drowning risk as a consequence of how males and females behaved in aquatic settings. For example, males consistently reported greater at-risk behaviour than females, especially with regard to alcohol consumption during aquatic activity, lifeguard supervision, obeying safety advice, and the wearing of lifejackets. Furthermore, the association of alcohol consumption and a cluster of other at-risk behaviours among young males are especially disconcerting given that a similar clustering of risky behaviours around alcohol use has been identified as a major contributor to drowning fatalities among older males (Bell et al., 2001; Howland et al., 1996). Thus, it would appear that many of the at-risk behaviours reported in drowning fatalities among older males are common practice in males at an earlier age. Because of this, early educational interventions that address entrenched practices such as mixing alcohol with aquatic recreation should be persisted with and intensified.

The study has identified clearly the nature of youth aquatic recreational practice, and especially what activities are popular within the youth population of New Zealand. Swimming, surfing, paddling, boating and fishing activities were popular among youth and programmes that specifically target these activities may provide youth with a better appreciation of safe participation in them. In addition, youth water safety education may also need to focus on the realistic demands of open water environments because most youth activities take place in open water locations such as surf beaches. Consequently, opportunity to learn about water safety in an open water environment may prove to be more valuable than pool-based activity. Surf beaches in particular have been shown to be popular sites of youth aquatic activity and learning about them on location may make young people's water safety education more meaningful and relevant. Furthermore, because much of youth aquatic activity is done without adult supervision, water safety education might also need to concentrate on empowering youth to make effective decisions about their own safety. Therefore, programmes that promote risk identification and risk-reduction management skills, both of which have been identified as lacking among many youth (Moran, 2006) may be effective in teaching youth how to look after themselves in the aquatic environment.

Finally, encouraging young people to take part in safe aquatic activity because of its potential benefits to the individual and to society should still be an essential part of every school health and physical education curriculum. Encouraging young and old alike to take part in a safe and considered manner through the application of sound principles of water safety has the potential to realise many of the pleasures traditionally associated with aquatic activity without the attendant pitfalls - for health professionals to advocate anything less is simply not an option.

REFERENCES

Ausport (2003). Participation in exercise, recreation and sport 2002. Retrieved August 28, 2007, from: http://www.ausport.gov.au/fulltext/2003/scors/ERASS.pdf

Baker, S.P., & Dietz, P.E. (1979). Injury prevention. In *Healthy people: The Surgeon General's report on health promotion and disease prevention, background papers.* Washington, DC: Government Printing Offices (no. 70-55071A).

Baker, S.P., O'Neil, B., Ginsburg, M.J., & Li, G. (1992). *The injury fact book.* New York: Oxford University Press.

Bell, N.S., Amoroso, P.J., Yore, M.M., Senier, L., Williams, J.O., Smith, G.S., & Theriault, A. (2001). Alcohol and other risk factors among male active duty U.S. army soldiers. *Aviation, Space and Environmental Medicine, 72,* 1086-1095.

Berger, B.G., & Owen, D.R. (1992). Preliminary analysis of a causal relationship between swimming and stress reduction: Intense exercise may negate effects. *International Journal of Sports Psychology, 23,* 70-85.

Berger, B.G., & Owen, D.R. (1988). Stress reduction and mood enhancement in four exercise modes: Swimming, body conditioning, Hatha yoga and fencing. *Research Quarterly for Exercise and Sport, 59,* 148-159.

Biro, M., Fugedi, B., & Revesz, L. (2007). The role of teaching swimming in the formation of a conscious healthy lifestyle. *International Journal of Aquatic Research and Education, 1*(3), 269-284.

Board of Education. (1919). *Syllabus of physical training for schools, 1919.* London: His Majesty's Stationery Office.

Brenner, R.A. (2002). Childhood drowning is a global concern. *British Medical Journal, 324*(7345), 1049-1050.

Brenner, R.A., Trumble, A.C., Smith, G. S., Kessler, E.P., & Overpeck, M.D. (2001). Where children drown, United States, 1995. *Pediatrics, 108*(1), 85-89.

British Marine Federation. (2006). Watersports and leisure participation survey 2006. Egham, Surrey: BMF.

Canadian Red Cross Society. (1998). *National drowning report: Visual surveillance report.* Gloucester, ON: Canadian Red Cross Society.

Centers for Disease Control and Prevention [CDC]. (1992). Behaviours related to unintentional and intentional injuries among high school students – United States, 1991. *Mortality and Morbidity Weekly Review, 41,* 760, 721.

Centers for Disease Control and Prevention [CDC]. (1996). *Physical activity and health: A report of the Surgeon-General.* Washington: CDC. Retrieved August 26, 2007 from http://www.cdc.gov/nccdphp/sgr/contents.htm

Centers for Disease Control and Prevention [CDC]. (2002). *Water-related injuries in NCIPC Injury Fact book,* 2001-2002. Washington: CDC. Retrieved 25 August, 2005, from http:// www.cdc.gov/ncipc/fact_book/30_waterRelated_Injuries.htm

Chalmers, D., McNoe, B., & Stephenson, S. (2004). *Drowning, near-drowning and other water-related injury: Literature review of national injury data.* A report to the Accident Compensation Corporation, May 2004. Wellington: ACC.

Child and Youth Mortality Review Committee [CYMR]. (2005). *Circumstances surrounding drowning in those under 25 in New Zealand (1980-2002).* A report to Water Safety New Zealand June 2005. Wellington, New Zealand: WSNZ.

Gulliver, P., & Begg, D. (2005). Usual water-related behaviour and 'near-drowning' incidents in young adults. *Australian and New Zealand Journal of Public Health, 29*(3), 238-243.

Harborview Injury Prevention and Research Centre. (2000). *Drowning: Research questions.* Retrieved August 13, 2007, from http://depts.washington.edu/hiprc/practices/topic/ drowning/research.html

Hillary Commission. (1998). *Young people and sport.* Wellington, New Zealand: Hillary Commission.

Hillary Commission. (1999). *Push Play facts.* Wellington, NewZealand: Hillary Commission.

Howland J., Hingson, R., Mangione, T.W., Bell, N., & Bak, S. (1996). Why are most drowning victims men? Sex differences in aquatic skills and behaviours. *American Journal of Public Health, 86,* 93-96.

Injury Prevention Research Unit. (2003). *Drowning-related deaths in New Zealand 1989-1998. IPRU Fact Sheet, 28.* Dunedin: IPRU, University of Otago.

Italian Statistical Institute (2000). Italian 2000 data on participation in single sports. Retrieved August 29, 2007, from: http://w3.uniroma1.it/compass/italy.htm

Lamprecht, M., & Stamm, H. (2002). Sports activity in Switzerland and the COMPASS framework. Retrieved August 29, 2007, from: http://w3.uniroma1.it/compass/switzerland. htm

Langley, J.D., Warner, M., Smith, G., & Wright, C. (2002). Drowning related deaths in New Zealand 1980-1994. *Australian and New Zealand Journal of Public Health, 25*(5), 451-457.

Langley, J.D., & Smeijers, J. (1997). Injury mortality among children and teenagers in New Zealand compared with the United States. *Injury Prevention, 3,* 195-199.

Lenček, L., & Bosker, G. (1999). *The beach: The history of paradise on earth.* London: Pimlico.

Levy, D.T., Mallone, S., Miller, T.R., Smith, G.S., Spicer, R.S., Romano, E.O., & Fisher, D.A. (2004). Alcohol involvement in burn, submersion, spinal cord, and brain injuries. *Medical Science Monitor, 10*(1), 17-24.

McKirnan, M.D., & Bloor, C.M. (1994). Clinical significance of coronary vascular adaptations to exercise training. *Medicine and Science in Sport and Exercise, 26*, 1262-1268.

Mackie, I.J. (1999). Patterns of drowning in Australia, 1992-1997. *Medical Journal of Australia, 171*, 587-590.

Marine Institute. (2004). A national survey of water-based leisure activities in Ireland 2003. Galway, Ireland: Marine Institute.

Matsumoto, I., Araki, H., Tsuda, K., Odajima, H., Nishima, S., Higaki, Y. et al. (1999). Effects of swimming training on aerobic capacity and exercise induced bronchoconstriction in children with bronchial asthma. *Thorax, 54*(3), 196-201.

Mohlberg, P.J., Hopkins, R.S., Paulson, J., & Gunn, R.A. (1993). Fatal incident risk factors in recreational boating in Ohio. *Public Health Reports, 108*(3), 340-346.

Moran, K. (1996). *Surf Survival*. Wellington, New Zealand: Surf Life Saving New Zealand.

Moran, K. (2003). *New Zealand youth water safety survey*. Wellington, New Zealand: WSNZ.

Moran, K. (2006). *Re-thinking drowning risk: The role of water safety knowledge, attitudes and behaviours in youth aquatic recreation*. Unpublished doctoral thesis. Palmerston North, New Zealand: Massey University.

Murase, T., Haramizu, S., Shimitoyodome, A., & Tokimitsu, I. (2005). Reduction of diet induced obesity by a combination of tea-catechin intake and regular swimming. *International Journal of Obesity, 30*, 561-568.

Netz, Y. (2003). Mood alterations in mindful versus aerobic exercise modes. *The Journal of Psychology, 137*(5), 405-419.

Ntoumanis, N. (2001). *A step-by-step guide to SPSS for sport and exercise studies*. London: Routledge.

Oda, S., Matsumoto, T., Nakagawa, K., & Moriya, K. (1999). Relaxation effects in humans of underwater exercise of moderate intensity. *European Journal of Applied Physiology and Occupational Physiology, 80*, 253-259.

Orlowski, J.P. (1987). Adolescent drownings: Swimming, boating, diving and scuba incidents. *Pediatric Annals, 17*(2), 125-132.

Pavlik, G., Olexo, Z., Osváth, Sidó, Z., & Frenkl, R. (2001). Echocardiographic characteristics of male athletes of different ages. *British Journal of Sports Medicine 35*, 95-99.

Quan, L., Bennett, E., Cummings, P., Trusty, M.N., & Treser, C.D. (1998). Are life vests worn? A multi-regional observational study of personal flotation device use in small boats. *Injury Prevention, 4*, 203-205.

Quan, L., Bennett, E., & Williams, K. (2002). *PFD's: The missing link to open water drowning prevention*. Book of Abstracts of the World Congress on Drowning, Amsterdam, 26-28 June 2002. Amsterdam: Stichting Foundation Drowning 2002.

Quan, L., & Cummings, P. (2003). Characteristics of drowning by different age groups. *Injury Prevention, 9*(2), 163-6.

Rasanathan, K., Craig, D., & Perkins, R. (2004). *Is "Asian" a useful category for health research in New Zealand?* In: Tse, S., Thapliyal, A., Garg, S., Lim, G., & Chatterji, M.

(Eds.), Proceedings of the Inaugural International Asian Health Conference: Asian health and wellbeing, now and into the future. The University of Auckland, School of Population Health, pp 8-17.

Reeder, A. I., Stanton, W.R., Langley, J.D., & Chalmers, D.J. (1991). Adolescents' sporting and leisure time physical activities during their 15th year. *Canadian Journal of Sports Science, 16*(4), 308-315.

Ross, J.G., & Gilbert, G.G. (1985). The national children's and youth fitness study: A summary of findings. *Journal of Physical Education, Recreation and Dance, 56*(1), 45-50.

Royal Society for the Prevention of Accidents [RoSPA]. (2002). *Drowning Statistics in the UK 2000*. Birmingham: RoSPA.

Rumuka, M., Abererga-Augskalne, L., & Upitis, I. (2007). Effects of a 12-week swimming training program on spirometric variables in teenage females. *International Journal of Aquatic Research and Education, 19*(2), 101-107.

Russell, D., & Wilson, N. (1992). *Life in New Zealand.* Wellington, New Zealand: Hillary Commission for Recreation and Sport.

Rychtecky, A. (2002). Lifestyle activities and participation in sports among Czech and German youth. *Acta Universitatis Carolinae Kinanthropologica, 38*(1), 39-49.

Smith, G.S., Keyl, P., Hadley, J.A., Bartley, C.L., Foss, R.D., Tolbert, W.G., & McKnight, J. (2001). Drinking and recreational boating fatalities: A population-based case control study. *Journal of the American Medical Association, 286*(23), 2974-2980.

Smith, G.S., & Brenner, R. (1995). The changing risks of drowning for adolescents in the U.S. and effective control strategies. *Adolescent Medicine: The State of the Art Reviews, 6*(2), 153-169.

Sport England (2006). The active people survey. Retrieved August 28, 2007, from: http://www.sportengland.org/index/get_resources/research/active_people/active_people_s urvey_headline_results.htm

Sport England. (2002). Participation in selected sports by young people outside lessons; by sex, 2002. *Social Trends 34.* Retrieved August 31, 2007, from http://www.statistics. gov.uk/CCI/SearchRes.asp?term=swimming

Sport Scotland (2001). Sports participation in Scotland 2000. Research Digest no.84 July 2001. Edinburgh: SportScotland.

Statistics Canada. (2000). A family affair: Children's participation in sports. *Canadian Socials Trends,* Autumn 2000. Catalogue No 11-008. Ottawa: Statistics Canada.

Surf Life Saving New Zealand. (2000). *Rescue statistics – trend analysis of incidents type.* Retrieved September 15, 2002, from https://www.slsnz.org.nz

Tomanek, R.T. (1994). Exercise induced coronary angiogenesis: A review. *Medicine and Science in Sports and Exercise, 26*, 1245-1477.

United States Coastguard (2003). *Boating statistics – 2001.* U.S. Department of Transportation Report No. 1-41. Washington: U.S. Department of Transportation.

University of Auckland. (2001). *Youth 2000: A profile of their health and wellbeing.* Auckland: University of Auckland, Adolescent Health Research Group.

Water Safety New Zealand. (2000). *Water safety – profile.* Wellington, New Zealand: Water Safety New Zealand.

Water Safety New Zealand. (2002). *Riversafe.* Retrieved 16 April 2006 from http://www. riversafe.org.nz/facts/index.html

Waxweiler, R.J., Harel Y., & O'Carroll, P.W. (1993). Measuring adolescent behaviours related to unintentional injuries. *Public Health Reports, 108*(Suppl. 1), 4-11.

Wells, G.D., Plyley, M., Thomas, S., Goodman, L., & Duffin, J. (2005). Effects of concurrent inspiratory and expiratory muscle training on respiratory and exercise performance in competitive swimmers. *European Journal of Applied Physiology, 94*, 527-540.

Welsh, L., Kemp, J.G., & Roberts, R.G.D. (2005). Effects of physical conditioning on children and adolescents with asthma. *Sports Medicine, 35*(2), 127-141.

In: Physical Activity and Children: New Research
Editor: N. P. Beaulieu, pp. 65-93

ISBN: 978-1-60456-306-1
© 2008 Nova Science Publishers, Inc.

Chapter 3

INTER-LIMB COORDINATION AND CONSTRAINTS IN SWIMMING: A REVIEW

Ludovic Seifert[*] and Didier Chollet

Centre d'Etudes des Transformations des Activités Physiques et Sportives, EA UPRES 3832, Faculty of Sport Sciences, University of Rouen, France

ABSTRACT

This review presents a new approach to assessing swimming skill through the analysis of the inter-limb coordination: inter-arm coordination in the alternate strokes (front crawl and backstroke) and arm-leg coordination in the simultaneous strokes (breaststroke and butterfly). Based on Newell's concept of constraints [27], for whom constraints may be viewed as features that reduce the degree of freedom of the human motor organisation, we aimed to identify the three types of constraint (organismic, environmental and task), all of which can serve as control parameters in experiments designed to determine how and why inter-limb coordination in swimming changes. The lag time between the propulsion of one limb and the other, or one set of limbs and the other, has often been considered a mistake, but this type of experiment has shown that lag time can be an adaptation to a relative constraint. Scientists, coaches and instructors are invited to revisit the theoretical knowledge of biomechanics and motor control in the contexts of competitive swimming, swim training programs and instructions to beginners. Practical applications are proposed to improve inter-limb coordination in children and/or unskilled swimmers.

[*] Address for correspondence: Ludovic Seifert, CETAPS, EA UPRES 3832, Faculté des Sciences du Sport, Boulevard Siegfried, Université de Rouen, 76130 Mont-Saint-Aignan, France. Tel: +33 232 10 77 84; Fax : +33 232 10 77 95; E-mail : ludovic.seifert@univ-rouen.fr

1. INTRODUCTION

This review presents a new perspective for the assessment of swimming skill, with a motor control approach based on the dynamical theory of inter-limb coordination [15]. Swim performance has traditionally been analysed from the race components (start time, swim time, turn time, final time), particularly swim time (i.e. in the central part of the pool and thus not affected by the dive start or turn-in and turn-out). During this time, changes in velocity, stroke rate, distance per stroke and stroke index can be calculated [8]. Moreover, biomechanical research on active drag, power output and propelling efficiency [30, 31, 55, 56], as well as hand kinematics and kinetics during the underwater path [38], has greatly improved our understanding of what constitutes swimming skill, but nevertheless little attention has been given to motor organization. In fact, the classic variables provide an indirect indication of how humans coordinate limb movements to attain high performance and overcome different types of constraints. This review therefore presents the recent findings on inter-limb coordination in the four competitive swimming strokes (front crawl, back stroke, butterfly and breaststroke). For each stroke, three aspects are considered:

i)   The nature of the inter-limb coordination (or order parameter) is highlighted using concepts and principles of dynamical theory, notably with reference to the findings of fundamental studies on bimanual, walking-running and lower-upper limb tasks.

ii) The control parameters of the inter-limb coordination are analysed using the concept of constraints developed by Newell [27]. Considerable research has been conducted on the front crawl, the most popular and fastest stroke, documenting the influence of three types of constraint (organismic, environmental and task, Newell, 27]. For the other alternate stroke (backstroke) and the two simultaneous strokes (butterfly and breaststroke), the review presents the influence of organismic constraints, particularly skill level, which includes expertise, experience and age effects. Breaststroke is presented last because it is the slowest, the most resistive, and the most regulated stroke.

iii) Practical applications are presented for swimmers, coaches, instructors and scientists. Recommendations about monitoring the relevant constraints are given. These applications are aimed particularly at improving the inter-limb coordination of children and/or unskilled swimmers.

2. INTER-LIMB COORDINATION IN FRONT CRAWL

2.1. Order Parameters and Attractors: Specific Parameters of Coordination

The dynamical approach to inter-limb coordination hypothesizes that behaviour can be characterized at a macroscopic level by *collective variables*, also called *order parameters*. An order parameter is specific and qualitatively defines the coordination. The values of the order parameter are used to identify stable states of coordination, called *attractors*. In bimanual coordination tasks of flexion/extension finger movements, the order parameter that defines the inter-finger coordination is the relative phase [14]. The relative phase calculation could be conducted throughout the cycle, frame by frame, from angle and angular velocity of the fingers to obtain the continuous relative phase or by using a discrete method which calculates the point-estimated relative phase from relative timing of key events [10, 11, 59]. When the fingers flex (or extend) simultaneously, the relative phase value is 0° and the coordination mode is in-phase. Conversely, when one finger flexes while the other finger extends, this is phase shifting, which in the present example is 180°; thus, the coordination mode is anti-phase.

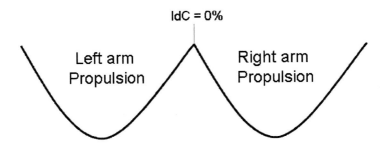

Figure 1a. Opposition coordination mode showing a continuity between the propulsive phases of the two arms.

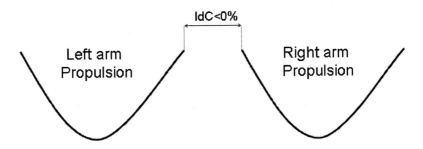

Figure 1b. Catch-up coordination mode showing a lag time between the propulsive phases of the two arms.

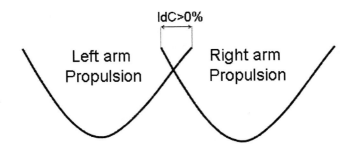

Figure 1c. Superposition coordination mode showing an overlap between the propulsive phases of the two arms.

Front crawl and backstroke are considered to be alternate swimming strokes because the inter-arm coordination is globally in anti-phase [28], i.e. one arm propels underwater while the other recovers aerially. However, the hand velocity during an arm cycle is not constant because of the time spent catching the water forward and downward. Therefore, closer analysis of inter-arm coordination was conducted to determine more exactly the inter-arm coupling in front crawl. The index of coordination (IdC) [4] is an interesting order parameter based on the time gap between the start of the propulsion of one arm and the end of propulsion of the other arm. As indicated above, this discrete method corresponds to the punctual estimation of the inter-arm coordination from relative timing of key events (and not angle and angular velocity, as regularly done to calculate the continuous relative phase), which is expressed in percentage of an arm cycle duration. Based on the degree of continuity between the propulsive actions, three theoretical modes of coordination exist: when IdC=0%, the mode is opposition (Figure 1a); when IdC<0%, the mode is catch-up (Figure 1b); and when IdC>0%, the mode is superposition (Figure 1c). However, in a functional point of view, it is reasonable to consider the opposition mode for -1%<IdC<1%.

Figures 2a, 2b and 2c show that at the start of right-arm propulsion, the left arm can be finishing its propulsive phase (Figure 2a), has already finished the propulsive phase and is re-entering in the water (Figure 2b), or has not finished its propulsive phase (Figure 2c).

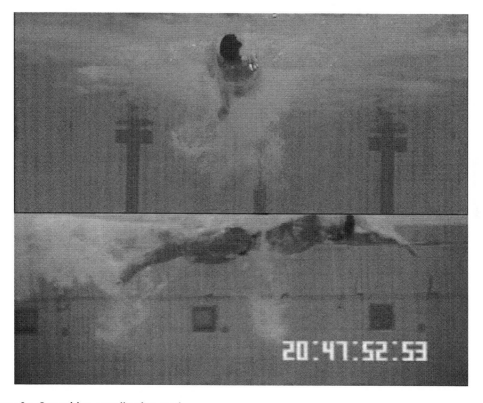

Figure 2a. Opposition coordination mode.

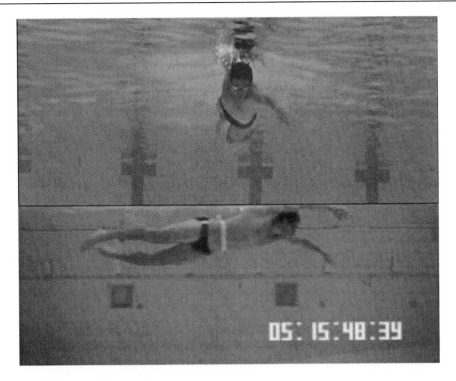

Figure 2b. Catch-up coordination mode.

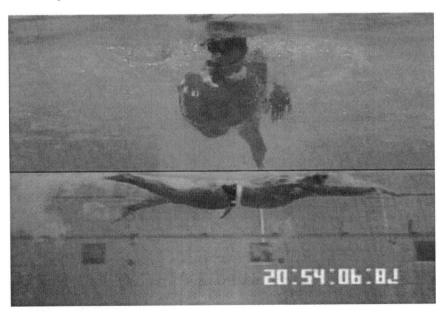

Figure 2c. Superposition coordination mode.

Catch-up coordination is usually considered to be a mistake by coaches and instructors. However, Seifert et al. [50] showed that this mode is useful for slow paces, whatever the skill level, because it favours the glide phase following propulsive actions. Propulsive actions instantaneously propel the body above its mean velocity. Therefore, at the same velocity, Seifert et al. [50] observed that elite swimmers had greater catch-up than did non-expert swimmers, because each propulsive action of the elite swimmers led to higher propulsive peaks. Conversely, lack of expertise led to smaller catch-up due to the weak sensation of the catch and to slippage through water. These swimmers then tended to compensate by increasing their stroke rate. A final point is that the coordination mode adopted - for example, catch-up mode - is not intrinsically efficient but is instead related to the inter-relation between the task (like speed), the environment (like active drag) and the organism (like gender) constraints [27] and, more generally, to the control parameters of the mode.

2.2. Control Parameters and Phase Transition

The *control parameters* are non-specific, i.e. they may lead to a change in the order parameter but do not define it. In bimanual coordination tasks, the frequency of finger oscillation is a control parameter because bi-stability (in-phase and anti-phase coordination modes) is observed at slow frequency oscillation, whereas an increase in oscillation above a critical value involves a shift to mono-stability in in-phase coordination mode [14]. The shift from one coordination mode to another does not occur progressively or continuously, but is abrupt, like the transition from walking to running [10], when a critical value of the control parameter is reached. This shifting of attractors occurs without any intermediary state and is called *phase transition*.

Similar to bimanual coordination tasks, in front crawl velocity, stroke rate and the ratio of stroke rate to distance per stroke are control parameters [47, 50]. They induce a qualitative change in the IdC, or a transition from catch-up to superposition mode. For example, high variability in the coordination mode is observed at low stroke rates because the environmental constraints (active drag that the swimmer must overcome) are low [34]. When the stroke rate increases above a critical value (a rate of 50 cycle.minute^{-1}), only the superposition mode occurs because the environmental constraints are high [34]. Moreover, when the velocity increases above a critical value (a velocity of 1.8 m.s^{-1}), a transition from catch-up mode to superposition mode is observed [50] (Figure 3).

One practical application of these findings concerns the risk that coaches and instructors will increase or decrease stroke rate and velocity to bring about a new coordination mode in unskilled swimmers or children, without automatically ensuring better propulsion. For example, these swimmers might try to increase their stroke rate, as requested, but could tire quickly and let their hand slip through the water instead of ensuring an effective hand sweep. Therefore, manipulating the control parameter "stroke rate" would induce a coordination mode that is not part of the swimmer's intrinsic dynamics but would not automatically ensure better propulsion. Conversely, a tether attached to the waist at one end and the starting block at the other (with the resistive force exerted by the tether permitting a 25-m lap) forces swimmers to correctly adapt coordination to reach the end of the pool. In semi-tethered swimming, glide time diminishes in favour of long propulsive phases and/or great peaks of force, which are often associated with high stroke rate. Therefore, non-expert swimmers who start this task with catch-up coordination adopt a superposition of arm propulsions to reach the end of the pool with effective propulsion.

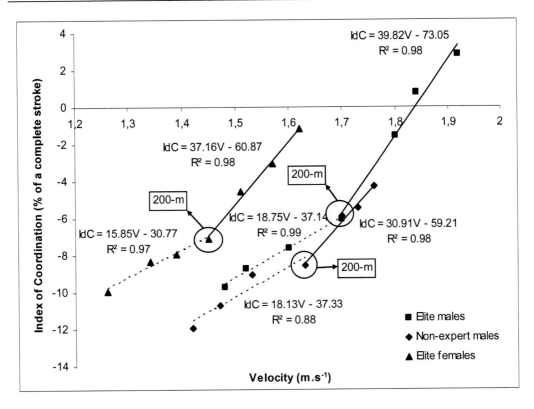

Figure 3. Change in the index of coordination when swim velocity increases from 1500 m to maximal velocity [50].

2.3. Relationships between Control Parameters and Constraints

According to the dynamical systems approach, coordination emerges not as a result of symbolic prescriptions of action patterns but rather as a consequence of the constraints imposed on action, reflecting a propensity towards self-organizing optimality in biological systems. Thus, constraints may be viewed as features that reduce the degree of freedom of the human motor organisation, i.e. that limit the number of possible of actions of the swimmer. Newell [27] presented three types of constraint (related to the environment, the task, and the organism) that can influence the order parameter. Environmental constraints reflect the ambient conditions of the task and are usually not manipulated by the experimenter. The environmental features can, however, be manipulated for a participant by changing the environment in which the activity takes place. Task constraints refer to the goal of the activity and have been classified into three categories: (i) the task goal inducing a coordination mode, (ii) the rules or instructions specifying the response dynamics, and (iii) the instruments or devices inducing a coordination mode. An interesting question is how these constraints are applied in front crawl. Organismic constraints are structural or functional constraints associated with the actor and influencing development of coordination. For example, body weight, height and shape are assumed to be structural constraints to the development of coordination because of their very slow rate of change with development.

2.3.1. Environmental Constraints

In swimming, the environmental constraints refer to water properties as the density of the fluid, the temperature of the water, the length of the pool (25 m, 33.3 m, 50 m) or the underwater visibility. Move in the aquatic environment naturally imposes forward resistance, and propulsive force and velocity are required to overcome it. The forward resistance is a function of the swimmer's hydrodynamic coefficient but mostly of the velocity squared [55, 56], suggesting that velocity could be considered as an indirect environmental constraint. Wearing a wet suit can artificially decrease friction drag by 5 to 7.5%, which explains the greater glide and catch-up coordination of triathletes swimming at an 800-m pace with a wet suit (IdC = -11.7%) as opposed to without (IdC = -9.6%) [13].

2.3.2. Task Constraints

Task constraints concern the goal of the activity and have been classified into three categories: (i) the task goal inducing a coordination mode, (ii) the rules or instructions specifying the response dynamics, and (iii) instruments or devices inducing a coordination mode.

(i) The goal of most experiments on inter-limb coordination in swimming is either to simulate individual race paces over 25 m in order to test coordination variability, with self-pacing to avoid fatigue effects, or to examine the fatigue effects on inter-limb coordination in a race or set of trials at maximum intensity, i.e. to test the stability of coordination.

- To test coordination variability, a "scanning task" where race pace, stroke rate, number of stroke per 25-m lap (i.e. distance per stroke) or velocity progressively increased from the minimal to the maximal individual value could be used. In fact, this type of task explores the range of the young swimmer's capabilities; that is to say, the different coordination modes that the young swimmer is capable of and the critical values of race pace, velocity and stroke rate that induce a non-linear change of coordination. For example, the task instruction could be to "swim at different race paces like slow, mid, fast"; the coordination adopted by the swimmer would then be analysed to determine the span of his coordination variability. Seifert et al. [50] asked elite and non-expert swimmers to simulate seven race paces (1500 m, 800 m, 400 m, 200 m, 100 m, 50 m, maximal speed) over 25 m (Figure 3). The results indicated that, whatever the expertise level or gender, the 200-m pace was the critical point for adapting coordination as it marked the separation between the mid- and long-distance paces and the sprint paces. Swimmers of course swim at different velocities for the same pace (some swimmers have a velocity of 1.5 m.s^{-1} for the 200-m pace whereas others have a velocity of 1.7 m.s^{-1}), which indicates clearly that the task is a major constraint, and not just the environment.
- A task constraint that leads to fatigue, like swimming at maximal speed for a given distance (for the 100-m event, see [40, 48] ; for the 200-m event, see [1] ; for the 400-m, see [39] ; for the 800-m, see [9]), can be used to evaluate the stability of coordination. High expertise is revealed by relatively stable IdC values over the course of a race, whereas lower expertise or great fatigue is

indicated by an increase; this increase thus does not indicate greater propulsive efficiency but rather greater time spent in the pull and push phases due to lower hand velocity and thus smaller mechanical power output [57].

(ii) The rules or instructions specify the response dynamics, in terms of the mode of coordination desired.

(iii) A task constraint may also be the requirement to swim at an imposed stroke rate as dictated by an instrument or device, such as a metronome. Similarly, velocity can be imposed by a luminous rail [25], a system by which the subject's passing over each pylon (placed at every 10-m at the bottom of the pool) has to coincide with an underwater audio signal [26], or a swimming flume [24]. Last, artificially applied resistance can be used with a tethered swimming system to assess force output [58] and to constrain inter-limb coordination.

Thus, using various task constraints, the instructor (and not the environment) tries to bring out the desired behaviour and can test the variability and stability of the adopted coordination.

2.3.3. Organismic Constraints

Organismic constraints refer to the swimmer's properties, notably anthropometric characteristics (like arm span, arm size, hand area, foot size, leg length and height), locomotor disabilities, passive drag and floatation parameters (hydrostatic lift, sinking force acting at the ankle), force and power, laterality (handedness and the preferred breathing side) which could be included in larger categories as age, gender, expertise, and the swimmer's specialty (sprint vs. mid-distance, swimmer vs. triathlete). Several studies have shown that these organismic constraints affected the inter-arm coordination and the coordination symmetry.

For example, Seifert et al. [41] showed that women have more coordination in catch-up than men because of their greater fat mass, a different distribution of this mass, lower arm strength, and greater difficulty in overcoming forward resistance.

Moreover, it is reasonable to assume that a swimmer with large hands and/or feet will have bigger propulsive surfaces and thus a greater yield for every action, on condition that these actions are efficient. This too should lead to more coordination in catch-up [52]. Thus, using fins or paddle, the instructor can artificially increase beginners' propulsive surfaces and induce new coordination, on condition that the quality of catch is monitored. Conversely, swimmers with locomotor disabilities, i.e. amputation, cerebral palsy, spinal cord injury or others, may have smaller propulsive surfaces than able-bodied swimmers or an unbalanced capacity for propulsion, both of which would influence their inter-arm coordination [37]. These authors showed that even if swimmers with locomotor disabilities vary the coordination mode in relation to their degree of impairment, correct coordination is fundamental to front crawl swimming, just as in able-bodied swimmers.

The swimmer's specialty also influences the coordination mode. Because the triathletes usually swim at small range of velocity (long distance paces), they have to overcome small range of active drag and adopted the constant coordination to do this. Thus, when velocity was increased from long distance paces to sprint paces, their inter-arm coordination was less flexible. Despite the velocity increase, competitive triathletes maintained a catch up coordination mode while the swimmers changed to a superposition mode [12]. In elite triathletes, when velocity increased, IdC decreased between 98 and 100% of their maximum velocity to relative catch-up (IdC = -1.7%) [23]. Conversely, the IdC of elite swimmers was shown to always increase until the superposition mode was reached (IdC = 2.3%) when the velocity increased [23].

Moreover, breathing caused catch-up coordination because the time spent inhaling leads to a lag time in propulsion [21], that occurred to the preferential breathing side [43, 46]. Throughout a 100-m race, Seifert et al. [46] then found that swimmers having unilateral breathing patterns (every 2, 4, or 6 arm strokes) showed an asymmetric coordination (rickety swimming), characterized in non-experts by a prolonged catch with the arms extended forward to facilitate head rotation during breathing and thus by catch-up to the breathing side.

Conversely, swimmers with bilateral breathing patterns (breath every 3 or 5 arm strokes) tended to balance the arm coordination by distributing the asymmetries [46]. The control of breathing laterality would help to bring about efficient inter-arm coordination. Seifert et al. [43] have voluntary disturbed the breathing laterality by imposing seven breathing patterns (each trial was swum on 25-m to avoid fatigue), divided in two categories: unilateral patterns and axed and bilateral patterns. The unilateral patterns corresponded to breathing every 2 strokes to the preferential breathing side, breathing every 2 strokes to the non-preferential breathing side, simulation of breathing every 2 strokes on the preferential breathing side, i.e. turning the head as if breathing but not breathing to analyse whether rolling the body affected the coordination symmetry, breathing every 2 strokes in a frontal snorkel. The axed and bilateral patterns were breathing freely in a frontal snorkel, breathing every 3 strokes (bilateral breathing) and apnoea. The results indicated that breathing to the preferential side led to an asymmetry, in contrast to the other breathing patterns, and the asymmetry was even greater when the swimmer breathed to his non-preferential side [43]. Moreover, coordination was symmetric in patterns with breathing that was bilateral, axed (as in breathing with a frontal snorkel) or removed (as in apnoea) [43]. The practical applications for the coach or the instructor could be: (i) to help children to determine their preferred side for unilateral breathing, (ii) to vary the learning situations to encourage symmetric coordination, i.e. alternating tasks with unilateral, bilateral and frontal snorkel breathing, and (iii) to adapt the breathing rate to the swim distance by inserting apnoea times (especially in sprint, by asking the swimmer to breathe only once or twice every 25 m).

Last, when Newell's three types of constraint [27] are used as control parameters to bring about the desired coordination mode, it is equally important to first analyse the environmental context of practice, to prepare the task instructions, and to take into account the diversity of the population.

3. INTER-LIMB COORDINATION IN BACKSTROKE

Like the front crawl, the backstroke's main propulsion comes from the alternating arm movements. The IdC is thus used to quantify the difference between the start of propulsion of one arm and the end of propulsion of the other arm. In front crawl, the wide range of race events (from the 1500-m to the 50-m) suggests that several coordination modes are possible. The three coordination modes (catch-up, opposition, superposition) are regularly observed, in relation to the individual profile (sprinter, mid- or long-distance). In backstroke, the range of events is smaller and, in any case, the organismic constraints greatly limit the choice of coordination mode. Indeed, the alternating body-roll, which could lead to 90° abduction of the shoulder during the mid-pull, and the low shoulder flexibility [35, 36] require an additional arm stroke phase to recover into the water surface (called clearing phase, Figure 4). Only one mode of coordination is thus possible: catch-up [19, 20].

3.1. Effects of Expertise and Velocity on Inter-arm Coordination

Whatever the race pace or level of expertise, backstrokers use a catch-up mode of coordination, with IdC varying from -25% to -5%. For example, at the 100-m pace, Chollet et al. [5] showed an IdC of -11.4% for elite swimmers (velocity = 1.56 m.s^{-1}), while Lerda and Cardelli [19] showed an IdC of -9.7% for the more expert backstrokers (velocity = 1.44 m.s^{-1}) and an IdC of -11.3% for the less expert (velocity = 1 m.s^{-1}).

However, although the coordination mode and IdC value do not seem to change with expertise, several studies have highlighted the effect of technical mistakes on arm coordination in backstroke, particularly (i) hand entry outside of the shoulder axis, (ii) head flexion on the thorax and (iii) hand lag time at the thigh [3, 5]. Head flexion on the thorax and particularly the entry of the hand outside of the shoulder axis lead to a decrease in the relative duration of the entry and catch phase. These mistakes prevent the deep hand sweep that prepares the propulsion and are regularly associated with a dorsal position without shoulder body roll. Beginners are often not aware that having the hand entry in the shoulder axis is important; they thus shorten the entry and catch phase to rest on the water (i.e. to maintain the upper body and the head on the surface) instead of plunging their hand deeper to find a resistive mass of water [3]. This mistake also leads to longer push and clearing phases and consequently to less marked catch-up coordination (less negative IdC), which does not indicate better propulsion, as commonly assumed, but rather a problem of hand sweep rhythm. In particular, the premature entry of the hand means that the hand stays in the water too long and has an upward path during the push phase instead of a backward and downward path with acceleration [3]. Last, having a long hand lag time at the thigh leads to propulsive discontinuity, which explains why elite swimmers limit their hand lag time to near 2% of the stroke cycle duration [5].

3.2. Practical Applications

The consequences of the mono-stability of catch-up coordination mode are such that three recommendations can be made to improve backstroke performance: (i) children and unskilled swimmers should minimise the clearing phase and the hand's lag time at the thigh, especially by increasing hand speed in this specific phase, which can be achieved by a bigger or faster shoulder roll; (ii) they should compensate the loss of speed in the clearing phase - which prevents propulsive continuity - by increasing the distance per stroke. Indeed, Pai et al. [29] compared the four strokes and showed that backstroke had the lowest stroke rate and backstroke and front crawl had the longest distance per stroke. These findings suggest that propulsive discontinuity can be minimised and that the lag time due to the clearing phase and the hand lag at the thigh can be compensated by greater distances per stroke.

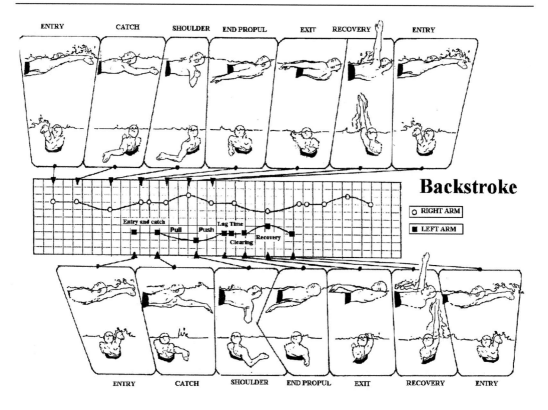

Figure 4. Inter-arm coordination in backstroke defined from the arm phases (entry and catch, pull, push, clearing and recovery) [5].

4. INTER-LIMB COORDINATION IN BUTTERFLY

Whereas inter-arm coordination is studied in the alternate strokes (front crawl and backstroke), arm-leg coordination is analysed in the simultaneous strokes (butterfly and breaststroke), so-called because the FINA rules impose simultaneous arm movements and simultaneous leg movements. The challenge is therefore to monitor the duration of the glide between the arm propulsion and the leg propulsion. The following section presents the influence of organismic constraints, particularly expertise level, and the most common mistakes.

4.1. Elite Coordination: Synchronisation of Arm and Leg Actions

Butterfly learners often imagine that this stroke is difficult because of the arm strength that it requires. The fear of being unable to bring the arms forward leads the novice to focus almost exclusively on the aerial recovery with far less attention given to the legs, and the result is a body position that is generally in the shape of a banana, with the head rising too high and the back arched. Conversely, efficient arm-leg coordination requires one arm cycle for two leg cycles or a ratio of 1:2, with the upward and downward phases of the leg kicks synchronised [6, 51] (Figure 5). The arm-leg coordination is assessed from four time gaps: T1 is the time difference between the start of the arms' catch phase and the start of the downward phase of the first leg kick; T2 is the time difference between the start of the arms' pull phase and the start of the upward phase of the first leg kick; T3 is the time difference between the start of the arms' push phase and the start of the downward phase of the second leg kick; and T4 is the time difference between the start of the arms' recovery and the start of the upward phase of the second leg kick. As in breaststroke, the total time gap (TTG) is defined as the sum of the absolute values of T1, T2, T3 and T4, and is used to assess the effectiveness of the global arm-leg coordination.

The TTG of expert butterflyers was shown to decrease from 30% at a velocity of 1.4 m.s^{-1} to 15% at a velocity of 1.8 m.s^{-1}, whereas the TTG of the non-expert swimmers decreased from 50% at a velocity of 1.4 m.s^{-1} to 30% at a velocity of 1.6 m.s^{-1} [45]. Therefore, as observed in breaststroke, at a velocity similar to that of expert swimmers (1.4 m.s^{-1}), non-expert swimmers have a TTG nearly two times greater, indicating mistakes in the arm-leg coordination. The analysis of each time gap (T1, T2, T3 and T4) indicates time lags in the phases of the beginners (Figure 6a), whereas the experts tend to synchronise the key points of the arm phases with those of the legs (Figure 6b), showing a coordination close to in-phase [51] as observed in hand-foot coupling tasks [16].

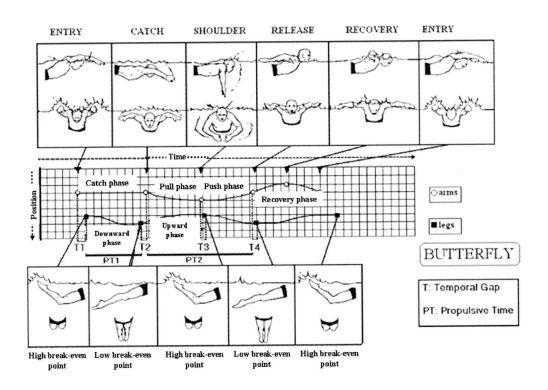

Figure 5. Arm-leg coordination in butterfly defined from the arm phases (catch, pull, push and recovery) and leg phases (upward and downward phases for each leg kick) [6].

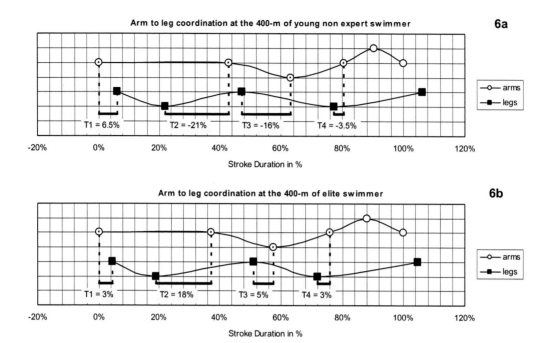

Figure 6. Arm-leg coordination in butterfly of a beginner (6a) and an expert (6b).

4.2. Time Lags in the Butterfly Phases of Beginners

4.2.1. Catch-up with Arms forward

Catch-up with the arms extended forward indicates a time lag or a glide time for the hands. This catch-up occurs when leg propulsion (beginning of downward phase of the kick) begins after the hands enter the water, and the arms remain extended forward (measured by T1). It also occurs when the downward phase of the kick ends early or the arm propulsion starts late (measured by T2). The smaller the T2, the greater the propulsive continuity is between the end of leg propulsion and the beginning of arm propulsion.

4.2.2. Ineffective Propulsion

When non-experts do not show "forward catch-up", it is often because they have begun leg propulsion before the arms have finished the recovery, which thus coincides with the "banana" form (i.e. highest drag) that does not lead to efficient stroke. Moreover, non-experts do not synchronise the beginning of the downward phase of the leg kick with the beginning of the push phase of the arms (measured by T3) whereas in elite swimmers, the superposition of these two propulsive phases provides the highest body acceleration in the stroke [22]. It should be noted that expert coordination is most probably only possible with a highly adapted muscular system. So the novice swimmer's problem is not only learning the proper coordination but also acquiring the required muscular capacity to bring about this type of coordination.

4.2.3. Aerial Arm Recovery: Late or Curtailed (Calculated by T4)

In extreme cases, a late arm recovery is associated with a head that is hyper-extended to enable long respirations and a flexed back, leading to the "banana" shape. Figure 6 shows clearly the difference in the relative duration of this phase, which is rapid and stiff in the non-expert (and often linked to a shorter push that ends with the arms flexed at the hips and relaxed at the thighs) and longer and more fluid in the expert.

The unsynchronised phases of the beginner can also lead to an arm-leg coordination that is completely ineffective, transforming the stroke into a genuine test of strength to the point where some beginners perform only one leg undulation or group two undulations together during the "forward catch-up" of the arms. In terms of control, it is easier to alternate the arm actions with those of the legs (anti-phase or out-of-phase), with a glide time between these two actions, than to avoid a lag time and achieve in-phase coordination. This explains the prevalence of this coordination mode in novice butterfly swimmers. An increase in stroke rate is thus recommended to bring about the emergence of in-phase arm-leg coordination, because it prevents any lag time during the limb cycles. However, although stroke rate can be used as a control parameter to obtain the desired coordination, it shouldn't automatically be used to permanently modify behaviour because a high stroke rate will provoke early fatigue in beginners. "Forward catch-up" occurs because the swimmer is catching downward to maintain buoyancy and prepare for raising the head out of the water to breathe. The catch, however, should be both downward and backward to prepare for arm propulsion. Moreover, the relative shortening of the push phase, with the hands leaving the water before passing the hip line, is associated with the beginner's major objective: to bring the arms violently forward.

4.3. Practical Applications: Coordination Implies Dissociation… but also Association

The instructor's task is thus to help change the beginner's "swim logic" so that swim behaviour can progress. This means giving information on the behaviours that specify the best-adapted coordination mode at key-points of the cycle. Obviously, all the information needed to obtain arm-leg effectiveness cannot be given at once. Achieving expert coordination will occur in steps, as in the following example: (i) A first step might be to increase both the spatial and temporal aspects of the two arm propulsive phases, pulling and pushing, by associating accelerations with the rhythm of hand sweep. An underwater recovery is recommended at this step. (ii) Raising the head at the end of propulsion to breathe can then be addressed, and most importantly the underwater recovery of the head should be verified as this prepares the arm recovery. (iii) A third step could focus on relaxing at the recovery phase, followed by (iv) work on developing maximal forward extension of the arms to develop a correct catch. (v) Initial work on synchronising the downward phase of leg kick (even if it means performing only one kick) during the push phase of the arms can begin, and this will lead to the upward phase synchronised with the arm pull phase. And only now can this last step be undertaken because it will be easier to integrate: (vi) another leg kick (although chronologically the first) should be introduced with the upward phase during the arm recovery and the downward phase (propulsive) during the catch phase (which is in fact the addition of arm extension, gliding and finding the correct catch).

5. INTER-LIMB COORDINATION IN BREASTSTROKE

The other simultaneous stroke is the breaststroke and the first challenge in this stroke is to monitor the duration of the glide time between the arm propulsion and the leg propulsion. Second, the breaststroke is strictly controlled, and the FINA rules impose underwater recoveries that imply synchronised arm and leg recoveries to minimise active drag. Third, the last challenge is to adopt a hydrodynamic position with one pair of limbs while the other pair of limbs is propelling. The following section presents the influence of organismic constraints, particularly the expertise effect.

5.1. The Elite Swimmer's Coordination

A breaststroke cycle is composed of three arm phases and three leg phases (propulsion, recovery and glide) (Figure 7). The recovery phases of the two limbs are considered to be negative because they provoke strong forward resistances in the opposite direction of movement. For this reason, the expert swimmer's coordination includes synchronised recovery phases to diminish this negative time. In other words, the first part of the cycle corresponds to in-phase coordination of the recoveries [7, 44]. In contrast, the limb propulsions are positive and the propulsion of one set of limbs should be performed while the other set is in neutral position (hydrodynamic position), as when the limbs are extended (the glide phase, which is neither negative nor positive). In fact, this second part of the cycle shows an anti-phase coordination of the propulsions [7, 44] to ensure propulsive continuity in two of the phases, whereas the third phase is devoted to recoveries (Figure 7).

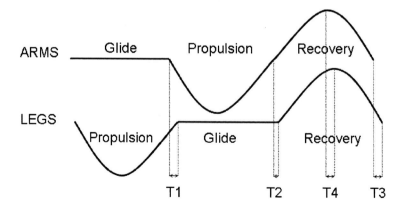

Figure 7. Arm – leg coordination for an expert breaststroker: Propulsive continuity between the leg propulsion and the arm propulsion, and in-phase of the leg and arm recoveries.

Given that a breaststroke cycle lasts about 2 seconds, it is difficult to achieve a motor organization combining two contrasting modes of coordination within the same cycle, one in-phase for the recoveries and the other anti-phase for the propulsions. For this reason, the beginner's coordination is quite different from that of the expert [17]. Four time gaps (T1, T2, T3, T4) are used to quantify the time lags between arm and leg actions (for further details, see [7]) (Figure 7): T1 is the time difference between the end of leg propulsion and the beginning of arm propulsion; T2 is the time difference between the beginning of arm recovery and the beginning of leg recovery; T3 is the time difference between the end of arm recovery and the end of leg recovery; and T4 is the time difference between 90° arm flexion in arm recovery and 90° leg flexion in leg recovery [32, 33]. Finally, the total time gap (TTG) is defined as the sum of the absolute values of T1, T2, T3 and T4, and is used to assess the effectiveness of the global arm-leg coordination [45]. The time gaps and TTG are expressed as the percentage of a complete cycle. The TTG of expert breaststrokers was shown to decrease from 60% at a velocity of 1.2 m.s^{-1} to 20% at a velocity of 1.8 m.s^{-1} [45].

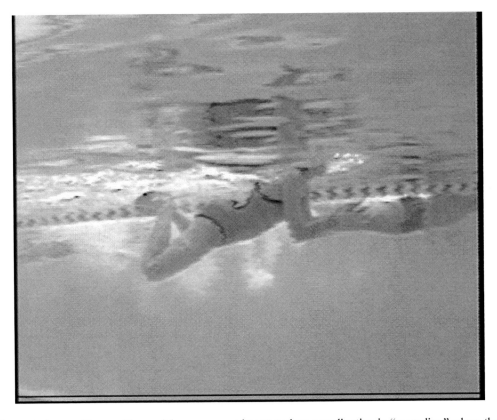

Figure 8. Arm and leg positions of the non-expert breaststroker: coordination in "accordion" where the leg propulsion is thwarted by the arm recovery.

5.2. The Beginner's Superposition Coordination: Between an Accordion and a Windscreen Wiper

The TTG of the breaststroke beginner was shown to decrease from 50% at a velocity of 1 m.s^{-1} to 30% at a velocity of 1.2 m.s^{-1} [17]. Therefore, at a velocity similar to that of expert swimmers (1.2 m.s^{-1}), beginners have a TTG two times greater, which indicates mistakes in the arm-leg coordination, notably the use of superposition coordination. Two types of superposition coordination, both often arising spontaneously, are seen in the beginner and can be explained by mechanical principles.

5.2.1. Superposition of Two Contradictory Phases

Some beginners opt for an ineffective coordination consisting of the superposition of two contradictory phases: leg propulsion during the arm recovery and arm propulsion during the leg recovery (Figure 8).

This superposition of contradictory actions can be complete and characterized as an "accordion" coordination in which no phase is effective because each propulsive action (positive) is thwarted by a recovery action (negative) (Figure 9a).

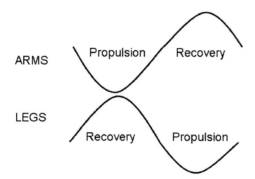

Figure 9a. Arm-leg coupling for non-expert breaststroker: « *accordion* » coordination where the leg propulsion *completely* overlaps the arm recovery.

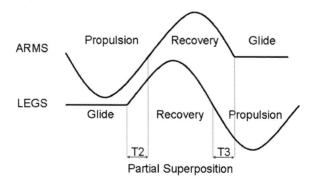

Figure 9b. Arm-leg coupling for non-expert breaststroker: « *accordion* » coordination where the arm propulsion *partially* overlaps the leg propulsion or/and the leg propulsion *partially* overlaps the arm recovery.

The superposition of contradictory actions can also be partial, occurring at two points in the cycle: the end of arm propulsion can be superposed at the beginning of leg recovery (evaluated by T2, Figure 9b) [17]. These gaps in coordination are generally linked to time lags in the cycle; for example, beginners regularly stop their hands at the chest at the end of arm propulsion, usually to take a long breath. By doing so, the arm recovery lags and overlaps with the leg push (evaluated by T1, Figure 9b). In contrast to the beginner, the expert's hands do not stop at the chest because this position causes strong forward resistances. Moreover, the elite swimmer adds a propulsive phase: when the hands have finished their propulsion up to the breast, the elbows then also sweep inward to the breast.

In non-experts, these mistakes of coordination cause velocity fluctuations of the hip which are detrimental to propulsion. In Figure 10, the beginner's arm propulsion led to reduced acceleration because the end of the arm propulsion overlapped the start of leg recovery (assessed by T2) [18]. Figures 10 and 11 show a great decrease in instantaneous velocity because the leg propulsion had started, whereas the arm recovery did not finish in a streamlined position (assessed by T3) [18].

Seifert and Chollet [44] showed that this partial superposition of the end of the arm recovery with the beginning of leg propulsion is also seen in sprint experts: It can be a motor solution to avoid too great a reduction in instantaneous velocity before beginning leg propulsion. However, even in elite swimmers it is advisable to ensure that this superposition of contradictory actions is not detrimental to performance.

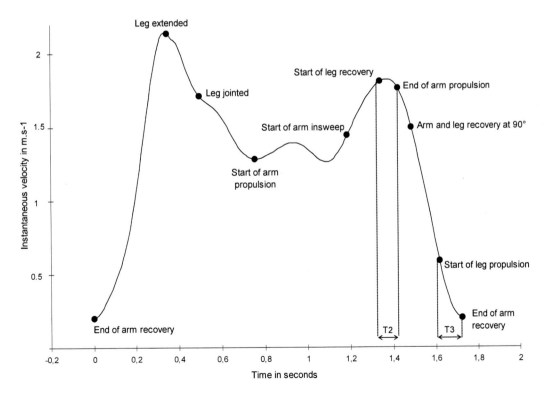

Figure 10. Key points of the leg and arm phases in relation to the instantaneous velocity fluctuations.

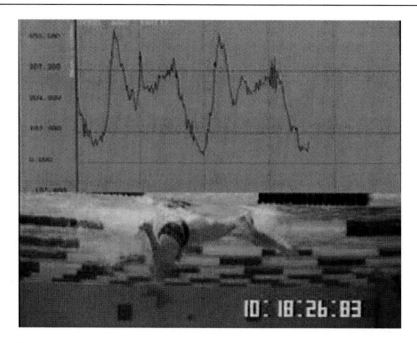

Figure 11. Video-velocity system showing two strokes with two acceleration peaks per stroke related to arm and leg propulsion. By freezing the frame, contradictory superposition can be observed.

The French national champion in 2004 for the 50-m, 100-m and 200-m breaststroke events, also the silver medallist in the Madrid European Championships in 2004 for the 100-m breaststroke, provides an illustration of the utility of regular evaluation. Seven evaluations were made over a two-year period, and four technical sessions were added to prepare the swimmer for the Athens 2004 Olympic Games [49]. We assumed a parallel between the evaluated performances and the competitive performances during the same period and thus monitored the arm-leg coordination for deterioration in technique (Figure 12). The evaluations at E1 and E2 were made during the period in which the swimmer was setting his personal record and were thus taken as references for correct arm-leg coordination. Then at E3 and E4, his coordination showed deterioration, with an increase in the relative duration of the contradictory superposed movements (T2: leg recovery before the end of arm propulsion; T3: beginning of leg propulsion before the end of arm recovery) that resulted in a shortened glide (T1). This motor change was inefficient because, despite a new French record in the World Championship of July 2003, for the first time his performance in the finals was not as good as in the semi-finals. Therefore, just after E4, four technical sessions were held to focus on the dissociation of the arms and legs and then on the continuity of propulsive movements (further details about the technical sessions are provided in section 5.3, Practical applications). These sessions led to greater glide time (T1) and less superposition of negative arm and leg movements (T2 and T3), and thus a better degree of recovery coordination was seen at E6 and E7. Better organization of the glide, propulsion and arm and leg recoveries, and then their coupling, enabled him to achieve a high velocity during the propulsive phases and to conserve this high velocity during the glide time [54]. The arm-leg coordination in both expert breaststrokers and breaststroke learners should thus be evaluated to determine whether it is efficient.

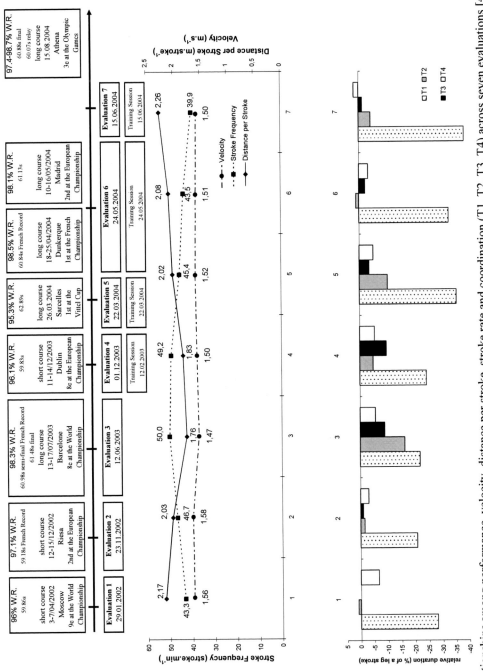

Figure 12. Relationships among performance, velocity, distance per stroke, stroke rate and coordination (T1, T2, T3, T4) across seven evaluations [49].

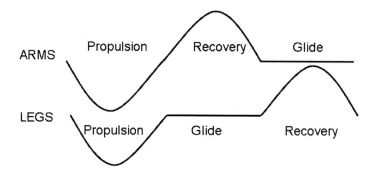

Figure 13a. Arm-leg coupling for non-expert breaststroker: « *windscreen wipers* » coordination where the arm propulsion *completely* overlaps the leg propulsion.

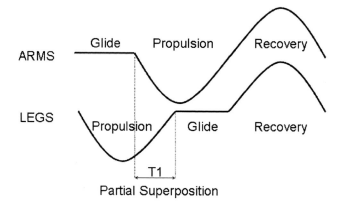

Figure 13b. Arm-leg coupling for non-expert breaststroker: « **X** » coordination where the arm propulsion *partially* overlaps the leg propulsion.

Accordion coordination is the least efficient but, mechanically, is the easiest to achieve, which explains its prevalence in beginners. Beginners synchronise the flexion movements of both arms and legs, as well as the extension movements. This control mode is based on the principle of iso-contraction (simultaneous flexions or simultaneous extensions) noted by Kelso [14] in bi-manual coordination, where in-phase mode seems more stable.

5.2.2. Superposition of Two Propulsions

Other beginners superpose two propulsions. A complete superposition of the propulsive phases of the arms and legs resembles the movement of "windscreen wipers", with in-phase coordination of propulsions and anti-phase of recoveries (Figure 13a).

The superposition of propulsions can be partial (evaluated by T1), with the body in an X position with arms and legs in complete extension (Figure 13b) [17]. This position can result from a lack of sensation in the forward-extended arms, with the beginner not performing a true catch but continuing the stroke by a lateral arm movement to maintain buoyancy (Figure 14]. In this case, the propulsive times are not cumulative, whereas the braking due to dissociated recoveries is. This results in inefficient coordination because two of the three The type of control in this coordination mode can seem complex because a flexion movement of one set of limbs occurs during the extension of the other set, which does not follow the principle of iso-contraction. In fact, in this case another principle is operative: iso-direction, which consists in making movements in the same direction (for example, forward or backward) without involving muscular iso-contraction [2, 53]. This type of behaviour is also inefficient in breaststroke because performing two propulsions simultaneously does not ensure the long propulsive time noted in experts. The use of X coordination might be explained by an analytic mode of teaching popular at the beginning of last century, where the scissor work of the legs was emphasized (and not beating) based on the traditional model of "bend, separate, squeeze together".

These coordination modes of beginners are not necessarily independent: some beginners manifest several mistakes at once. For example, the swimmer in Figure 15 displays the simultaneous recovery of both sets of limbs (iso-contraction), then a lag time of the hands at the chest at the end of propulsion. This causes an arm recovery that is prolonged into the third phase, with the superposition of two contradictory actions (beginning of leg propulsion superposed on the end of arm recovery). Following the absence of a glide time with the arms extended, a fourth key point shows that the arm propulsion catches up to the leg propulsion to superpose in the form of an X.

Last, good arm-leg coordination in the breaststroke is based on complex inter-segmental organization that occurs within a very brief time; the coordination is managed by iso-contraction and iso-direction principles and mechanical constraints are more implicated than central nervous system prescriptions. In the beginner, several attractor states emerge, whereas high performance implies only one mode of coordination with a single margin for manoeuvring: the glide time for each set of limbs and, moreover, with the body in full extension.

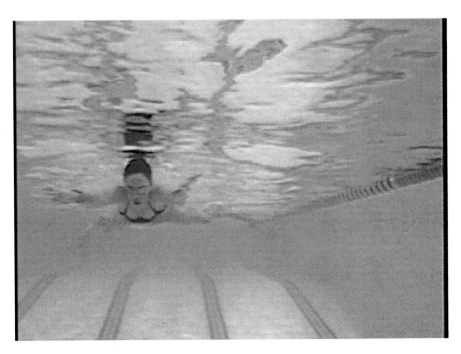

Figure 14. Arm-leg position of a non-expert breaststroke swimmer: **X** coordination where arm propulsion *partially* overlaps that of the legs.

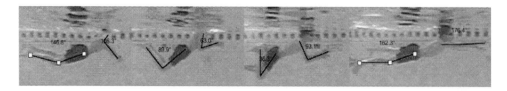

Figure 15. Angular position of the arms and legs at the four key points of the breaststroke cycle.

5.3. Practical Applications: Coordination Implies Dissociation

Given the complexity of breaststroke coordination, the classic drills of performing two arm actions for one leg action or one arm action for two leg actions are well-founded to bring about an adequate coordination in breaststroke. This requires dissociating the propulsive actions of the arms from those of the legs by integrating glide times. This is difficult for beginners because the lack of a sharp sensation of the catch causes them to omit the glide and instead focus on using their arms to maintain buoyancy. In contrast, the bronze medallist of the 100-m breaststroke in the 2004 Olympic Games spent 50% of the arm cycle time in gliding (thus, doing nothing), 42% of the leg cycle time doing nothing, and yet only 17% of the total cycle time was spent with the body in total extension. This indicated that he had partially associated the glide of one limb set with that of the other and that this organization was efficient since he was able to maintain a high mean swim velocity [49].

Coordination implies dissociation: it seems easier to perform one action after the other rather than two actions at the same time, especially when it concerns performing two contradictory actions simultaneously (anti-phase) rather than two identical actions (in-phase). In other words, in teaching the breaststroke, the arm actions should be dissociated from those of the legs actions, with "putting it all together" as a final step, because organizing the phases of propulsion, recovery and glide follows in inverse logic in the arms and legs. Gliding with the legs seems logical because the glide follows a propulsive action: thus, an efficient movement brings a brief velocity peak. In contrast, gliding with the arms does not seem logical because the glide follows a recovery and thus a braking movement. In fact, gliding after a recovery is rarely seen in beginners, who tend to let the hands lag at the chest after the arm propulsion. This is not a glide time, however, because the body is not in a hyrodynamic position.

The beginner should thus be taught to organize the phases of an arm cycle and a leg cycle, with emphasis placed on the importance of the glide time, the sine qua non of expert coordination. The drill of "two arm actions for one leg action" works to develop a glide time for the arms between two cycles and the drill of "one arm action for two leg actions" works to develop a glide time for the legs between two cycles.

Using a tether to pull or hold back the swimmer can amplify the behaviour that reflects poor coordination or a lack of dissociation. For example, pulling the swimmer leads to velocity peaks, situations in which the swimmer has to dissociate the actions of the arms and legs to optimise the glide. For example, the beginner should be in a hydrodynamic position with complete extension for a complete glide or have one set of limbs streamlined before beginning to streamline the other set. Last, using a tether, changing the swim velocity and/or stroke rate, and instructions to dissociate the limb actions by imposing a glide time are all control parameters for manipulating the beginner's coordination.

6. CONCLUSION

A dynamical approach to swim coordination provides insight into the inter-limb organization that is adopted in response to the constraints imposed by the environment (forward resistances, swim velocity), task (instructions on pacing, stroke rate and amplitude), and organism (expertise level, anthropometric characteristics, gender, specialty, etc.). By manipulating these three types of constraints, the coach or instructor can bring about desired behaviours. Several elements can be used: (i) the water environment can be modified (using tethers and kick boards) and the environmental constraints can be varied, (ii) propulsive surfaces can be modified (swim paddles or fins) and organismic constraints can be acted on, and (iii) inadequate coordination can be destabilized by acting on task constraints (stroke rate, amplitude and pace), in order to bring about a coordination mode not expected from the beginner's initial dynamics.

7. ACKNOWLEDGEMENTS

We thank Didier Delignières and Huub Toussaint for the review of this paper and their advices about inter-limb coordination in swimming.

8. REFERENCES

[1]   Alberty, M., Sidney, M., Huot-Marchand, F., Hespel, J.M. & Pelayo. P. (2005). Intracyclic velocity variations and arm coordination during exhaustive exercise in front crawl stroke. *International Journal of Sports Medicine,* 26, 471-475.

[2]   Baldissera, F., Cavalleri, P. & Civaschi, P. (1982). Preferential coupling between voluntary movements of ipsilateral limbs. *Neuroscience Letters,* 74, 95-100.

[3]   Chollet, D., Carter, M. & Seifert L. (2006). Effect of technical mistakes on arm coordination in backstroke. *Portuguese Journal of Sport Sciences,* 6 (Supl. 2), 30-32.

[4]   Chollet, D., Chalies, S. & Chatard J.C. (2000). A new index of coordination for the crawl: description and usefulness. International Journal of Sports Medicine, 21, 54-59.

[5]   Chollet, D., Seifert, L. & Carter, M. (in press). Arm coordination in elite backstroke swimmers. *Journal of Sports Sciences.*

[6]   Chollet, D., Seifert, L., Boulesteix, L. & Carter, M. (2006). Arm to leg coordination in elite butterfly swimmers. *International Journal of Sport Medicine,* 27, 322-329.

[7]   Chollet, D., Seifert, L., Leblanc, H., Boulesteix, L. & Carter M. (2004). Evaluation of the arm-leg coordination in flat breaststroke. *International Journal of Sport Medicine,* 25, 486-495.

[8]   Costill, D.L., Kovaleski, J., Porter, D., Kirwan, J., Fielding, R. & King, D. (1985). Energy expenditure during front crawl swimming: predicting success in middle-distance events. *International Journal of Sports Medicine,* 6, 266-270.

[9]   Delaplace C. (2004). Contribution à l'analyse du crawl du nageur non-expert: étude des paramètres spatio-temporels, des parties nagées et non nagées et de la coordination de nage en fonction du niveau d'expertise, de la distance et du genre [Front crawl analysis

in the non-expert swimmer: spatial-temporal parameters, swimming and non-swimming segments, and coordination in relation to skill, distance swum and gender], *PhD thesis,* University of Montpellier, France.

[10] Diedrich, F.J. & Warren, W.H. (1995). Why change gaits? Dynamics of the walk-run transition. *Journal of Experimental Psychology: Human Perception and Performance,* 21, 183-202.

[11] Hamill, J., Haddad, J.M. & McDermott, W.J. (2000). Issues in quantifying variability from a dynamical systems perspective. *Journal of Applied Biomechanics,* 16, 407-418.

[12] Hue, O., Benavente, H., & Chollet, D. (2003). Swimming skill in triathletes and swimmers using the index of coordination. *Journal of Human Movement Studies,* 44, 107-120.

[13] Hue, O., Benavente, H., & Chollet, D. (2003). The effect of wet suit use by triathletes: an analysis of the different phases of arm movement. *Journal of Sports Sciences,* 21, 1025-1030.

[14] Kelso, J.A.S. (1984). Phase transitions and critical behavior in human bimanual coordination. *American Journal of Physiology, Regulatory, Integrative and Comparative Physiology,* 246, R1000-R1004.

[15] Kelso, J.A.S. (1995). *Dynamic patterns: The self-organization of brain and behavior.* Cambridge: MIT Press.

[16] Kelso, J.A.S. & Jeka, J.J. (1992). Symmetry breaking dynamics of human multilimb coordination. *Journal of Experimental Psychology: Human Perception and Performance,* 18, 645-668.

[17] Leblanc, H., Seifert, L., Baudry, L. & Chollet, D. (2005). Arm-leg coordination in flat breaststroke: a comparative study between elite and non-elite swimmers. *International Journal of Sports Medicine,* 26, 787-797.

[18] Leblanc, H., Seifert, L., Tourny-Chollet, C. & Chollet, D. (2007). Velocity variations in breaststroke swimmers of different competitive levels. *International Journal of Sports Medicine,* 28, 140-147.

[19] Lerda, R. & Cardelli, C. (2003). Analysis of stroke organization in the backstroke as a function of skill. *Research Quarterly in Exercise and Sport,* 74, 215-219.

[20] Lerda, R., Cardelli, C. & Coudereau, J.P. (2005). Backstroke organization in physical education students as a function of skill and sex. *Perceptual and Motor Skills,* 100, 779-790.

[21] Lerda, R., Cardelli, C. & Chollet D. (2001). Analysis of the interactions between breathing and arm actions in the front crawl. *Journal of Human Movement Studies,* 40, 129-144.

[22] Mason, B. R., Tong, Z., & Richards, R. J. (1992). Propulsion in the butterfly stroke. In D. MacLaren, T. Reilly, & A. Lees (Eds.), *Swimming science* VI (pp. 81-86), London, E, & FN Spon.

[23] Millet, G., Chollet, D., Chalies, S. & Chatard, J.C. (2002). Comparison of coordination in front crawl between elite swimmers and triathletes. *International Journal of Sports Medicine,* 23, 99-104.

[24] Monteil, K.M., Rouard, A.H., & Troup, J.P. (1994). Etude des paramètres cinétiques du nageur de crawl au cours d'un exercice maximal dans un flume [Kinetic parameters in front crawl swimmers during maximal exercise in a flume]. *Revue STAPS,* 33, 57-68

[25] Montpetit, R., Cazorla, G., & Lavoie, J.M. (1988). Energy expenditure during front crawl swimming: a comparison between males and females, In B.E. Ungerechts, K. Wilke & K. Reischle (Eds.), *Swimming Science V* (pp. 229-235), Champaign, Illinois: Human Kinetics Publishers.

[26] Montpetit, R., Léger, L.A., Lavoie, J.M., & Cazorla, G. (1981). VO2 peak during free swimming using backward extrapolation of the O2 recovery curve. *European Journal of Applied Physiology, 47*, 385-91.

[27] Newell, K.M. (1986). Constraints on the development of coordination. In M.G. Wade & H.T.A. Whiting (Eds.), *Motor development in children: aspect of coordination and control* (pp. 341-360), Dordrecht, Nijhoff.

[28] Nikodelis, T., Kollias, I. & Xatzitaki, V. (2005). Bilateral inter-arm coordination in freestyle swimming: effect of skill level and swimming speed. *Journal of Sports Sciences, 23*, 737-745.

[29] Pai, Y.C., Hay, J.G. & Wilson, B.D. (1984). Stroking techniques of elite swimmers. *Journal of Sports Sciences, 2*, 225-239.

[30] Pendergast, D.R., Capelli C., Craig, A.B., di Prampero, P.E., Minetti, A.E., Mollendorf, J., Termin, A. & Zamparo, P. (2006). Biophysics in swimming. *Portuguese Journal of Sport Sciences, 6* (Supl. 2), 185-189.

[31] Pendergast, D.R., Mollendorf, J., Zamparo, P., Termin, A., Bushnell, D. & Paschke, D. (2005). The influence of drag on human locomotion in water. *Undersea and Hyperbaric Medicine, 32*, 45-58.

[32] Persyn, U.J.J., Colman, V. & Van Tilborgh, L. (1992). Movement analysis of the flat and undulating breaststroke pattern. In D. MacLaren, T. Reilly & A. Less (Eds.), *Swimming Science VI* (pp. 75-80), London: E & FN SPON.

[33] Persyn, U.J.J., Hoeven, R.G.C. & Daly D.J. (1979). An evaluation procedure for competitive swimmers. In J. Terauds, Bedingfield E.W. (Eds.), *Swimming Science III* (pp. 182-195), Baltimore: University Park Press.

[34] Potdevin, F., Delignières, D., Dekerle, J., Alberty, J., Sidney, M. & Pelayo P. (2003). Does stroke frequency determine swimming velocity values and coordination? In J.C. Chatard (Ed.), *Biomechanics and Medicine in Swimming IX* (pp. 163-167), Saint Etienne, France: University of Saint Etienne.

[35] Richardson, A.B. (1986). The biomechanics of swimming: the shoulder and knee. *Clinics Sports Medicine, 5*, 103-113.

[36] Richardson, A.B., Jobe, F.W. & Collins, H.R. (1980). The shoulder in competitive swimming. *American Journal of Sports Medicine, 8*, 159-163.

[37] Satkunskiene. D., Schega. L., Kunze. K., Birzinyte. K. & Daly, D. (2005). Coordination in arm movements during crawl stroke in elite swimmers with a loco-motor disability. *Human Movement Science, 24*, 54-65.

[38] Schleihauf, R.E. (1979). A hydrodynamic analysis of swimming propulsion. In J.Terauds & E.W. Bedingfield (Eds.), Swimming Science III (pp. 71-109), Baltimore: University Park Press.

[39] Schnitzler, C., Ernwein, V., Seifert, L. & Chollet, D. (2006). The stability of IdC during maximal and submaximal swim trials questioned. *Portuguese Journal of Sport Sciences, 6* (Supl. 2), 255-257.

[40]   Seifert, L., Boulesteix, L., Carter, M., & Chollet D. (2005). The spatial-temporal and coordinative structure in elite men 100-m front crawl swimmers. *International Journal of Sports Medicine, 26*, 286-293.

[41]   Seifert, L., Boulesteix, L. & Chollet D. (2004). Effect of gender on the adaptation of arm coordination in front crawl. *International Journal of Sport Medicine, 25*, 217-223.

[42]   Seifert, L., Boulesteix, L., Chollet, D. & Vilas-Boas, J.P. (in press). Difference in spatial-temporal parameters and arm to leg coordination in butterfly stroke regarding race pace, skill and gender. *Human Movement Science.*

[43]   Seifert, L., Chéhensse, A., Tourny-Chollet, C., Lemaitre, F. & Chollet D. (in press). Effect of breathing pattern on arm coordination symmetry in front crawl. *Journal of Strength and Conditioning Research.*

[44]   Seifert, L. & Chollet, D. (2005). A new index of flat breaststroke propulsion: comparison between elite men and elite women. *Journal of Sports Sciences, 23*, 309-320.

[45]   Seifert, L., Chollet, D. (in press). Modelling spatial-temporal and coordinative parameters in swimming. *Journal of Science and Medicine in Sport.*

[46]   Seifert, L., Chollet, D. & Allard, P. (2005). Arm coordination symmetry and effect of breathing in front crawl. *Human Movement Science, 24*, 234-256.

[47]   Seifert, L., Chollet, D. & Bardy, B. (2004). Effect of swimming velocity on arm coordination in front crawl: a dynamical analysis. *Journal of Sports Sciences, 22*, 651-660.

[48]   Seifert, L., Chollet, D. & Chatard, J.C. (2007). Changes in coordination and kinematics during a 100-m front crawl. *Medicine and Science in Sports and Exercise, 39*, 1784-1793.

[49]   Seifert, L., Chollet, D., Papparadopoulos, C., Guerniou, Y. & Binet G. (2006). Longitudinal evaluation of breaststroke spatial-temporal and coordinative parameters: preparing of the 100-m breaststroke bronze medallists of the Athena 2004 Olympic Games. *Portuguese Journal of Sport Sciences, 6* (Supl. 2), 260-262.

[50]   Seifert, L., Chollet, D. & Rouard, A. (2007). Swimming constraints and arm coordination. *Human Movement Science, 26*, 68-86.

[51]   Seifert, L., Delignières, D., Boulesteix, L. & Chollet D. (2007). Effect of expertise on butterfly stroke coordination. *Journal of Sports Sciences, 25*, 131-141.

[52]   Sidney, M., Paillette, S., Hespel, J.M., Chollet, D., & Pelayo, P. (2001). Effect of swim paddles on the intra-cyclic velocity variations and on the arm coordination of front crawl stroke. In J.R. Blackwell & R.H. Sanders (Eds.) *XIX International Symposium on Biomechanics in Sports* (pp. 39-42), San Francisco, ISBS.

[53]   Swinnen, S.P., Jardin, K., Meulenbroek, R., Douskaia, N. & Hofkens-Van Den Brandt R. (1997). Egocentric and allocentric constraints in the expression of patterns of inter-limb coordination. *Journal of Cognitive Neuroscience, 9*, 348-377.

[54]   Takagi, H., Sugimoto, S., Nishijima, N. & Wilson, B. (2004). Differences in stroke phases, arm-leg coordination and velocity fluctuation due to event, gender and performance level in breaststroke. *Sports Biomechanics, 3*, 15-27.

[55]   Toussaint, H.M. & Beek, P.J. (1992). Biomechanics of competitive front crawl swimming. *Sports Medicine, 13*, 8-24.

[56]   Toussaint, H.M., & Truijens, M. (2005). Biomechanical aspects of peak performance in human swimming. *Animal Biology, 55*, 17-40.

[57]   Toussaint, H.M., A. Carol, H. Kranenborg & M. Truijens. (2006). Effect of fatigue on stroking characteristics in an arms-only 100-m front-crawl race. *Medicine and Science in Sports and Exercise,* 38, 1635-1642.

[58]   Yeater, R.A., Martin, R.B., White, M.K. & Gilson, K.H. (1981). Tethered swimming forces in the crawl, breast and back strokes and their relationship to competitive performance. *Journal of Biomechanics,* 14, 527-537.

[59]   Zanone, P.G. & Kelso, J.A.S. (1992). Evolution of behavioral attractors with learning: Nonequilibrium phase transitions. *Journal of Experimental Psychology: Human Perception and Performance,* 18, 403-421.

In: Physical Activity and Children: New Research
Editor: N. P. Beaulieu, pp. 95-116

ISBN: 978-1-60456-306-1
© 2008 Nova Science Publishers, Inc.

Chapter 4

Exercise Capacity and Exercise Training in Children with Cyanotic Congenital Heart Disease: With Special Reference to Children with a Fontan Circulation or Repaired Tetralogy of Fallot

Tim Takken[1],* and A. Christian Blank[2]
[1]Department of Pediatric Physical Therapy and Exercise Physiology,
[2]Department of Pediatric Cardiology,
Wilhelmina Children's Hospital, University Medical Center Utrecht, The Netherlands

Abstract

The purpose of this chapter is to describe the exercise capacity of children with cyanotic congenital heart disease (Fontan circulation and Tetralogy of Fallot) and secondly to summarize the available evidence on exercise training in these patients. Eleven patients with a Fontan circulation (5 males and 6 females) with a mean age of 9.5 ± 3.5 years (range 6.4-16.5) and 12 patients with Tetralogy of Fallot (7 males and 5 females) with a mean age of 12.6 ± 3.7 years (range 6.7-18.8) underwent a maximal exercise test. The results were compared to reference values for Dutch children matched for age and sex. Data were expressed as Z-scores. Moreover, based on current literature, best evidence guidelines on physical activity and exercise training will be provided.

Z-score of $\dot{V}_{o2peak}$/kg in Fontan patients was -3.17 ± 1.22 (p<0.001) and in Tetralogy of Fallot patients -1.22 ± 0.94 (p<0.01). Z-score of peak heart rate was -5.90 ± 3.28 in

---

* Address correspondence to: Dr Tim Takken, MSc, PhD, Department of Pediatric Physical Therapy & Exercise Physiology, Wilhelmina Children's Hospital, University Medical Center Utrecht, Room KB2.056.0, PO Box 85090, NL 3508 AB Utrecht, The Netherlands. E-mail: t.takken@umcutrecht.nl

Fontan patients and -2.10 ± 1.98 in patients with Tetralogy of Fallot. Peak work load (p=0.009), duration of test (p=0.008), $\dot{V}O_{2peak}$/kg (p<0.001), peak heart rate (p=0.002), oxygen pulse (p=0.008), ventilation (p=0.002) and oxygen saturation (p=0.003) were all significant lower in the Fontan group compared to the Tetralogy of Fallot patients.

Conclusion: A reduced exercise capacity in patients with a Fontan circulation and patients with Tetralogy of Fallot is observed compared to reference values. Exercise capacity in Fontan patients was significantly lower compared to Tetralogy of Fallot patients. Best-evidence guidelines for physical activity and exercise training are provided.

Keywords: Fontan circulation, Tetralogy of Fallot, children, exercise capacity, maximal oxygen uptake

INTRODUCTION

In every 1000 live births, there are 4 to 50 children born with congenital heart disease [1]. Some of these patients have only mild disease with relatively little need for medical care, but others have complicated problems and require the services of an array of people with great expertise in the field [1]. The goal of surgical correction of congenital heart defects in children is not only to ensure survival but also to enable a life as normal as possible [2].

Hypoplastic left heart syndrome has an incidence of 226 per 1 million live births. Hypoplastic right heart syndrome occurs in 222 cases per 1 million live births, which includes tricuspid atresia (79 cases) and pulmonary atresia with an intact ventricular septum (132 cases) [1]. In 1971, Fontan & Baudet described an operation for separation of the systemic and pulmonary venous return in patients with tricuspid atresia [3]. In a so called Fontan circulation the systemic venous return is connected to the pulmonary arteries without the interposition of an adequate ventricle, and all shunts on the venous, atrial, ventricular and arterial level are interrupted [4]. During the last three decades, the principles of the Fontan operation have been applied to all forms of congenital heart disease characterized by a single ventricle [5].

Tetralogy of Fallot is the most common form of cyanotic congenital heart disease [6]. It occurs in 421 cases per 1 million live births [1]. Fallot described the four cardinal features of the anomaly in 1888, namely pulmonary stenosis, ventricular septal defect, a shift of the aorta to the right and hypertrophy of the wall of the right ventricle [7]. The current standard of its treatment is reparative operation in early infancy [6]. Early repair is advocated in these patients to allow for non-restricted cardiopulmonary development, as well as to avoid possible complications involving other organs and systems [8].

Several studies found that children with congenital heart disease have a very low physical activity level [9, 10]. However, this is not significantly related to physical function [10], indication that probably the physical inactivity might be a result of sedentary behavior.

In exercise physiology terms, inactivity is associated with a loss of maximal oxygen uptake ($\dot{V}O_{2peak}$), or aerobic capacity. The $\dot{V}O_{2peak}$ attained during a graded maximal exercise to volitional exhaustion is considered by the World Health Organization as the single best indicator of exercise tolerance [11].

A significantly reduced aerobic capacity in patients with congenital heart disease is worrisome, as health outcome and survival may be directly related to exercise capacity [12]. Moreover, exercise capacity is an important predictor of health outcome and survival in adult patients with cardiovascular disease [12] or congenital heart disease [13], children with pulmonary disease [14], as well as in healthy subjects [12, 15].

Patients with unoperated single ventricle or Tetralogy of Fallot have severely reduced exercise tolerance. Although surgical correction of Tetralogy of Fallot and the Fontan operation lead to a dramatic improvement in exercise tolerance, most patients have a subnormal exercise tolerance, especially the patients with a Fontan circulation [16, 17]. However, the individual variations in exercise tolerance in patients with Tetralogy of Fallot are large [18-20]. Previous studies have investigated the reduced exercise capacity in both patient groups [17, 20], however this is one of the only studies comparing the exercise capacity in the same laboratory.

The purpose of this chapter is to describe the exercise capacity of these two groups and secondly to summarize the available evidence on exercise training in these two patient groups.

MATERIALS AND METHODS

Study Population

The group of patients with a Fontan circulation consisted of 11 patients (5 males and 6 females) with an age range of 6.4 to 16.5 years. Six patients had a hypoplastic left ventricle and 5 patients a hypoplastic right ventricle.

Twelve patients with Tetralogy of Fallot (7 males and 5 females) with an age range of 6.7 to 18.8 years participated. All patients had total correction of Tetralogy of Fallot. Three patients had a transannular patch and three patients a right ventricular outflow tract patch. The patient characteristics are given in table 1 and 2. Patients were tested in the Pediatric Exercise Physiology Laboratory of the Wilhelmina's Children Hospital, Utrecht, the Netherlands. All procedures were approved by the local ethics committee, all patients and/or parents provided informed consent.

Exercise Testing

Maximal exercise tests were performed on a treadmill or cycle ergometer, depending on the height of the patient. Cycle ergometer protocol was a continuous ramp protocol with increments of 10, 15 or 20 Watt each minute [21]. The test started with 1 minute rest period, followed by a warm-up of 1 minute. Pedaling rate was 60-80 revolutions per minute. The used treadmill protocol was a modified Bruce protocol [22]. The test started with 1 minute rest period, followed by 1.5 minutes warm-up. The subject continued to exercise until the limit of his tolerance has been reached, despite verbal encouragement of the test leader.

Data from the exercise tests were used to determine maximal oxygen consumption, peak heart rate, oxygen saturation and ventilatory indexes. During the test, patients breathed through a face mask (Hans Rudolph Inc, Kansas City, MO, USA), which was connected to a calibrated gas analyzer (Oxycon Pro, Jaeger, Viasys BV, Bilthoven, the Netherlands). Breath-by-breath measurements were analyzed by the Jaeger Oxycon Software (Windows 98, Jaeger, Viasys BV, Bilthoven, the Netherlands). Oxygen uptake ($\dot{V}O_2$; ml/min), carbon dioxide production ($\dot{V}CO_2$; ml/min), respiratory exchange ratio (RER; $= \dot{V}CO_2/\dot{V}O_2$), ventilation ($\dot{V}_E$; breaths/min), ventilatory equivalent for oxygen ($\dot{V}_E/\dot{V}O_2$) and the ventilatory equivalent for carbon dioxide ($\dot{V}_E/\dot{V}CO_2$) were measured. Heart rate (HR; beats/min) was monitored continuously throughout exercise by means of a 10-channel ECG-equipment connected to the system. Oxygen pulse was calculated as the ratio between $\dot{V}O_2$ and HR [23]. Blood oxygen saturation ($SaO_2\%$) was measured by means of a pulse oximeter at the index finger (Nellcor 200 E, Breda, the Netherlands). Ventilatory anaerobic threshold (VAT) was determined using the ventilatory equivalents method [24].

The values given at maximal exercise are the mean of 20 seconds. Maximal exercise was defined as the highest heart rate at the highest achieved workload. The results were compared to reference values of Dutch children matched for sex and age [25]. Data were expressed as Z-scores or as percentage of predicted. The Z-score was calculated as the difference between the observed and the predicted values for a given patient divided by the standard deviation.

Best-evidence Synthesis

Literature was selected from 1966 until July 2007 using Medline, Embase and SportDiscus databases. Search terms were "physical fitness", "exercise training", "cardiac rehabilitation" "exercise", "exercise capacity", "exercise tolerance", "Fontan", "univentricular" or "Tetralogy of Fallot". References of the selected publications were tracked to find additional publications on this subject. Inclusion criteria consisted of studies with at least a 3 week training period and a minimum of 6 training sessions.

Statistical Analyses

Independent sample T-tests were done to test differences between patients and reference values and between the two patient groups. Z-scores were used to test between the two groups. Statistical analyses were performed using the Statistical Package for the Social Sciences for Windows (version 12.0.2, SPSS Inc, Chicago, Ill). Alpha level was set at $p < 0.05$ for all analyses.

RESULTS

Patients

Patient characteristics can be found in table 1 (Fontan) and in table 2 (Tetralogy of Fallot). There were some significant differences between the two patient groups; patients with

Tetralogy of Fallot were significantly older (p = 0.044), had a higher body mass (p = 0.005), stature (p = 0.008), and a longer time since operation (p = 0.003).

Exercise Capacity

The results of the maximal exercise tests are provided in table 3 and 4. In the children with a Fontan circulation, 4 children performed a cycling test and 6 children a treadmill test. In the children with Tetralogy of Fallot, 8 children performed a cycling test and 4 children a treadmill test. All patients had a RER above 1.0 except for two children with a Fontan circulation and one child with Tetralogy of Fallot.

The mean Z-scores of maximal workload, duration of test and $\dot{V}O_{2peak}$ of both groups were significantly lower compared to reference values. When the two patient groups were compared, the outcome of the children with a Fontan circulation was significant worse compared to the children with Tetralogy of Fallot (p < 0.05). There was no correlation between age at test and Z-score for $\dot{V}O_{2peak}$ or $\dot{V}O_{2peak}/kg$.

Hemodynamics

Both groups had a significant reduced HR_{peak} to healthy children. The HR_{peak} was significantly lower in children with a Fontan circulation compared to children with Tetralogy of Fallot (Table 3).

The oxygen pulse in patients with a Fontan circulation was significantly lower compared to children with Tetralogy of Fallot, who had an almost normal oxygen pulse.

In the Fontan group, 3 patients had a $SaO_2\%$ of $\leq 80\%$ at peak exercise.

Ventilatory Indexes

Z-score for RER_{max} in patients with a Fontan circulation was lower compared to children with Tetralogy of Fallot (p=0.031; table 3). Minute ventilation ($\dot{V}_E$) in children with a Fontan circulation was significantly lower compared to children with Tetralogy of Fallot (Table 3); both groups differed significantly compared to reference values. Respiratory rate was not significantly different between the two groups (p = 0.118).

VAT was at a significantly higher percentage of $\dot{V}O_{2peak}$ in children with a Fontan circulation compared to children with Tetralogy of Fallot (p = 0.002; table 4).

$\dot{V}_E/\dot{V}O_2$ and $\dot{V}_E/\dot{V}CO_2$ in children with a Fontan circulation were significantly higher compared to children with Tetralogy of Fallot (p = 0.056 and p = 0.0001 respectively, Table 4).

Table 1. Characteristics of the patients with a Fontan circulation

Sub-ject	Sex	Diagnosis	Previous palliation	Systemic ventricle	Type of Fontan operation	Age at Fontan operation (yr)	Age at test (yr)	Length (cm)	Weight (kg)
1	M	HRV, ccTGA, PS, DC	PCPC	LV	TCPC/IAB	3.1	8.6	129	27
2	M	HLHS	NW, PCPC	RV	TCPC/EC	2.8	6.7	126	25
3	F	TA	APS, PCPC	LV	TCPC/IAB	2.3	7.8	128	23
4	F	HLHS	NW, PCPC	RV	TCPC/LT	3.7	6.4	108	19
5	F	HLHS	NW, PCPC	RV	TCPC/IAB	3.3	16.5	141	38
6	M	DILV, PS	PCPC	LV	TCPC/EC	4.0	7.9	132	30
7	F	TA, TGA, IAA	DKS, PCPC	LV	TCPC/EC	3.5	6.6	117	20
8	M	HLV, DORV, TGA	PAB, DKS	RV	TCPC/IAB	2.2	13.5	152	37
9	M	TPA	APS, PCPC	LV	TCPC/LT	2.5	14.0	155	47
10	F	HRV, PS	PCPC	LV	TCPC/EC	2.0	11.7	145	37
11	F	HLV, PA, TGA	APS, PCPC	RV	TCPC/EC	4.0	6.4	118	22
Mean ± sd						3.0 ± 0.7	9.6 ± 3.5	131.9 ± 15.0	29.5 ± 9.0

Abbreviations: APS: aorto-pulmonary shunt; DC: dextrocardia; DKS: Damus Kay Stansel; DORV: double outlet right ventricle; HLHS: hypoplastic left heart syndrome; HLV: hypoplastic left ventricle; HRV: hypoplastic right ventricle; IAA: interrupted aortic arch; NW: Norwood 1; PCPC: partial cavopulmonary connection; PA: pulmonary atresia; PS: pulmonary stenosis; TA: tricuspid atresia; TCPC/IAB: total cavopulmonary connection with an intraatrial baffle; TCPC/ECC: total cavopulmonary connection with a extracardiac conduit; TCPC/LT: total cavopulmonary connection with a lateral tunnel; TGA: transposition of the great arteries; ccTGA: congenitally corrected transposition of the great arteries; TPA: tricuspid and pulmonary atresia; PAB: pulmonary artery banding.

Table 2. Characteristics of the patients with Tetralogy of Fallot

Subject	Sex	Previous palliation	Type of operation	Age at operation (yr)	Age at test (yr)	Time from operation (yr)	Length (cm)	Weight (kg)
1	M		TC, TP	3.2	13.5	10.3	146	37
2	F		TC	1.0	13.6	12.6	167	52
3	M		TC, TP	1.1	13.4	12.3	165	51
4	M		TC	1.0	13.0	12.0	158	45
5	F		TC	1.2	17.4	16.2	170	56
6	F		TC	0.7	18.8	18.1	169	50
7	M	APS	TC, RVOTP	1.0	10.5	9.5	140	40
8	M	APS	TC, RVOTP	1.2	8.0	6.8	132	27
9	M		TC, RVOTP	0.8	6.7	5.9	128	26
10	M		TC	1.3	16.0	14.7	165	45
11	F		TC	0.7	12.0	11.3	159	41
12	F		TC, TP	0.7	8.5	7.8	121	22
Mean ± SD				1.2 ± 0.7	12.6 ± 3.7	11.5 ± 3.7	151.7 ± 17.5	41 ± 11.1

Abbreviations: APS: aorto-pulmonary shunt; RVOTP: right ventricular outflow tract patch; TC: total correction; TP: transannular patch.

Table 3. Maximal exercise performance in children with a Fontan circulation and Tetralogy of Fallot compared to reference values

	Fontan	Z-score Fontan	Tetralogy of Fallot	Z-score Tetralogy of Fallot	p
$\dot{V}O_{2peak}$ (ml/min)	812 ± 248	-3.3 ± 0.9***	1572 ± 418	-1.21 ± 1.00*	0.000
$\dot{V}O_{2peak}$ (ml/min/kg)	28.67 ± 6.95	-3.2 ± 1.28***	38.96 ± 5.67	-1.22 ± 0.94**	0.000
RER_{peak}	1.07 ± 0.09	-1.4 ± 1.1**	1.19 ± 0.15	0.18 ± 2.01	0.031
HR_{peak} (beats/min)	151 ± 26.7	-5.6 ± 3.2***	179 ± 16.21	-2.10 ± 1.98**	0.002
O_2 pulse (ml/beat)	5.6 ± 2.16	73.77 ± 12.3% of predicted	9.92 ± 3.57	98.30 ± 21.00% of predicted	0.008
$\dot{V}_{E\ peak}$ (L/min)	32.33 ± 6.70	-2.76 ± 0.62***	55.58 ± 18.63	-1.28 ± 1.26*	0.002

Abbreviations: HR_{peak}: peak heart rate; RER: Respiratory exchange ratio; $\dot{V}_E$: Ventilation; $\dot{V}O_{2peak}$: maximal oxygen uptake.* = P<0.05; ** = P<0.01 ; *** = P<0.001 compared to reference values.

Table 4. Maximal exercise test data compared between the two groups

	Fontan	Tetralogy of Fallot	p
SaO_2 (%)	88.0 ± 6.6	95.80 ± 4.6	0.003
VAT (% of $\dot{V}O_{2peak}$)	90.5 ± 8.0	74.80 ± 13.9	0.002
VAT (% of predicted $\dot{V}O_{2peak}$)	50.2 ± 12.1	60.46 ± 11.7	0.08
Respiratory rate (breaths/min)	50.6 ± 6.4	46.58 ± 8.7	0.118
$\dot{V}_E/\dot{V}O_2$	37.1 ± 5.9	32.94 ± 5.0	0.05
$\dot{V}_E/\dot{V}CO_2$	34.9 ± 4.9	27.73 ± 2.7	0.0001

Abbreviations: SaO_2: O_2 saturation; VAT: ventilatory anaerobic threshold; $\dot{V}_E/\dot{V}O_2$: ventilatory equivalent for oxygen; $\dot{V}_E/\dot{V}CO_2$: ventilatory equivalent for carbon dioxide.

Exercise Training

Fontan Patients

Six studies were identified in the literature, one of which was a case-report. Two of the studies included children with congenital heart diseases other than Fontan circulation [26-28]. The characteristics of the six studies are displayed in Table 5, and the results in table 6 and Figure 1.

Exercise response in Fontan circulation

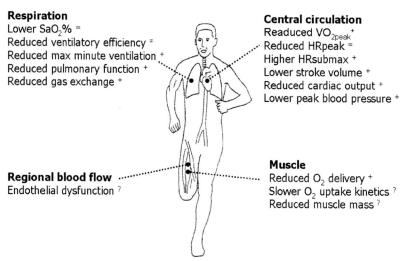

Abbreviations: SaO_2%: arterial oxygen saturation, HRpeak: peak heart rate, HRsubmax: heart rate during submaximal exercise, +: indicates improvement after exercise training, =: indicates no change after exercise training, ?: indicates no data available.

Figure 1. Limitations of $\dot{V}O_{2peak}$ in patients with a Fontan circulation and the effects of exercise training. Modified after [29].

McCall and Humphrey were the first to document training effects of a formal exercise program in a single patient with a Fontan circulation [30]. The patient attended in-hospital cardiopulmonary training sessions 2 to 3 times a week for 22 weeks at a moderate intensity. Training sessions consisted of a combination of cardiovascular exercise, both treadmill and stationary cycle, and light resistance training with weights (see Table 5). The patient was unable to complete formal exercise testing prior to the training program, however, formal exercise testing was successfully conducted on the patient following the exercise training program. As expected, exercise capacity was still much lower than normal values after the training program.

Minamisawa et al. [31] studied exercise programs in 11 patients with Fontan circulation, each subject entered an exercise program that was individually prescribed. The exercise program consisted of 3 supervised training sessions in the first three weeks of the program, thereafter the training was continued using home-based exercise training sessions. The exercise training was performed 2 to 3 days a week for 2 to 3 months. Patients underwent fast walking or jogging for 20 to 30 minutes at a moderate intensity (Table 5). After the training program, there was a significant improvement in peak oxygen uptake ($\dot{V}O_{2peak}$; Table 2), however, the improvement was lower when compared to the results of the other studies. Lower $\dot{V}O_{2peak}$ values obtained in the Minamisawa study might be explained by the use of a bicycle ergometer test to evaluate a running-based exercise training program. Training effects are exercise mode specific with only a small transfer effect to other exercise modalities.[32, 33]

Opocher et al. [34] studied the effects of an eight month training program in 10 children with a Fontan circulation. Supervised training sessions were held twice a week for the first three weeks (10 sessions) and then once a month for the next four months of the training program (Table 5). Home training sessions were held at each child's home twice a week for 30 to 45 minutes. The exercise level during training was designed to range from low to moderate intensity (Table 5).

A clinically important increase in $\dot{V}O_{2peak}$ was noted (Table 6), as well as a decrease in the heart rate curve and an increased oxygen pulse (the ratio of oxygen uptake and heart rate) during submaximal exercise.

In the study by Rhodes et al. [27], 16 children with congenital heart disease (11 Fontan patients, 5 with other congenital heart disease) participated in an exercise training program. The program consisted of a twice a week one hour supervised aerobic and light weight resistance exercise for 12 weeks (see Table 5). The sessions were held in a clinic facility. Patients were encouraged to exercise at a heart-rate that was equivalent to their ventilatory anaerobic threshold measured during their baseline exercise test, moreover they were encouraged to exercise at least 2 times per week at home. There was no specific program supplied for the home exercise, nor was compliance monitored.

They reported a significant increase in $\dot{V}O_{2peak}$ (Table 6) and other physiological parameters during exercise upon completion of the exercise rehabilitation program. The peak exercise systolic blood pressure was not affected by the program. However, the patients' peak exercise diastolic blood pressure was significantly higher after rehabilitation. Also a rise in peak minute ventilation (22%) was reported, which resulted in an insignificant decline in the breathing reserve. Exercise rehabilitation had no effect on peak exercise oxygen saturation.

The authors suggested that the improvements were related, at least in part, to an exercise-induced increase in muscle strength, muscle mass, and pumping capacity of the skeletal muscles [27].

In a recent study by Brassard et al. [35] five Fontan patients were enrolled in an 8 week trial of combined aerobic and resistance training programs. Two patients exercised in-hospital and three patients exercised at home. Aerobic training consisted of exercise on a cycle ergometer, 20-30 minutes/session, twice a week. The training program was individually prescribed to allow the subjects to work progressively at 50%-80% of their $\dot{V}_{O2peak}$ throughout the 8 weeks (see Table 5). Resistance training exercises were also performed and consisted of an 8 exercises circuit training program without rest between the exercises (see Table 5). Brassard et al, included resistance exercise because they found a strong significant correlation between muscle strength and $\dot{V}_{O2peak}$ [35], suggesting a role for peripheral muscle strength as one of the causes of exercise intolerance. However, they did not find significant changes in $\dot{V}_{O2peak}$, $\dot{V}_{O2peak}$/kg and skeletal muscle strength after exercise training (Table 6).

Table 5. Characteristics of the exercise training studies

Author	Age	Number of patients	Type of exercise	Duration Training	Frequency	Intensity	Time
McCall & Humphrey [30]	18	1	Aerobic exercise (bicycle, treadmill)	22 weeks	2-3/ week	50-70% $\dot{V}_{O2peak}$	20-30 min
			Resistance exercise			12-15 repetitions, light exercises	
Minamisawa et al. [31]	19 ± 4	11		8-12 weeks	2-3 / week	60-80% HR_{peak}	20-30 min
Opocher et al. [34]	8.7 ±0.6	10	Aerobic training (cycling)	8 months	2 / week	50-70% $\dot{V}_{O2peak}$	30-45 min
Rhodes et al. [27]	11.9 ± 2.1	11 Fontan, 5 other CHD	Aerobic training	12 weeks	2/ week*	55-58% $\dot{V}_{O2peak}$	60 min
			Resistance exercises		2/ week	Light resistance	
Moalla et al [26, 28]	13.0 ± 1.4	2 Fontan, 8 other CHD	Aerobic training (cycling)	12	3/week	62% $\dot{V}_{O2peak}$	45 min
Brassard et al. [35]	16 ± 5	5	Aerobic exercise Resistance Exercise	8 weeks	3 / week	50-80% $\dot{V}_{O2peak}$	20-30 min
						12-15 repetitions	

Abbreviations: * patients were encouraged to exercise an additional 2x / week at home.

Table 6. Used outcome instruments and reported results of exercise training

Study	Outcome measure	Results
McCall & Humphrey [30]	Exercise capacity (Treadmill exercise test)	Improvement in exercise capacity
Minamisawa et al. [31]	Exercise capacity (Bicycle ergometer test)	7% improvement in $\dot{V}O_{2peak}$
Opocher et al. [34]	Exercise capacity (Treadmill exercise test)	19% improvement in $\dot{V}O_{2peak}$
Rhodes et al. [27]	Exercise capacity (Bicycle ergometer test)	22% improvement in $\dot{V}O_{2peak}$
Rhodes et al. [27]	Pulmonary function	7% improvement in FEV1
Moalla et al. [26, 28]	Exercise capacity (Bicycle ergometer)	8.1% improvement in $\dot{V}O_{2peak}$
Moalla et al. [26]	Six minute walk	13% improvement in walking distance
Moalla et al. [28]	Oxygenation respiratory muscles (NIRS)	28% improvement respiratory muscle oxygenation
Moalla et al. [28]	Pulmonary function	Non-significant improvements in FEV1 (7.5%), FVC (6.2%), TLC (4.2) and MVV (5.7%)
Brassard et al. [35]	Exercise capacity (Bicycle ergometer test)	No significant improvement in $\dot{V}O_{2peak}$.
Brassard et al. [35]	Muscle strength	No significant improvement in MVC.
Brassard et al. [35]	Blood pressure	Significant improvement in ergoreflex

Abbreviations: NIRS: Near Infrared Spectroscopy, FEV1: Forced expiratory volume in 1 second, FVC: forced vital capacity, TLC: total lung capacity, MVV: maximum voluntary ventilation, MVC: maximum voluntary contraction.

Moalla et al [26, 28] also studied a home-based training program in children with congenital heart disease. The training program was 12 weeks in duration with three exercise training sessions per week, 45 minutes per session (see Table 5). The children were instructed to perform their exercise on a supplied cycle ergometer. A six minute walk test was used in this study to measure the outcome of the program as well as a maximal cycle ergometer test. After the training program the mean distance walked improved significantly (+62 meters). An increase in ventilatory anaerobic threshold, $\dot{V}O_{2peak}$, heart rate and minute ventilation were also reported (Table 6). No significant difference for SaO_2% were found before or after training.[26]

Tetralogy of Fallot Patients

Six studies were identified in the literature concerning the effects of training in 56 patients with Tetralogy of Fallot [18, 36-38], of which one was conducted in adult patients [38]. Several studies included children with congenital heart diseases other than Tetralogy of Fallot. Only the data of the patients with Tetralogy of Fallot was included in this review. The characteristics of the studies are displayed in Table 7, the results are displayed in Table 8 and in Figure 2. None of the studies reported adverse events during or after the exercise sessions, however the studies only included hemodynamically stable patients.

In the study of Bradley et al. [36] 4 children with repaired Tetralogy of Fallot participated in a supervised exercise training program. They trained twice a week for 12 weeks in a hospital-based gymnasium. Each session commenced with a 15 minute warm-up period of stretching and flexibility exercises. Thereafter 15-30 minutes of aerobic activities were performed. Activities consisted of walking, running, rope jumping, and aerobic dance at a submaximal intensity. The children with Tetralogy of Fallot showed a significant improvement in $\dot{V}O_{2peak}$ after the training program (Table 8).

Goldberg et al. [18] included 16 children with Tetralogy of Fallot in their study. The children performed a 6 week home based cycling program on a ergometer. Cycling sessions were scheduled on a alternate day base. After the exercise program a small non-significant improvement in $\dot{V}O_{2peak}$ was observed.

Ruttenberg et al. [37] included 8 children with Tetralogy of Fallot in their study. Their training program consisted of 3 times per week held jogging sessions, for 9 weeks during the summer in local gymnasiums. In this study there was a considerable drop-out of patients. Of the initial 50 children who participated in the study (several different patient groups), only 12 patients and 9 controls successfully completed the study. After the program an improvement in $\dot{V}O_{2peak}$ was observed, although they found a considerable improvement in endurance time.

Exercise response in Tetralogy of Fallot

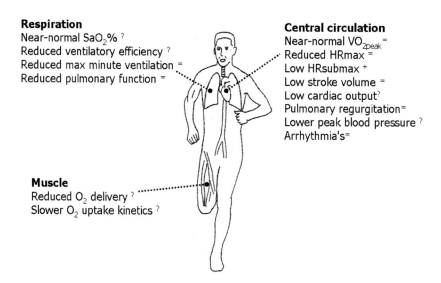

Respiration
Near-normal $SaO_2\%$?
Reduced ventilatory efficiency ?
Reduced max minute ventilation =
Reduced pulmonary function =

Central circulation
Near-normal VO_{2peak} =
Reduced HRmax =
Low HRsubmax +
Low stroke volume =
Low cardiac output?
Pulmonary regurgitation =
Lower peak blood pressure ?
Arrhythmia's =

Muscle
Reduced O_2 delivery ?
Slower O_2 uptake kinetics ?

Abbreviations: $\dot{V}O_{2peak}$: peak oxygen uptake, $SaO_2\%$: arterial oxygen saturation, HR_{peak}: peak heart rate, HRsubmax: heart rate during submaximal exercise, +: indicates improvement after exercise training, =: indicates no change after exercise training, ?: indicates no data available.

Figure 2. Limitations of $\dot{V}O_{2peak}$ in patients with Tetralogy of Fallot and the effects of exercise training.

Therrien et al. [38] performed the only randomized trial on this topic. However, this study was performed in clinically stable young adults with Tetralogy of Fallot. Supervised training sessions were held in a cardiac rehabilitation department once a week. Moreover, the participants were instructed to perform 2-weekly exercise sessions at home consisting of 30 minutes sub maximal brisk walking. They found after a 3 months exercise training program, significant improvements in $\dot{V}O_{2peak}$ (Table 8).

Sklansky et al. [39] et al performed a 8 week exercise intervention in 11 asymptomatic children after repair for Tetralogy of Fallot. The exercise training consisted of supervised sessions held three times per week in a in-hospital exercise room. The program lasted 8 weeks. After this program, the authors found no improvement in $\dot{V}O_{2peak}$, the occurrence of arrhythmia's or cardiac function (Table 8). However, there was a significant improvement in endurance time.

Calzolari et al. [40] performed an 3 month exercise training intervention in 9 children after repair for Tetralogy of Fallot. Supervised training sessions were held in a hospital gymnasium three times per week. The sessions gradually increased to 1 hour. After the training program no significant improvements in maximal exercise capacity or pulmonary function were observed. Only improvements in submaximal exercise capacity were observed (Table 8).

Table 7. Characteristics of the exercise training studies in patients with Tetralogy of Fallot

Author	Age (years)	Number of patients	Type of exercise	Duration Training	Frequency	Intensity	Time
Bradley et al. [36]	8 ± 3.4	4	Aerobic training	12 weeks	2x/ week	60-80% of HR_{peak}	45-60 min
Goldberg et al. [18]	14 ± 3.1	16	Cycling at home	6 weeks	Alternate day	50-70% of $\dot{V}O_{2peak}$	45 min
Ruttenberg et al. [37]	12.75 ± 4.4	8	Walking/ jogging	9 weeks	3x/ week	65-75% HR_{peak}	5 to ~30 minutes
Therrien et al. [38]	35 ± 9.5	18 (9 Ex, 9 Con)	Walking/ cycling	12 weeks	3x/ week	60-85% of $\dot{V}O_{2peak}$	30 –50 minutes*
Sklansky et al. [41]	8.7	10	Walking/ cycling	8 weeks	3x/ week	60 to >70% of HR_{peak}	30 minutes
Calzolari et al. [40]	9.9 ± 3.7	18 (9 Ex, 9 Con	Breathing exercises, stretching, aerobic exercises	3 months	3x/ week	60 to >70% of HR_{peak}	Increasing to 60 minutes

Abbreviations: * patients were instructed to walk 2 times per week for 30 minutes, once a week a hospital based training session of 50 minutes was held. Ex: exercise, Con: control. HR_{peak}: peak heart rate. $\dot{V}O_{2peak}$: peak oxygen uptake.

Table 8. Used outcome instruments and reported results of exercise training patients with Tetralogy of Fallot

Study	Outcome measure	Results
Bradley et al. [36]	Exercise capacity (Treadmill exercise test)	29% improvement in $\dot{V}O_{2peak}$
Goldberg et al. [18]	Exercise capacity (Bicycle ergometer test)	5% improvement in $\dot{V}O_{2peak}$ (NS)
Ruttenberg et al. [37]	Exercise capacity (Treadmill exercise test)	0% improvement in $\dot{V}O_{2peak}$ 21% improvement in endurance time
Therrien et al. [38]	Exercise capacity (Bicycle ergometer test)	10 % improvement in $\dot{V}O_{2peak}$
Therrien et al. [38]	Pulmonary function	No improvement in FEV_1 and FVC
Sklansky et al. [39]	Exercise capacity (Treadmill exercise test)	No improvement in $\dot{V}O_{2peak}$ 15% improvement in endurance time
Sklansky et al. [39]	Arrhytmia's (Holter monitoring and exercise ECG)	No change in atrial or ventricular ectopy
Sklansky et al. [39]	Cardiac function (Echocardiography)	No change in resting left ventricular end-diastolic dimensions or posterior wall thickness
Calzolari et al. [40]	Exercise capacity (Bicycle ergometer test)	No significant improvement in exercise capacity (total workload) and endurance time
Calzolari et al. [40]	Submaximal Exercise performance	11% improvement in running distance
Calzolari et al. [40]	Pulmonary function	No significant improvement in FVC, FEV, MMEF

Abbreviations: $\dot{V}O_{2peak}$: peak oxygen uptake, ECG: electrocardiogram.

DISCUSSION

The purpose of this chapter was firstly to describe the exercise capacity of children with a Fontan circulation and Tetralogy of Fallot and secondly to summarize the available evidence on exercise training in these patients.

Previous studies have investigated the reduced exercise capacity in both patient groups [17, 20], however this is one of the only studies comparing the exercise capacity in the same laboratory. We found a significantly reduced exercise capacity in children with a Fontan circulation or Tetralogy of Fallot compared to reference values. Children with a Fontan circulation had significantly lower outcome in all variables, except for respiratory rate, compared to children with Tetralogy of Fallot.

Our findings are in accordance with a previous study in adolescents with a Fontan circulation or Tetralogy of Fallot [42]. Rhodes et al [42] found a significantly larger reduction in $\dot{V}O_{2peak}$ in children with a Fontan circulation compared to children with Tetralogy of Fallot.

According to Fick's equation [43]; $\dot{V}O_{2peak}$ is the product of cardiac output (heart rate x stroke volume) and arterio-mixed venous O_2 extraction. The reduced $\dot{V}O_{2peak}$ can be caused by a combination of several factors. First of all chronotropic incompetence may partly explain the diminished $\dot{V}O_{2peak}$ in both patient groups. Moreover, cardiac stroke volume might also be a limiting factor for these patients, as has been found previously [42, 44]. Oxygen pulse, a surrogate index of stroke volume, was more reduced in the patients with a Fontan circulation, and might be explained by a limited diastolic return to the systemic ventricle [45], or by a chronic volume overload [46]. Oxygen pulse in children with Tetralogy of Fallot was almost normal, suggesting a near normal stroke volume in children with Tetralogy of Fallot [42].

Peak minute ventilation was decreased in both patient groups. This has been observed in other studies as well [47, 48]. In patients with a Fontan circulation the non-pulsatile pulmonary blood flow might lead to a deterioration in gas exchange in the lungs [47]. Patients with Tetralogy of Fallot have a diminished minute ventilation during exercise [49]. The reduced ventilation might be explained by a low pulmonary blood flow. In patients with Tetralogy of Fallot, right ventricular outflow tract obstruction is associated with a low pulmonary blood flow [50]. Moreover, an increased pulmonary vascular resistance with is observed in congenital heart disease, might contribute to a reduced pulmonary blood flow, and hence a reduced cardiac output and impaired gas exchange in both groups [51].

$\dot{V}_E/\dot{V}CO_2$ was higher in Fontan patients compared to Tetralogy of Fallot patients, which is an indication of a gas-exchange abnormality. Ventilation/perfusion mismatching has been identified as a major factor contributing to an increase in physiologic dead space in Fontan patients [52]. Moreover, patients with a Fontan circulation have small lungs [47], requiring a higher breathing frequency to obtain an certain minute ventilation. A reduced pulmonary function has been shown to be related with $\dot{V}O_{2peak}$ in patients with a Fontan circulation [48]. Patients with Tetralogy of Fallot might also have an persistent ventilation-perfusion mismatch and/or the inability to increase pulmonary blood flow appropriately with exercise [53], moreover just as in Fontan patients, the velocity of the increase of oxygen uptake at the onset of exercise is slowed [54], increasing the dependency on anaerobic energy sources.

In both patient groups a reduction in $SaO_2\%$ was observed during exercise, showing the reduced arterial oxygen saturation and hence limitations in oxygen transport. Since patients with a Fontan circulation have a larger arterio-venous O_2 difference during exercise (to compensate the reduced cardiac output)[44], a reduced $SaO_2\%$ contributes to a limitation in $\dot{V}O_{2peak}$.

Moreover, recent studies have suggested skeletal muscle impairment in patients with a congenital heart disease. Inai et al [55] found a reduced muscle blood flow during exercise in children with a Fontan circulation as measured with near-infrared spectroscopy. Furthermore, Brassard et al [35] found a significant correlation between muscle strength and $\dot{V}O_{2peak}$ in patients with a Fontan circulation, indicating that peripheral muscle mass might also be related to exercise capacity. These observations indicate that peripheral oxygen extraction might be a limiting factor during exercise in patients with congenital heart disease.

A limitation of our study was that both patient groups differed in some characteristics. Patients with Tetralogy of Fallot were older compared to the patients with a Fontan circulation. Their weight and height also were significantly different. However, we calculated Z-scores matched for age and gender, to correct for these differences. Another potential source of variation is the use of two different exercise modalities. Some of the younger children were tested on the treadmill since they did not fit our cycle ergometer due to their small stature. A reduced body height is frequently observed in congenital heart disease [56]. However, our results compare well with the literature [57].

To summarize, a reduced exercise capacity in patients with a Fontan circulation and patients with Tetralogy of Fallot is observed compared to reference values. Exercise capacity in Fontan patients was significantly lower compared to Tetralogy of Fallot patients. Moreover, this study shows that cardiopulmonary exercise testing can be a valuable tool in the management of children with congenital heart disease. The results of the measurement of gas exchange during exercise can be used to record the function of cardiac, pulmonary and muscular system during exercise stress.

Best-evidence Guideline for Exercise Training

Studies of the effect of exercise training on patients with a Fontan circulation have only been recently performed. Only six small studies have been conducted that focus on outcomes of physical performance measures such as $\dot{V}O_{2peak}$ and pulmonary function. One study incorporated a functional outcome measure, the 6 minute walk test [26].

The improvements in $\dot{V}O_{2peak}$ after exercise training in patients with a Fontan circulation could be explained by improvements on several factors. As described above, $\dot{V}O_{2peak}$ is dependent on cardiac, pulmonary and muscular function. On all three domains improvements have been reported after exercise training in patients with a Fontan circulation (See Figure 1), however the effects of exercise training on muscular function in patients with a Fontan circulation are yet not well established [17].

During submaximal exercise heart-rates of children with a Fontan circulation were decreased, whereas oxygen uptake did not change, increasing the oxygen pulse. A increased oxygen pulse is a reflection of an increased stroke volume and/or an increased peripheral oxygen extraction. Exercise training did not improve arterial oxygen saturation, or peak heart rate.

Most of the studies performed in Tetralogy of Fallot were performed 1 to 2 decades ago, during a time when research designs were not so rigorous as today's standards. Most of the studies consisted of small sample sizes, had large drop-out rates and only one study had a randomized control group. Therefore the outcomes of these studies are likely to be biased. The single randomized study performed by Therrien et al [38], which was performed in adult patients, found a significant improvement in $\dot{V}O_{2peak}$. Studies in children with Tetralogy of Fallot found mixed results, ranging from improvements in $\dot{V}O_{2peak}$ from 0 –29%. Additionally improvements in submaximal exercise capacity and endurance time were observed in three studies (Table 6).

Practical Implications

Almost all studies showed that exercise training could improve (submaximal) exercise capacity in patients with a Fontan circulation and to al lesser degree in patients with Tetralogy of Fallot. However, the included patients in the studies were patients with a stable hemodynamic condition. It is preferable to screen patients for abnormalities and possible contra-indications during an exercise test (e.g., exercise-induced arrhythmias, ST-depression, hypertension, hypotension, cardiac chest pain, or systemic desaturation < 80%) before they start participating in exercise training [27, 58].

A study in adults with a congenital heart disease found that only one third of the patients asked a doctor about how much exercise they could do safely [59]. The most common reason for not seeking advice was the assumption that all exercise was safe, including several patients with a severe cardiac disease [59]. Of those given instruction it was more common to receive prohibitive advice (30%) than to be encouraged to take more exercise (19%) [59]. This shows the need for a individualized exercise prescription based on (exercise) physiological data.

The prescribed exercise intensity should be low to moderate (i.e. 50-80% of $\dot{V}O_{2peak}$), the sessions should last between 20-45 minutes, should be performed 2 to 3 times per week, and a training program should persist at least two to three months. The additive effect of light resistance exercise is unclear. It is advisable to start with in-hospital / supervised training sessions. After several sessions patients and parents become more confident and home-based training sessions become more feasible. Several programs have supplied exercise equipment (e.g. cycle ergometers and heart rate monitors) to participating children for exercise training at home, however even a more simpler program with exercises with simply using the own body weight as mode of resistance supervised by the parents has been effective in children with (mild) congenital heart disorders [60]. For patients with severe heart failure (e.g. patients on listed for transplant), it is advised to perform a supervised in-hospital exercise training program with monitoring of heart rate, rhythm and blood pressure during exercise sessions [61].

Patients with a Fontan circulation who are in good hemodynamic condition should be encouraged to only take part in aerobic, low-intensity sport activities [62].

Patients with repaired Tetralogy of Fallot can generally be given permission for non-competitive sports with moderate cardiovascular involvement [62]. Only in a few selected cases with exceptionally good results, can eligibility for competitive sports be granted [62].

All operated patients should be re-evaluated rather frequently (e.g. every 6–12 months) to assess the eligibility for participation in physical activity and non-competitive sports [62].

Directions for Further Research

For both patient groups, studies with a more rigorous research design (i.e. larger sample size, randomized control group, blinded observers, etc) and a longer follow-up are indicated. In addition, the effects of exercise training on cardiac function (i.e. indices of cardiac strain such as atrial and brain natriuretic peptide (ANP/BNP), or cardiac damage such as cardiac troponins), peripheral muscle function, perceived competence, self esteem, physical activity, and health-related quality of life, needs further study.

Next to safety issues (exercise might be unsafe for patients with an unstable hemodynamic condition), not every body will benefit as much from an exercise program. Therefore the patients who will benefit most should be identified and, if indicated, carry out such a exercise program [63].

CONCLUSION

Reduced exercise capacity is observed in patients with congenital heart disease such as patients with a Fontan circulation and in patients with Tetralogy of Fallot when compared to healthy children. When the two groups were compared, patients with Fontan circulation had a more reduced capacity than patients with Tetralogy of Fallot. Possible explanations for this reduction are chronotropic incompetence, diminished lung function, low pulmonary blood flow, cardiac output and arterial desaturation. But also inactivity and deconditioning plays a role in this reduction. It is therefore important that patients become more active in daily life so effects of an exercise program remain sustained.

Based on the available evidence, training programs in Fontan and Tetralogy of Fallot patients with a stable hemodynamic status are safe, can result in an improved (submaximal) exercise capacity, and can be performed without adverse effects. No significant effects of exercise training on oxygen saturation and peak heart rate were reported in these studies. After training, exercise capacity was still significantly lower than those reported in healthy children. More research is needed to establish the optimal exercise mode, and the effects of exercise training on cardiac and peripheral muscle function, physical activity, and health-related quality of life.

REFERENCES

[1]   Hoffman, J. I., Kaplan, S. (2002) The incidence of congenital heart disease. *J Am Coll Cardiol, 39*, 1890-1900.

[2]   Norozi, K., Gravenhorst, V., Hobbiebrunken, E., Wessel, A. (2005) Normality of cardiopulmonary capacity in children operated on to correct congenital heart defects. *Arch Pediatr Adolesc Med, 159*, 1063-1068.

[3]   Fontan, F., Baudet, E. (1971) Surgical repair of tricuspid atresia. *Thorax, 26*, 240-248.

[4]   Gewillig, M. (2005) The Fontan circulation. *Heart, 91*, 839-846.

[5]   Cilliers, A., Gewillig, M. (2002) Fontan procedure for univentricular hearts: have changes in design improved outcome? *Cardiovasc J S Afr, 13*, 111-116.

[6]   Sarubbi, B., Pacileo, G., Pisacane, C., Ducceschi, V., Iacono, C., Russo, M. G., Iacono, A., Calabro, R. (2000) Exercise capacity in young patients after total repair of Tetralogy of Fallot. *Pediatr Cardiol, 21*, 211-215.

[7]   Blalock, A., Hanlon, C. R., Scott, H. W. (1949) The surgical treatment of congenital cyanotic heart disease. *The Scientific Monthly, 69*, 360-367.

[8]   James, F. W., Kaplan, S., Schwartz, D. C., Chou, T. C., Sandker, M. J., Naylor, V. (1976) Response to exercise in patients after total surgical correction of Tetralogy of Fallot. *Circulation, 54*, 671-679.

[9]   Lunt, D., Briffa, T., Briffa, N. K., Ramsay, J. (2003) Physical activity levels of adolescents with congenital heart disease. *Aust J Physiother, 49*, 43-50.

[10] McCrindle, B. W., Williams, R. V., Mital, S., Clark, B. J., Russell, J. L., Klein, G., Eisenmann, J. C. (2007) Physical activity levels in children and adolescents are reduced after the Fontan procedure, independent of exercise capacity, and are associated with lower perceived general health. *Arch Dis Child, 92*, 509-514.

[11] Shephard, R. J., Allen, C., Benade, A. J., Davies, C. T., Di Prampero, P. E., Hedman, R., Merriman, J. E., Myhre, K., Simmons, R. (1968) The maximum oxygen intake. An international reference standard of cardiorespiratory fitness. *Bull World Health Organ*, *38*, 757-764.

[12] Myers, J., Prakash, M., Froelicher, V., Do, D., Partington, S., Atwood, J. E. (2002) Exercise capacity and mortality among men referred for exercise testing. *N Engl J Med*, *346*, 793-801.

[13] Giardini, A., Specchia, S., Tacy, T. A., Coutsoumbas, G., Gargiulo, G., Donti, A., Formigari, R., Bonvicini, M., Picchio, F. M. (2007) Usefulness of cardiopulmonary exercise to predict long-term prognosis in adults with repaired tetralogy of Fallot. *Am J Cardiol*, *99*, 1462-1467.

[14] Nixon, P. A., Orenstein, D. M., Kelsey, S. F., Doershuk, C. F. (1992) The prognostic value of exercise testing in patients with cystic fibrosis. *N Engl J Med*, *327*, 1785-1788.

[15] Gulati, M., Black, H. R., Shaw, L. J., Arnsdorf, M. F., Merz, C. N., Lauer, M. S., Marwick, T. H., Pandey, D. K., Wicklund, R. H., Thisted, R. A. (2005) The prognostic value of a nomogram for exercise capacity in women. *N Engl J Med*, *353*, 468-475.

[16] Driscoll, D. J., Durongpisitkul, K. (1999) Exercise testing after the Fontan operation. *Pediatr Cardiol*, *20*, 57-59; discussion 60.

[17] Brassard, P., Bedard, E., Jobin, J., Rodes-Cabau, J., Poirier, P. (2006) Exercise capacity and impact of exercise training in patients after a Fontan procedure: a review. *Can J Cardiol*, *22*, 489-495.

[18] Goldberg, B., Fripp, R. R., Lister, G., Loke, J., Nicholas, J. A., Talner, N. S. (1981) Effect of physical training on exercise performance of children following surgical repair of congenital heart disease. *Pediatrics*, *68*, 691-699.

[19] Mulla, N., Simpson, P., Sullivan, N. M., Paridon, S. M. (1997) Determinants of aerobic capacity during exercise following complete repair of tetralogy of Fallot with a transannular patch. *Pediatr Cardiol*, *18*, 350-356.

[20] Wessel, H. U., Paul, M. H. (1999) Exercise studies in tetralogy of Fallot: a review. *Pediatr Cardiol*, *20*, 39-47.

[21] Godfrey, S. Exercise testing in children. London: W.B. Saunders Company Ltd.; 1974.

[22] Bruce, R. A., Blackmon, J. R., Jones, J. W., Strait, G. (1963) Exercise testing in adult normal subjects and cardiac patients. *Pediatrics*, *32*, 742-756.

[23] Wasserman, K., Hansen, J. E., Sue, D. Y., Casaburi, R., Whipp, B. J. Principles of Exercise Testing and Interpretation. 3rd Edition ed. Baltimore, MD, USA: Lippincott, Williams & Wilkins; 1999.

[24] Caiozzo, V. J., Davis, J. A., Ellis, J. F., Azus, J. L., Vandagriff, R., Prietto, C. A., McMaster, W. C. (1982) A comparison of gas exchange indices used to detect the anaerobic threshold. *J Appl Physiol*, *53*, 1184-1189.

[25] Binkhorst, R. A., van 't Hof, M. A., Saris, W. H. M. Maximale inspanning door kinderen; referentiewaarden voor 6-18 jarige meisjes en jongens [Maximal exercise in children; reference values girls and boys, 6-18 year of age]. Den-Haag: Nederlandse Hartstichting; 1992.

[26] Moalla, W., Gauthier, R., Maingourd, Y., Ahmaidi, S. (2005) Six-minute walking test to assess exercise tolerance and cardiorespiratory responses during training program in children with congenital heart disease. *Int J Sports Med*, *26*, 756-762.

[27] Rhodes, J., Curran, T. J., Camil, L., Rabideau, N., Fulton, D. R., Gauthier, N. S., Gauvreau, K., Jenkins, K. J. (2005) Impact of cardiac rehabilitation on the exercise function of children with serious congenital heart disease. *Pediatrics, 116*, 1339-1345.

[28] Moalla, W., Maingourd, Y., Gauthier, R. M., Cahalin, L. P., Tabka, Z., Ahmaidi, S. (2006) Effect of exercise training on respiratory muscle oxygenation in children with congenital heart disease. *Eur J Cardiovasc Prev Rehabil, 13*, 604-611.

[29] Takken, T., Hulzebos, H. J., Blank, A. C., Tacken, M. H., Helders, P. J., Strengers, J. L. (2007) Exercise prescription for patients with a Fontan circulation: current evidence and future directions. *Neth Heart J, 15*, 142-147.

[30] McCall, R., Humphrey, R. (2001) Exercise training in a young adult late after a fontan procedure to repair single ventricle physiology. *J Cardiopulm Rehabil, 21*, 227-230.

[31] Minamisawa, S., Nakazawa, M., Momma, K., Imai, Y., Satomi, G. (2001) Effect of aerobic training on exercise performance in patients after the Fontan operation. *Am J Cardiol, 88*, 695-698.

[32] Baquet, G., van Praagh, E., Berthoin, S. (2003) Endurance training and aerobic fitness in young people. *Sports Med, 33*, 1127-1143.

[33] Stromme, S. B., Ingjer, F., Meen, H. D. (1977) Assessment of maximal aerobic power in specifically trained athletes. *J Appl Physiol, 42*, 833-837.

[34] Opocher, F., Varnier, M., Sanders, S. P., Tosoni, A., Zaccaria, M., Stellin, G., Milanesi, O. (2005) Effects of aerobic exercise training in children after the Fontan operation. *Am J Cardiol, 95*, 150-152.

[35] Brassard, P., Poirier, P., Martin, J., Noel, M., Nadreau, E., Houde, C., Cloutier, A., Perron, J., Jobin, J. (2006) Impact of exercise training on muscle function and ergoreflex in Fontan patients: a pilot study. *Int J Cardiol, 107*, 85-94.

[36] Bradley, L. M., Galioto, F. M., Jr., Vaccaro, P., Hansen, D. A., Vaccaro, J. (1985) Effect of intense aerobic training on exercise performance in children after surgical repair of tetralogy of Fallot or complete transposition of the great arteries. *Am J Cardiol, 56*, 816-818.

[37] Ruttenberg, H. D., Adams, T. D., Orsmond, G. S., Conlee, R. K., Fisher, A. G. (1983) Effects of exercise training on aerobic fitness in children after open heart surgery. *Pediatr Cardiol, 4*, 19-24.

[38] Therrien, J., Fredriksen, P., Walker, M., Granton, J., Reid, G. J., Webb, G. (2003) A pilot study of exercise training in adult patients with repaired tetralogy of Fallot. *Can J Cardiol, 19*, 685-689.

[39] Sklansky, M. S., Pivarnik, J. M., Smith, E. O., Morris, J., Bricker, J. T. (1994) Exercise training hemodynamicsand the prevalence of arrhytmias in children following tetralogy of Fallor repair. *Pediatric Exercise Science, 5*, 188-200.

[40] Calzolari, A., Turchetta, A., Biondi, G., Drago, F., De Ranieri, C., Gagliardi, G., Giambini, I., Giannico, S., Kofler, A. M., Perrotta, F., et al. (1990) Rehabilitation of children after total correction of tetralogy of Fallot. *Int J Cardiol, 28*, 151-158.

[41] Sklanski, M. S., Pivarnik, J. M., Smith, E. O., Morris, J., Bricker, J. T. (1994) Exercise training hemodynamicsand the prevalence of arrhytmias in children following tetralogy of Fallor repair. *Pediatric Exercise Science, 5*, 188-200.

[42] Rhodes, J., Garofano, R. P., Bowman, F. O., Jr., Grant, G. P., Bierman, F. Z., Gersony, W. M. (1990) Effect of right ventricular anatomy on the cardiopulmonary response to exercise. Implications for the Fontan procedure. *Circulation, 81*, 1811-1817.

[43] Fick, A. (1870) Ueber die Messung des Blutquantums in den Herzventrikeln. *Sitx. der Physik-Med. Ges. Wurzburg*, *2*, 16.

[44] Stromvall Larsson, E., Eriksson, B. O. (2003) Haemodynamic adaptation during exercise in fontan patients at a long-term follow-up. *Scand Cardiovasc J*, *37*, 107-112.

[45] Cortes, R. G., Satomi, G., Yoshigi, M., Momma, K. (1994) Maximal hemodynamic response after the Fontan procedure: Doppler evaluation during the treadmill test. *Pediatr Cardiol*, *15*, 170-177.

[46] Driscoll, D. J., Danielson, G. K., Puga, F. J., Schaff, H. V., Heise, C. T., Staats, B. A. (1986) Exercise tolerance and cardiorespiratory response to exercise after the Fontan operation for tricuspid atresia or functional single ventricle. *J Am Coll Cardiol*, *7*, 1087-1094.

[47] Stromvall-Larsson, E. S., Eriksson, B. O., Sixt, R. (2003) Decreased lung function and exercise capacity in Fontan patients. A long-term follow-up. *Scand Cardiovasc J*, *37*, 58-63.

[48] Matthews, I. L., Fredriksen, P. M., Bjornstad, P. G., Thaulow, E., Gronn, M. (2006) Reduced pulmonary function in children with the Fontan circulation affects their exercise capacity. *Cardiol Young*, *16*, 261-267.

[49] Norgard, G., Bjorkhaug, A., Vik-Mo, H. (1992) Effects of impaired lung function and pulmonary regurgitation on maximal exercise capacity in patients with repaired tetralogy of Fallot. *Eur Heart J*, *13*, 1380-1386.

[50] Ercisli, M., Vural, K. M., Gokkaya, K. N., Koseoglu, F., Tufekcioglu, O., Sener, E., Tasdemir, O. (2005) Does delayed correction interfere with pulmonary functions and exercise tolerance in patients with tetralogy of fallot? *Chest*, *128*, 1010-1017.

[51] Schulze-Neick, I., Hartenstein, P., Li, J., Stiller, B., Nagdyman, N., Hubler, M., Butrous, G., Petros, A., Lange, P., Redington, A. N. (2003) Intravenous sildenafil is a potent pulmonary vasodilator in children with congenital heart disease. *Circulation*, *108 Suppl 1*, II167-173.

[52] Grant, G. P., Mansell, A. L., Garofano, R. P., Hayes, C. J., Bowman, F. O., Jr., Gersony, W. M. (1988) Cardiorespiratory response to exercise after the Fontan procedure for tricuspid atresia. *Pediatr Res*, *24*, 1-5.

[53] Rhodes, J., Dave, A., Pulling, M. C., Geggel, R. L., Marx, G. R., Fulton, D. R., Hijazi, Z. M. (1998) Effect of pulmonary artery stenoses on the cardiopulmonary response to exercise following repair of tetralogy of Fallot. *Am J Cardiol*, *81*, 1217-1219.

[54] Mocellin, R., Gildein, P. (1999) Velocity of oxygen uptake response at the onset of exercise: A comparison between children after cardiac surgery and healthy boys. *Pediatr Cardiol*, *20*, 17-20; discussion 21.

[55] Inai, K., Saita, Y., Takeda, S., Nakazawa, M., Kimura, H. (2004) Skeletal muscle hemodynamics and endothelial function in patients after Fontan operation. *Am J Cardiol*, *93*, 792-797.

[56] Witzel, C., Sreeram, N., Coburger, S., Schickendantz, S., Brockmeier, K., Schoenau, E. (2006) Outcome of muscle and bone development in congenital heart disease. *Eur J Pediatr*, *165*, 168-174.

[57] Takken, T., Tacken, M. H., Blank, A. C., Hulzebos, E. H., Strengers, J. L., Helders, P. J. (2007) Exercise limitation in patients with Fontan circulation: a review. *J Cardiovasc Med (Hagerstown)*, *8*, 775-781.

[58] Paridon, S. M., Alpert, B. S., Boas, S. R., Cabrera, M. E., Caldarera, L. L., Daniels, S. R., Kimball, T. R., Knilans, T. K., Nixon, P. A., Rhodes, J., Yetman, A. T. (2006) Clinical stress testing in the pediatric age group: a statement from the American Heart Association Council on Cardiovascular Disease in the Young, Committee on Atherosclerosis, Hypertension, and Obesity in Youth. *Circulation, 113*, 1905-1920.

[59] Swan, L., Hillis, W. S. (2000) Exercise prescription in adults with congenital heart disease: a long way to go. *Heart, 83*, 685-687.

[60] Longmuir, P. E., Turner, J. A., Rowe, R. D., Olley, P. M. (1985) Postoperative exercise rehabilitation benefits children with congenital heart disease. *Clin Invest Med, 8*, 232-238.

[61] McBride, M. G., Binder, T. J., Paridon, S. M. (2007) Safety and Feasibility of Inpatient Exercise Training in Pediatric Heart Failure: A PRELIMINARY REPORT. *Journal of Cardiopulmonary Rehabilitation and Prevention, 27*, 219-222.

[62] Picchio, F. M., Giardini, A., Bonvicini, M., Gargiulo, G. (2006) Can a child who has been operated on for congenital heart disease participate in sport and in which kind of sport? *J Cardiovasc Med (Hagerstown), 7*, 234-238.

[63] Driscoll, D. J. (1990) Exercise Rehabilitation Programs for Children With Congenital Heart Disease: A Note of Caution. *Pediatric Exercise Science, 2*, 191-196.

In: Physical Activity and Children: New Research
Editor: N. P. Beaulieu, pp. 117-135

ISBN: 978-1-60456-306-1
© 2008 Nova Science Publishers, Inc.

Chapter 5

CHILDREN'S MUSCULOSKELETAL SYSTEM: NEW RESEARCH PERSPECTIVES

Sébastien Ratel[1] and Craig Williams[2]

[1] Laboratory of Exercise Biology (BAPS, EA 3533),
University of Blaise Pascal, UFR STAPS, 63172 Aubière, France
[2] Children's Health and Exercise Research Centre,
University of Exeter, Exeter, Devon, United Kingdom

ABSTRACT

The development of musculoskeletal system is one of the major features of childhood and adolescence. Although growth and maturation of the cardiovascular and skeletal systems have been the focus of important research activities in recent years, the muscle system has received relatively little attention and the results were somewhat controversial. This lack of information on the musculoskeletal system during growth is mainly attributable to ethical and methodological constraints associated with paediatric testing. Besides the limited use of muscle biopsies, 31-phosphorus magnetic resonance spectroscopy (^{31}P-MRS) and Magnetic Resonance Imaging (MRI) are potent tools to investigate the musculoskeletal system. In adults, MRI and ^{31}P-MRS have been used for the non-invasive estimation of muscle fibre type composition. It has been shown that MRI-derived longitudinal and transversal relaxation times were positively correlated to the relative percentage of slow-twitch muscle fibres. Also, it has been shown that the resting phosphocreatine-inorganic phosphate ratio (PCr/Pi) measured by ^{31}P-MRS could be considered as a good indicator of muscle fibre type composition. For instance, the PCr/Pi ratio in the type I muscle was shown to be clearly lower than in the type II muscle. In addition, mapping of muscles activated during exercise is another interesting issue which can be addressed using MRI. Exercise-induced transversal relaxation time changes have been used in order to locate activated muscles and also as a quantitative index of exercise intensity. This approach, along with surface electromyography, provides an interesting avenue of investigation into the changes of muscle recruitment pattern during growth. In conclusion, the advent of technologies which are non-invasive, ethical for use on children and allow muscle bioenergetics to be measured during exercise will significantly enhance scientists understanding of children's physical activity.

1. Introduction

The development of the musculoskeletal system is one of the major features of childhood and adolescence. Although growth and maturation of the cardiovascular and skeletal systems have been the focus of important paediatric research activity in recent years, the muscle system has received relatively little attention. This lack of information on the skeletal muscle tissue during growth is mainly attributable to ethical and methodological constraints associated with muscles biopsies. The aim of this chapter is to examine the development of musculoskeletal system during growth and maturation and to describe new research perspectives through the use of non-invasive technologies such as [31]Phosphorus Magnetic Resonance Spectroscopy (^{31}P-MRS) and Magnetic Resonance Imaging (MRI).

2. Muscle Characteristics During Growth

2.1. Is child a 'Metabolic-Specialist'?

Following the earlier work of Bar-Or (1983), Bar-Or and Rowland (2004) suggested that children might be considered as "metabolic non-specialists" in reference to sports performance. What was inferred from this statement was that children appeared not to specialize in one sprint or endurance type event but often could be successful in both events. This observation is unlike adult athletes where clearly the best sprinter was not also the best endurance runner. These performance observations were then translated to the physiological pathways which can simplistically be categorized into the anaerobic (typified as short duration, high power but limited capacity systems) and aerobic (typified as long duration, lower power and extensive capacity systems) systems. Since the early "metabolic non-specialist" proposition in the 1980s a number of children's studies have found significant positive correlations between anaerobic and aerobic performance variables (Falk and Bar-Or, 1993; Falgairette et al., 1993). Whilst correlations do not establish causality, growth and maturational factors must also be added as a confounding variable, the biological significance of this relationship has yet to be determined. It is known that the ratio of peak anaerobic power to peak aerobic power is less than 2 at age 8 years and increases to approximately 3 by 13-14 years in girls and 14-15 years in boys (Bar-Or and Rowland, 2004). This indicates that the largest improvements are found in the anaerobic systems of children and adolescents and that the improvements are not synchronous between aerobic and anaerobic power. Although dimensionality theory is important to consider when investigating variables pertaining to children, it is clear that muscle composition and biochemical profiles are an important determinant of the metabolic characteristics and thus have an effect on performance. It is therefore all the more important that more research is focused on the musculoskeletal system to understand these changes with growth and maturation.

The notion of children as "metabolic non-specialists" has become such an established "fact" that it is rarely challenged. Eriksson et al. (1973) in his classical biopsy studies of young boys concluded on the existence of an attenuated anaerobic metabolism in children compared to adults. The results from Eriksson's studies although not designed to test the "metabolic non-specialist" concept have been used to support the "fact". This is despite the fact that the study was not designed to evaluate this proposition and the small sample size used in this study. Without doubt this is now an accepted paradigm in the paediatric literature.

However established the above paradigm, there is still much to investigate about the muscle metabolic profiles of children and adolescents. Most importantly, to investigate the metabolic non-specialist concept, the biological systems that comprise the aerobic and anaerobic metabolism need to be studied concurrently. Because firstly there is an *integrated* (our italics) metabolic response at the onset of exercise not separate responses and that the flux through all three metabolic pathways occur simultaneously. And finally, the control of each pathway depends on the regulated response of the whole system to a change in ATPase rate. In the paediatric literature the investigations of the notion of a "metabolic non-specialist" has focused on separate metabolic investigations of either an aerobic or anaerobic nature (Williams et al., 2006).

2.2. Muscle Fibre and Enzymatic Profile

Much research has tended to concentrate on the central circulation, therefore resulting in a discrepancy of knowledge related to peripheral factors such as muscle function. The invention of the needle biopsy in 1962 (Bergstrom) has helped but there are still many limitations in the knowledge of paediatric metabolism. This has partly been as a result of the invasive nature of the procedure and hence ethical concern, especially with regards to children. It was not until ten years later when the first studies were conducted with children (Eriksson et al., 1971).

The needle biopsy technique has a large variability of samples and comparisons of fibre composition must be interpreted carefully. The coefficients of variation (CV) found between repeated analyses on the same sample are 15-20 % (Nygaard and Hede, 1987). Similar CV values were also found from the site within the muscle which provided the sample (McMahon et al., 1984). The CV has been reduced if samples were taken from 3-5 sites as the mean value CV was only ± 5 % (Elder et al., 1982).

When interpreting muscle biopsy results between children and adults, it is important to have subjects matched for age and exercise background. This point is especially important if the study involves a period of training, pre- and post biopsy. The relative occurrence of type I and type II fibres in the medial *vastus lateralis* has been reported as approximately 50 % for both adolescents and sedentary adults (Hedberg and Jansson, 1976). In another study similar conclusions were reported for type I fibres but type IIa accounted for one-third while type IIb accounted for two-thirds (Nygaard, 1981). However, one problem when comparing children to adults is how to define what constitutes "normal" activity for a child.

Muscle fibre types have been studied in children as young as six years old (Bell et al., 1980). The specific objective of this study was to collect normative data on skeletal muscle structure for six year old boys and girls. A total of seven female and six male Swiss children, average age 6.4 years, were biopsied for muscle samples of the vastus lateralis. The fibres were classified as slow twitch oxidative (type I), fast twitch glycolytic (type IIb) and fast twitch oxidative glycolytic (type IIa) according to Peter et al. (1976). Also, VO$_2$ max tests were conducted on the subjects. Table 1 shows the muscle fibre types and VO$_2$ max values for the six year old children.

Table 1. Mean (SD) fibre type and VO$_2$ max measurements for six year old children (n=13). Data taken from the study of Bell et al. (1980)

Group	Type IIa (%)	Type IIb (%)	Type I (%)	VO$_2$max (mL·kg^{-1}·min^{-1})
Females (n=7)	22.1 (8.78)	22.3 (8.40)	55.6 (8.46)	43.1 (5.80)
Males (n=6)	17.3 (10.28)	20.6 (9.84)	62.1 (14.24)	47.2 (3.03)
All subjects (n=13)	21.5	19.7	58.8	45.2

There were no significant differences for muscle fibre types and VO$_2$ max values between males and females. Also, stereological analysis of muscle fibres (i.e. volume density of the central mitochondria) showed no statistical differences between males and females. A significant correlation was found between mitochondrial volume density and percentage of type I fibres (r = 0.69). The correlations between VO$_2$max and mitochondrial volume density (r=0.39) and VO$_2$max and percent type I fibres (r =0.24) were not statistically significant. As compared with normal adult tissue, Bell et al. (1980) concluded that the fibre type distribution pattern and ultrastructure of skeletal muscle in six-year-old children were not different. These results are in line with those of Elder and Kakulas (1993) indicating that less than 10% of fibres would be immature in the prepubertal period. Furthermore, according to Oertel (1988), the normal type II to type I transformation during development could be completed within the first two postnatal years.

In contrast, several more recent studies have found a significant and negative relationship between type I fibres and age (Lexell et al., 1992). According to Lexell et al. (1992), the proportion of slow-twitch fibres (type I) would decrease from around 65 % at the age of 5 years, to 50 % at the age of 20 (Lexell et al., 1992). The decrease in proportion of type I fibres would most likely be caused by a transformation of slow-twitch fibres to fast-twitch fibres (type II). This muscle fibre type composition would also be characterized by a higher percentage of type I fibres in young trained children (Dahlstrom et al., 1997). In the only longitudinal study investigating the relationship between age and % type I fibres, Glenmark et al. (1992) conducted biopsy samples on 66 males and 45 females at age 16 and then at follow up four years later. The percentage of type I fibres was shown to significantly decrease with age but only for the males. These conflicting findings could be related to the action of the gross muscle studied, the micro sample of the studied muscle, the limited number of samples investigated, biopsy sample errors and the training status of individuals. Further studies are therefore required to examine the morphological properties of different muscles groups in both children and adults (see section 4).

For enzymatic profiles, Haralambie (1979) reported quotient ratios between lactate dehydrogenase (LDH) and citrate synthase (CS) in the vastus lateralis for 11-14 year old females. The LDH/CS ratio was 11.5. The medial deltoid for 15-16 year old females was also examined and a LDH/CS ratio of 11.7 was found. It appeared that when LDH/CS ratios were compared with female and male adult and female adolescent data, differences were greater between muscle groups rather than the sexes. Significant differences were found in 11-14 year old girls and male and female adults for two citrate cyclus enzymes and aspartate aminotransferase. It was postulated that these significant findings may reflect an enhanced oxidation of substrate from amino acids of the 11-14 year old age group. An alternative explanation could be due the fact that a higher LDH activity in children suggests a daily activity pattern which is directed towards more intensity than endurance type exercise in this sample group. Haralambie (1982) in a later study comparing adolescent boys and girls and adult men and women found significantly higher oxidative enzyme activities in adolescents. However, there were no significant differences in the enzymatic activities related to free fatty acids between the groups.

Therefore, in summary, although muscle fibre biopsy data is fraught with methodological concerns, there does appear to be a trend towards decreases in the proportion of type I muscle fibres (mainly in the vastus lateralis) with age in healthy children and adolescents (Glenmark et al., 1992; Lexell et al., 1992). However, these findings need to be confirmed. For the enzymatic data, the observation by Eriksson's that prepubertal children possess glycolytic activity which is lower than older children and adults may hold true. This observation might be because of the enhanced oxidative enzyme activities of children which points to the possibility of children being able to oxidize pyruvate and free fatty acids at a higher rate than adolescents or adults. More definitive studies using acceptable techniques and pre, during and post exercise would help to resolve these issues. There are still too few biopsy studies on females to conclude about sex differences between boys and girls for fibre typing and enzymatic profiles.

2.3. Energy Stores

Results from the early work of Eriksson and colleagues in the 1970s and 1980s are shown in table 2. In this table, it is shown that the phosphocreatine (PCr) rather than the ATP increases with age from 11 to 15 years of age. Eriksson (1980) concluded that the depletion of the phosphagens was the same for both adults and children when expressed as a percentage of VO_2 max.

Eriksson (1980) has also reported marked differences in the muscle substrate levels in children with some diseases. In one study of 14 infants with heart failure due to left-right ventricular shunts, lower muscle concentrations of ATP and PCr were found. In the study, standard deviation (SD) for ATP concentration was found to be greater than 1 in 10 out of 14 infants as compared with normal children. For PCr concentration, SD was greater than 1 in 6 out of 14 as compared with healthy children. Further research showed, in two of the infants, that 6-12 months later after the heart failure, the muscle substrate levels were back to normal. In another study, 17 children aged 5-13.8 years with coarctation of the aorta were compared to 15 control patients aged 2.1-15.8 years. Both groups were biopsied under general anesthesia prior to surgery. Muscle biopsies were taken from the deltoid and vastus lateralis. Biopsy data revealed significantly higher levels of ATP, PCr, glucose and glycogen in the legs compared with the arms both in normal children and children with coarctation of the aorta. It was concluded that there is a qualitative metabolic difference between arms and legs in normal and disease children.

Table 2. Resting values for ATP, PCr and Glycogen in muscle of adults, and 11-15 year old boys

Group	ATP	PCr	Glycogen
Adults	5	17	80
Children #			
11.6 years	4	15	55
12.6 years	5	20	70
13.5 years	5	17	70
15.5 years	5	24	85

All values are mmol·kg^{-1} wet weight
Values taken from Eriksson, 1980.

The phosphagens are inefficient for storing energy because of their high molecular weight and relatively small energy store per unit weight (Gollnick, 1982). It is still unclear as to whether the total capacity stored as phosphagens is increased to any significant degree with training. In one study (Eriksson et al., 1973), increased ATP and PCr concentration values were reported with training. One of the difficulties with measuring these variables is that the kinetics of the chemical reactions are extremely fast, and the available techniques such as biopsies take seconds to sample the chemical events. The rate of turnover of ATP for adult sprinting has been approximated as a peak anaerobic rate of 15 mmol·s^{-1}·kg^{-1}dm (Glaister, 2005). The turnover rates for the PCr, anaerobic glycolytic (after ~5 s) and mean rate of aerobic ATP (first 6 s of a 30 s maximal sprint) are estimated at 9, 6-9 and 1.32 mmol·s^{-1}·kg^{-1}dm respectively (Glaister, 2005). To estimate values for children and adolescents more work needs to be conducted. However, as the above results were obtained by biopsy studies it is likely that these techniques will not result in increased data within the near future, therefore more "child-friendly" techniques must be sought.

3. ^{31}P-MRS INVESTIGATION OF MUSCLE BIO-ENERGETICS DURING GROWTH

3.1. ^{31}P-MRS Technique

^{31}Phosphorus Magnetic Resonance Spectroscopy (^{31}P-MRS) offers the opportunity of measuring non-invasively and continuously with high-time resolution the concentration of phosphorylated compounds involved in muscle energetics. Multiple tests are possible as its magnetic effects are harmless and there are no ionizing radiation effects unlike Computed Tomography (CT) scans. When subjects are placed inside a MR scanner, the magnetic field is activated and the nuclei of atoms within the body align with the magnetic field. Another oscillating magnetic field is applied and the ensuing nuclear transitions of the muscular region of interest capture a spectral analysis. As different molecules produce different spectra, any changes in the spectra can be detected and interpreted. The most common nuclei used for metabolic studies are ^{31}P, a naturally occurring phosphorus nucleus, ^{1}H, a hydrogen nucleus and ^{13}C, a carbon nucleus. Typical ^{31}P-MRS spectra exhibit six peaks, corresponding to PCr, inorganic phosphate (Pi), the three phosphate groups of ATP (in positions α, β and γ) and phosphomonoesters (PME) (figure 1). The decrease in PCr and the increase in Pi are clearly shown during exercise. Intracellular pH can also be measured from the chemical shift of the Pi peak (Moon and Richards, 1973). Indeed, at physiological pH, myoplasmic Pi (pK of 6.75) exists as mono- and diprotonated form (respectively $H_2PO_4^-$ and HPO_4^{2-}). These two forms are exchanging so fast that only a single Pi signal is detected. However, the chemical shift of this single signal is weighted by the contribution of each form, making it sensitive pH. Figure 2 shows the movement from left to right of the Pi peak towards the PCr peak during exercise. Furthermore, skeletal muscle oxidative capacity can be assessed from phosphocreatine resynthesis rates (Roussel et al., 2000). Overall, the contribution of the different metabolic pathways involved in energy production, i.e. ATP production from (i) phosphocreatine degradation, (ii) anaerobic glycolysis and (iii) mitochondrial phosphorylation, can be quantified due to advances in ^{31}P-MRS data analysis (Kemp and Radda, 1994). The detailed quantitative analysis can also provide information about buffering capacity and proton efflux during recovery (Kemp and Radda, 1994).

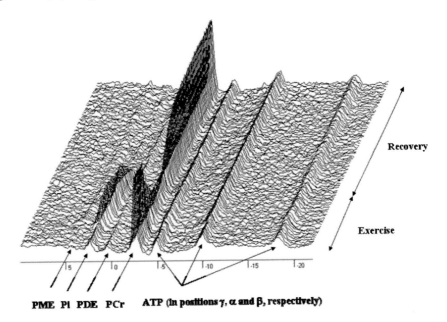

Figure 1. Spectra for calf exercise with PME, Pi, PDE, PCr and ATP peaks identified.

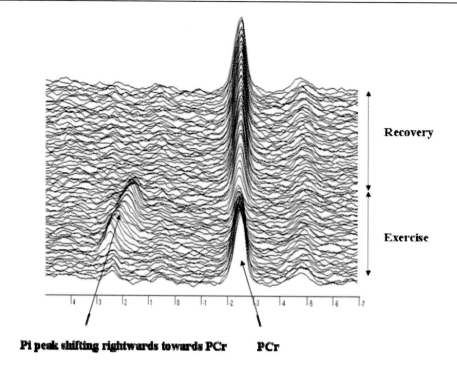

Recovery

Exercise

Pi peak shifting rightwards towards PCr   **PCr**

Figure 2. MRS spectra for calf ergometry showing a significant rightward shift of the Pi spectra towards the PCr peaks, indicative of an acidification of the muscle.

Although exercise is constrained by the size of the bore of the magnet, whole body scanners are able to accommodate either arm or leg contractions comfortably. The key methodological concern is to synchronize the muscle contraction with the timings of the data acquisition. Pilot testing in our laboratory have shown this to be problematic but which has been overcome in two ways. Firstly, we have built to scale a mock up of the MR scanner in which we thoroughly habituate the children to exercising in a 60 cm bore tube (figure 3). This dramatically reduces the anxiety of the children prior to the real tests but more importantly gives them an opportunity to practice the one legged quadriceps flexion and extension exercises. And secondly, the practice enables the children to synchronize the rate of the muscle leg actions to that of the data acquisition from the MR scanner which is pre-set at 40 repetitions per minute.

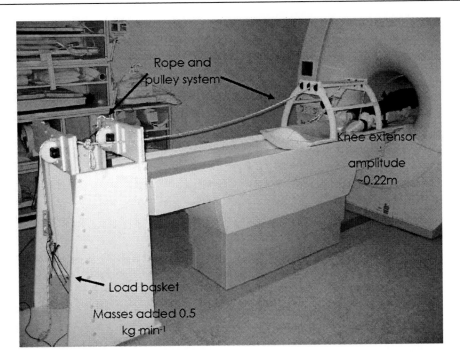

Figure 3. MR set up with ergometer system.

3.2. ^{31}P-MRS Studies in Children

Very few ^{31}P-MRS studies have been performed with child participants (Kuno et al., 1995; Zanconato et al., 1993; Taylor et al., 1997; Petersen et al., 1999). Although these early studies were clearly pioneering, the relatively small sample sizes, mixed sex and age groups, differing exercise protocols and inappropriate normalization of data make interpretation difficult. For example, both Taylor et al (1997) and Zanconato et al. (1993) chose calf muscle exercise. This modality presents two problems. Firstly, because of the size of the children's calf muscles, there is a lower signal to noise ratio which makes it difficult to curve fit the spectra. Secondly, the calf muscles consist of both the *gastrocnemius* and the *soleus* which differ in their proportion of type I and II fibres. This varying proportion of fibres in these two muscle groups will bias the response of the muscle metabolism during exercise, particularly when compared to adults performing the same exercise type.

Despite these differences in experimental protocols and the different types of muscles investigated, the study of Zanconato et al. (1993) support those found by Kuno et al. (1995). Zanconato et al. concluded that there were similar mitochondrial oxidative metabolism rates during low-intensity exercise between children (aged 7 to 10 years-old) and adults (aged 20 to 42 years-old). However, when exercise intensity was significantly increased, the slope of the Pi/PCr ratio and decline in pH were steeper in adults than in children, thus predicting a superior glycolytic activity in adults. The adult final pH value was also significantly lower than the children who could only achieve an end-of-exercise Pi/PCr ratio comparable to 27 % of the adult values. Kuno et al. (1995) also found that adult values for pH at the end of exercise were lower than 12 to 17 year children/adolescents and that adults exhibited a higher Pi/PCr ratio at exhaustion. These authors also reported similar rates of PCr resynthesis in children/adolescents as compared with adults following an incremental exercise protocol. On this basis, they suggested that muscle oxidative capacity was not different between children and adults. Taylor et al. (1997) essentially confirmed the lower ratio of PCr/ATP in children at rest compared to adults, as well as, the higher pH values during exercise which they interpreted as indicating a lower glycolytic contribution to metabolism. Contrary to the results of Kuno et al. (1995), these authors also indicated from non invasive measurements of post-exercise PCr resynthesis rates that muscle oxidative capacity was higher in 6-12 yr-old children as compared to adults. Petersen et al. (1999) investigated the effects of maturational differences in muscle metabolism between 10 year old prepubertal and 15 year pubertal female swimmers. Both submaximal (defined as 40 % of maximal work capacity) and supramaximal (defined as 140 % maximal work capacity) exercise bouts of two minutes were completed. At the end of the supramaximal exercise bout, pH was lower and Pi/PCr was higher, but these values were not statistically different between the prepubertal and pubertal girls. The authors concluded that the results could be interpreted as maturity not being dependent on glycolytic metabolism, however further work is needed to replicate these findings as the sample size was small and the discernible differences between the groups could be biologically significant and/or statistically significant with a larger sample size.

Recent reliability work from our centre has found that the coefficients of variation (CVs) for the power output at the subjectively determined intra-cellular threshold point for Pi/PCr and intra-cellular threshold for pH were 10.6 % and 10.3 %, respectively. Objective identification of the intra-cellular Pi/PCr had a CV of 16.3 %. CVs for end exercise pH and Pi/PCr values were 0.9 % and 50.0 %, respectively (Barker et al., 2006). The reliability data of our initial preliminary work has therefore allowed our group the confidence to begin to investigate some of these intra-cellular ratios and regression slopes. Although previous work by Chance et al. (1985) and Kent-Braun et al. (1993) have considered that the initial slow slope of Pi/PCr can be used to indicate mitochondrial oxidative metabolism, and that the second slope of Pi/PCr or pH may provide insight into 'anaerobic' or glycolytic energy metabolism, there is a distinct lack of paediatric reliability data for the Pi/PCr slope estimates. For both detection procedures caution must be applied before evaluations are made concerning the muscle metabolic response to exercise in children (Barker et al., 2006).

3.3. Relationship between O_2 Uptake Kinetics and ^{31}P-MRS Studies

At the onset of exercise, the oxygen uptake at the muscle does not increase in direct synchrony with ATP demand, but lags behind; therefore additional ATP must be generated anaerobically. The cost of O_2 derived anaerobically is termed the O_2 deficit. The response differs according to which exercise intensity domain (moderate, heavy or severe) the subject is exercising. However, in each domain, a rapid cardiodynamic phase I response is followed by an exponential rise in VO_2 (phase II) which results in a steady state (phase III). The inverse of the rate constant of a single exponential curve is represented by the time constant, τ. If the subject is exercising in the heavy exercise intensity domain (between the anaerobic threshold and peak VO_2), the steady state may be delayed and elevated due to what is termed the slow component. If the subject is exercising at higher exercise intensity i.e., the severe intensity domain, the response of the VO_2 and the possible achievement of peak VO_2 may curtail the exercise period prematurely. Although the oxygen uptake kinetics literature has expanded considerably in recent years for adults (Jones and Poole, 2005), relatively little is known for children. Overall, there appears to be a trend for a faster primary time constant and higher overall gain in VO_2 in children as compared to adults (Fawkner and Armstrong, 2003a). A number of authors have used this finding as evidence of a faster mobilisation of the aerobic energy system at the onset of exercise (Armon et al., 1991; Fawkner and Armstrong, 2003b). Similarly, Cooper and Barstow (1996) indicated that during high intensity exercise, at the same absolute work performed, the oxygen cost is higher for children compared to adults. This finding was interpreted as supporting the proposition that children rely more on aerobic metabolism and less on anaerobic compared to adults. For a more detailed review the reader should read the review publications by Fawkner and Armstrong (2003a; 2007).

The association between oxygen uptake kinetics and ^{31}P-MRS studies is such that the ^{31}P-MRS may be used as a proxy for muscle VO_2 dynamics (Mahler, 1985; Meyer, 1988; Rossiter et al., 2005). Recent unpublished work from our centre has established that phase II oxygen uptake kinetics during moderate intensity domain exercise is a close approximation of PCr utilisation during quadriceps exercise. Therefore, those without access to ^{31}P-MRS could use on-line respiratory gas analysis systems to infer muscle metabolism dynamics. Further work both with oxygen uptake kinetics and ^{31}P-MRS with children is required.

4. MR ASSESSMENT OF FIBRE TYPING DURING GROWTH

As previously indicated, muscle fibre type composition was poorly documented both in children and adolescents and the results were controversial (Bell et al., 1980; Elder and Kakulas, 1993; Glenmark et al., 1992; Lexell et al., 1992; Oertel, 1988). This lack of information on fibre typing during growth is mainly attributable to ethical constraints associated with pediatric testing. Muscle biopsies cannot be often used in young children because measurements have to be relatively non-invasive and certainly must carry minimal or no risk to health.

Besides the limited use of muscle biopsies, Magnetic Resonance Imaging (MRI) has been shown to be a potent tool for the non-invasive estimation of muscle fibre composition. A number of studies indicated in adults that the assessment of fibre typing is possible from longitudinal (T1) and transversal (T2) relaxation times (Houmard et al., 1995; Kuno et al., 1988; Kuno et al., 1990). T1 and T2 relaxation times refer to the time required for the tissue to dissipate energy received after radiofrequency pulses. Kuno et al. (1988) showed in 16 male physical education students that the proportion of fast-twitch fibres in the *vastus lateralis* was positively correlated to T1 and T2 relaxation times, indicating that fast-twitch fibres have a longer relaxation time than slow-twitch fibres (figure 4).

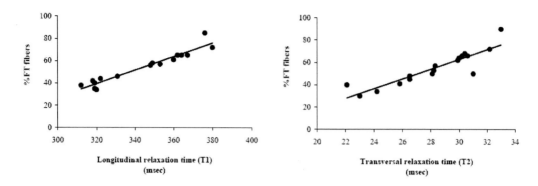

Figure 4. Relationships between MRI-derived relaxation times (T1 and T2) and the percentage of fast-twitch fibres (%FT) for a group of 16 male physical education students aged 22- to 28 yr-old. Data redrawn from Kuno et al. (1988).

In addition, it has been reported in 5 individuals that after a 20-week period of strength training, muscle fibre composition exhibited a significant shift to a predominance of fast-twitch fibres and prolonged T1 and T2 relaxation times (Kuno et al., 1990). Further evidence for a relationship between human muscle fibre composition and MRI-derived relaxation time was provided by Houmard et al. (1995). However, in contrast to the studies of Kuno et al., Houmard et al. (1995) showed a positive relationship between T1 and type I fibre percentage in the lateral *gastrocnemius* and no relationship between T2 and muscle fibre composition. Whilst the mechanism of the relationship between MRI relaxation times and fibre type composition is not known, it is possible that the length of the relaxation time of fast-twitch fibres may be associated with their water content. Kuno et al. (1988) suggested that fast-twitch fibres have a smaller extent of structuralization of the water around the protein than do slow-twitch fibres, thus indicating a larger amount of free water in fast twitch fibres than in slow-twitch fibres. However, Sjogaard and Saltin (1982) reported that total water content was not related to muscle fibre type composition in humans. Factors other than the total water content inherent in muscle may thus influence relaxation time. The nature (positive or negative) and mechanisms for the relationship between MRI-derived relaxation time and fibre composition are thus unclear and remain to be demonstrated.

Noninvasive assessment of fibre typing in children might be also possible using ^{31}P-MRS. It has been shown that the resting phosphocreatine-inorganic phosphate ratio (PCr/Pi) could be considered as a good indicator of muscle fibre type composition. For instance, the comparative analysis of Meyer et al. (1985) between cat *biceps brachii* (greater than 75% fast-twitch fibres) and *soleus* (greater than 92% slow-twitch fibres) muscles, indicated that the PCr/Pi ratio in the type I muscle was clearly lower than in the type II muscle (1.7 vs. 11 respectively). This could be related to a lower inorganic phosphate content and a higher phosphocreatine concentration in fast-twitch fibres compared to slow-twitch fibres. Clark et al. (1988) also showed *in vivo* that chronic stimulation of dog muscles was linked to muscle fibre types conversion (from type II to type I) and to a significant PCr/Pi decrease at rest. More recently, in adults, Vandenborne et al. (1995) showed a moderate positive relationship between the basal Pi/PCr ratio (the inverse of PCr/Pi) and the relative content of type I fibres and succinate dehydrogenase activity.

Clearly, MRI and ^{31}P-MRS can be considered as potent tools for assessing non-invasively the morphological properties of different muscles groups in children and adolescents. The increasing availability of these technologies should provide pediatric scientists more insights in the assessment of children's fibre type composition.

5. MR Investigation of Muscle Recruitment Pattern During Growth

Muscle recruitment pattern has also received little attention in children. This is certainly attributable to the difficulty of measuring muscle activation of small muscle groups. Surface electromyography (SEMG) has been commonly used to determine the activation level of skeletal muscle during contraction but, in a lesser extent, to provide insights into muscle recruitment patterns and neuromuscular control. The methodological issue commonly used for measuring muscle activation timing was to detect the onset (ON) and offset (OFF) of the EMG burst (Dorel et al., 2007). Besides, the intensity of muscle activation was measured from the amplitude of EMG signal. It has been shown that the within-session variability of the ON-OFF pattern of EMG timing was approximately two-fold higher in normally developing children as compared to adults especially for complex dynamic tasks as gait (Granata et al., 2005). Implications of this pediatric EMG variability suggest thus cautious interpretation of data from limited trial samples (Granata et al., 2005) and provoke in the use of complementary tools for evaluating muscle recruitment pattern in developing children.

Mapping of muscles activated during exercise is an interesting issue which can be addressed using MRI. Indeed, the acute effects of exercise on muscle MRI contrast obtained from transversal relaxation time (T2) changes were first reported in 1988 by Fleckenstein et al. From that time, muscle functional MRI has been shown to be valid for evaluating the muscle activity and the intensity of contraction (Hug et al., 2004; Kinugasa and Akima, 2005; Kinugasa et al., 2006). As shown in figure 5, changes in proton signal intensity cause exercised muscles to appear 'light-up' in the T2-weighted ^{1}H MR image. Hyper intense signals clearly indicate the different muscle activated during exercise, thereby providing a mapping of muscles activation.

The mechanisms of the T2 increase underlying muscle functional MRI is still poorly understood. Some studies reported that changes in T2 accounting for the discrimination between active and inactive muscles would result from the redistribution of body water (Fullerton et al., 1982). Given that T2 changes affect exclusively muscle and neither fat nor bone marrow, the signal changes would arise from one or more of the water compartments in muscle, i.e. from intra- and extra-cellular spaces. Changes in either intra- or extra-cellular water would be expected to alter the relaxation characteristics of the excited nuclei in the muscle (Fullerton et al., 1982). This redistribution of body water during exercise could be attributed to increased perfusion and the production and translocation of ionic species, which could alter the osmotic behavior of muscle cells (Rowell, 1988). However, Fisher et al. (1990) showed that venous occlusion had little effect on T2 despite significant changes in muscle volume, thereby indicating that exercise-induced enhanced MRI contrast does not result from the simple increase in fluid volume linked to increased perfusion. Probably more complex intracellular events would be responsible for exercise-induced contrast enhancement.

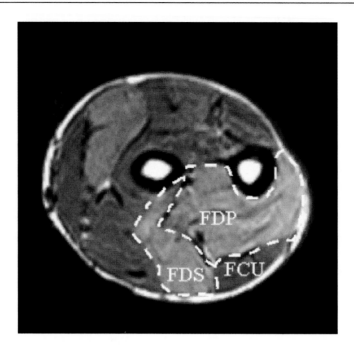

Figure 5. Typical T2-weighted ^{1}H MR image representing a transverse section of the forearm recorded after a finger-flexion exercise in an adult. Hyper intense signals indicate activated muscles i.e. the flexor digitorum profundus (FDP) and flexor digitorum superficialis (FDS). The flexor carpi ulnaris (FCU) located at the bottom was not activated. This MR image was provided by the Medical and Biological Magnetic Resonance Center (UMR CNRS 6612) from the University of Méditerranée (Marseille, France).

Besides these observations, it has been clearly showed that T2 changes were graded with exercise intensity (Fisher et al., 1990), thereby indicating that T2 changes during exercise are dependent on the force generated. In addition, changes in osmotically active metabolites such as hydrogen ions and inorganic phosphate have been correlated with the extent of T2 changes (Kerviler et al., 1991; Weidman et al., 1991), indicating that they are likely related to osmotically driven fluid shift. Further evidence for a relationship between T2 changes and the intensity of muscle contraction was provided by Kinugasa and Akima (2005). A remarkable correspondence between the changes in T2 values and integrated EMG activity has been shown under three different workloads for individual *triceps surae* muscles. Similarly, Price et al. (2003) showed a narrow relationship between MRI-derived T2 changes and integrated EMG activity for *triceps surae* muscles during plantar flexion activity at different knee angles.

However, in order to exploit MRI as either a mapping tool or an index of exercise intensity, one has to address the issue of normalizing the T2 changes between different muscles and different individuals. Indeed, heterogeneous exercise-induced T2 changes have been reported among subjects with different training status or among muscles within the same subject, with no clear interpretation regarding the underlying mechanisms (Weidman et al., 1991; Le Rumeur et al., 1994).

To conclude, MRI produce similar results as surface EMG thereby indicating that these tools are complementary for evaluating muscle activity. Although the exact nature of mechanisms underlying the T2 changes sill remains to be precisely determined, it is clear that the use of muscle functional MRI associated with surface EMG will provide in the future new insights in muscle recruitment patterns during single or complex tasks both in children and adolescents.

6. CONCLUSION

The majority of children's muscle metabolism is determined from a range of indirect sources e.g., measurements of mechanical power or oxygen uptake measurements. Direct measures from muscle biopsies indicated that prepubertal children have a trend towards higher oxidative and lower glycolytic enzyme activity than adolescents. The blood lactate/pyruvate ratio increases in age related manner which may be indicative of greater glycolytic activity in adults. The faster PCr resynthesis demonstrated in children has so far been interpreted as a result of a higher oxidative capacity. In regard to oxygen uptake kinetics, children's faster primary time constant, greater O_2 cost and smaller slow component appear indicative of enhanced oxidative function. Although not studied as extensively as it should, the findings from the interplay of anaerobic and aerobic exercise metabolism supports a relatively higher oxidative capacity in childhood. This finding is coupled with a glycolytic activity that increases with age into adolescence.

Undoubtedly, ^{31}P-MRS and MRI will also give us more information regarding the fibre typing in skeletal muscles and metabolic (aerobic and anaerobic) capabilities of the growing child. Furthermore, mapping of muscles activated during exercise is an interesting issue which can be addressed using MRI. This approach, along with surface electromyography, provides interesting avenues of investigation into the changes of muscle recruitment pattern during growth that was previously unobtainable with children and adolescents. The advent of ^{31}P-MRS and MRI technologies which are non-invasive, ethical for use on children and allow muscle function to be investigated during exercise will significantly enhance scientists understanding of children's physical activity.

ACKNOWLEDGEMENTS

We would like to thank colleagues with whom this work would not be possible Prof. Neil Armstrong, Assoc. Prof. Jo Welsman, Mr Alan Barker and Dr Jon Fulford. Also, colleagues at Michigan State University (Professors Bob Wiseman, Ron Meyer and James Potchen) and at the University of Méditerranée (Dr David Bendahan, Miss Anne Tonson, Prof. P. Cozzone).

REFERENCES

Armon, Y; Cooper, DM; Flores, R; Zanconato, S; Barstow, TJ. Oxygen uptake dynamics during high-intensity exercise in children and adults. *J. Appl. Physiol.* 1991 70, 841-848.

Astrand, P.O., and Rodahl, K. (1986). *Textbook of Work Physiology.* New York, McGraw-Hill.

Barker, AR; Welsman, JR; Fulford, J; Welford, D; Williams, CA; Armstrong, N. Reproducibility of muscle energetics using ^{31}P-magnetic resonance spectroscopy during exhaustive exercise test in children. *Pediatr. Exerc. Sci.* 2006 18, 137-138.

Bar-Or, O. (1983). Pediatric Sports Medicine for the Practitioner. From Physiologic Principles to Clinical Applications. New York, Springer-Verlag.

Bar-Or, O., and Rowland, T. (2004). Pediatric exercise medicine: from physiological principles to health care application. Champaign (IL), Human Kinetics.

Bell, RD; MacDougall, JD; Billeter, R; Howald, H. Muscle fibre types and morphometric analysis of skeletal muscle in six year old children. *Med. Sci. Sports Exerc.* 1980 12, 28-31.

Bergström, J. Muscle electrolytes in man. *Scand. J. Clin. Lab. Med.* 1980 14, 511-513.

Chance, B; Leigh, JS; Jr; Clark, BJ; Maris, J; Kent, J; Nioka, S; Smith, D. Control of oxidative metabolism and oxygen delivery in human skeletal muscle: a steady-state analysis of the work/energy cost transfer function. *Proc. Natl. Acad. Sci. USA.* 1985 82, 8384-8388.

Clark, BJ 3rd; Acker, MA; McCully, K; Subramanian, HV; Hammond, RL; Salmons, S; Chance, B; Stephenson, LW. In vivo 31P-NMR spectroscopy of chronically stimulated canine skeletal muscle. *Am. J. Physiol.* 1988 254, C258-C266.

Cooper, DM; Barstow, TJ. Magnetic resonance imaging and spectroscopy in studying exercise in children. *Exerc. Sport Sci. Rev.* 1996 24, 475-499.

Dahlstrom, M; Liljedahl, ME; Gierup, J; Kaijser, L; Jansson, E. High proportion of type I fibres in thigh muscle of young dancers. *Acta Physiol. Scand.* 1997 160, 49-55.

Dorel, S; Couturier, A; Hug, F. Intra-session repeatability of lower limb muscles activation pattern during pedaling. *J. Electromyogr. Kinesiol.* 207, in press.

Elder, GC; Kakulas, BA. Histochemical and contractile property changes during human muscle development. *Muscle Nerve.* 1993 16, 1246-1253.

Eriksson, BO. Muscle metabolism in children: a review. *Acta Paediat. Scand. (Suppl)*, 1980 283, 20-27.

Eriksson, BO; Karlsson, J; Saltin, B. Muscle metabolites during exercise in pubertal boys. *Acta Paediat. Scand.* 1971 217, 57-63.

Eriksson, BO; Gollnick, PD; Saltin, B. Muscle metabolism and enzyme activities after training in boys 11-13 years old. *Acta Physiol. Scand.* 1973 87, 485-97.

Falgairette, G; Duche, P; Bedu, M; Fellmann, M; Coudert, J. Bioenergetic characteristics in prepubertal swimmers; comparisons with active and non active boys. *Int. J. Sports Med.* 1993 14, 444-448.

Falk, B; Bar-Or, O. Longitudinal changes in peak aerobic and anaerobic mechanical power of circumpubertal boys. *Pediatr. Exerc. Sci.* 1993 5, 318-331.

Fawkner, S; Armstrong, N. Oxygen uptake kinetic response to exercise in children. *Sports Med.* 2003a 33, 651-669.

Fawkner, S; Armstrong, N. The slow component response of VO_2 to heavy intensity exercise in children. *Kinanthropometry.* 2003b VIII, 105-113.

Fawkner, S; Armstrong, N. Can we confidently study VO_2 kinetics in young people? *J. Sports Sci. Med.* 2007 6, 277-285.

Fisher, MJ; Meyer, RA; Adams, GR; Foley, JM; Potchen, EJ. Direct relationship between proton T2 and exercise intensity in skeletal muscle MR images. *Invest. Radiol.* 1990 25, 480-5.

Fleckenstein, JL; Canby, RC; Parkey, RW; Peshock, RM. Acute effects of exercise on MR imaging of skeletal muscle in normal volunteers. *AJR Am. J. Roentgenol.* 1988 151, 231-7.

Fullerton, GD; Potter, JL; Dornbluth, NC. NMR relaxation of protons in tissues and other macromolecular water solutions. *Magn. Reson. Imaging.* 1982 1, 209-26.

Glaister, M. Multiple sprint work. Physiological responses; mechanisms of fatigue and the influence of aerobic fitness. *Sports Med.* 2005 35, 757-777.

Glenmark, B; Hedberg, G; Kaijser, L; Jansson, E. Muscle strength from adolescence to adulthood-relationship to muscle fibre types. *Eur. J. Appl. Physiol.* 1994 68, 9-19.

Gollnick, PD. Peripheral factors as limitations to exercise capacity. *Can. J. Appl. Sports Sci.* 1982 7, 14-21.

Granata, KP; Padua, DA; Abel, MF. Repeatability of surface EMG during gait in children. *Gait Posture.* 2005 22, 346-50.

Haralambie, G. Skeletal muscle enzyme activities in female subjects of various ages. *Bull. Eur. Physiopathol. Resp.* 1979 15, 259-267.

Haralambie, G. Enzyme activities in skeletal muscle of 13-15 years old adolescents. *Bull. Eur. Physiopathol. Resp.* 1982 18, 65-74.

Hedberg, G; Jansson E. Skelettmuskel fiber komposition kapacitat och intresse for olika fysiska aktiviterterbland elever in gymnasieskolan. Pedagogiska Rapporter, Umea, 1976. Cited in Komi, PV; Karlsson, J. Skeletal muscle fibre types; enzyme activities and physical performance in young males and females. *Acta Physiol. Scand.* 1978 103, 210-218.

Houmard, JA; Smith, R; Jendrasiak, GL. Relationship between MRI relaxation time and muscle fibre composition. *J. Appl. Physiol.* 1995 78, 807-9.

Hug, F; Bendahan, D; Le Fur, Y; Cozzone, PJ; Grelot, L. Heterogeneity of muscle recruitment pattern during pedaling in professional road cyclists: a magnetic resonance imaging and electromyography study. *Eur. J. Appl. Physiol.* 2004 92, 334-42.

Jones, A.M., and Poole, D.C. (2005). *Oxygen uptake kinetics in sport; exercise and medicine.* Oxon, Routledge.

Kemp, GJ; Radda, GK. Quantitative interpretation of bioenergetic data from 31P and 1H magnetic resonance spectroscopic studies of skeletal muscle: an analytical review. *Magn. Reson. Q.* 1994 10, 43-63.

Kent-Braun, JA; Miller, RG; Weiner, MW. Phases of metabolism during progressive exercise to fatigue in human skeletal muscle. *J. Appl. Physiol.* 1993 75, 573-580.

Kerviler, E de; Leroy-Willig, A; Jehenson, P; Duboc, D; Eymard, B; Syrota, A. Exercise-induced muscle modifications: study of healthy subjects and patients with metabolic myopathies with MR imaging and P-31 spectroscopy. *Radiology.* 1991 181, 259-64.

Kinugasa, R; Akima, H. Neuromuscular activation of triceps surae using muscle functional MRI and EMG. *Med. Sci. Sports Exerc.* 2005 37, 593-8.

Kinugasa, R; Kawakami, Y; Fukunaga, T. Quantitative assessment of skeletal muscle activation using muscle functional MRI. *Magn. Reson. Imaging.* 2006 24, 639-44.

Kuno, S; Katsuta, S; Inouye, T; Anno, I; Matsumoto, K; Akisada, M. Relationship between MR relaxation time and muscle fibre composition. *Radiology.* 1988 169, 567-8.

Kuno, S; Katsuta, S; Akisada, M; Anno, I; Matsumoto, K. Effect of strength training on the relationship between magnetic resonance relaxation time and muscle fibre composition. *Eur. J. Appl. Physiol. Occup. Physiol.* 1990 61, 33-6.

Kuno, S; Takahashi, H; Fujimoto, K; Akima, H; Miyamaru, M; Nemoto, I; Itai, Y; Katsuta, S. Muscle metabolism during exercise using phosphorus-31 nuclear magnetic resonance spectroscopy in adolescents. *Eur. J. Appl. Physiol.* 1995 70, 301-304.

Le Rumeur, E; Carre, F; Bernard, AM; Bansard, JY; Rochcongar, P; De Certaines, JD. Multiparametric classification of muscle T1 and T2 relaxation times determined by magnetic resonance imaging. The effects of dynamic exercise in trained and untrained subjects. *Br. J. Radiol.* 1994 67, 150-6.

Lexell, J; Sjostrom, M; Nordlund, AS; Taylor, CC. Growth and development of human muscle: a quantitative morphological study of whole vastus lateralis from childhood to adult age. *Muscle Nerve.* 1992 15, 404–409.

Mahler, M. First-order kinetics of muscle oxygen consumption; and an equivalent proportionality between QO2 and phosphoryl-creatine level. Implications for control of respiration. *J. Gen. Physiol.* 1985 86, 135-165.

Meyer, RA. A linear model of muscle respiration explains monoexponential phosphocreatine changes. *Am. J. Physiol.* 1988 254, C548-553.

Meyer, RA; Brown, TR; Kushmerick, MJ. Phosphorus nuclear magnetic resonance of fast- and slow-twitch muscle. *Am. J. Physiol.* 1985 248, C279-C287.

Moon, RB; Richard, JH. Determination of intracellular pH by 31P magnetic resonance. *J. Biol. Chem.* 1973 248, 7276-7278.

Nygaard, E. (1981). Women and exercise with special reference to muscle morphology and metabolism. In J. Poortmans and G. Niset (Eds.), *Biochemistry and Exercise.* (pp. 161-175). Baltimore, University Park Press.

Nygaard, E., and Hede, K. (1987). Physiological profiles of the male and female. In D. Macleod, R. Maughan, M. Nimmo, T. Reilly, and C. Williams (Eds.), *Exercise: benefits, limitations and adaptations.* (pp. 289-307). London, E and FN Spon.

Oertel, G. Morphometric analysis of normal skeletal muscles in infancy; childhood and adolescence An autopsy study. *J. Neurol. Sci.* 1988 88, 303-313.

Peter, JB; Barnard, RJ; Edgerton, VR; Gillespie, CA; Stempel, KE. Metabolic profiles of three fibre types of skeletal muscle in guinea pigs and rabbits. *Biochem.* 1972 11, 2627-2633.

Petersen, SR; Gaul, CA; Stanton, MM; Hanstock, CC. Skeletal muscle metabolism during short-term; high-intensity exercise in prepubertal and pubertal girls. *J. Appl. Physiol.* 1999 87, 2151-2156.

Price, TB; Kamen, G; Damon, BM; Knight, CA; Applegate, B; Gore, JC; Eward, K; Signorile, JF. Comparison of MRI with EMG to study muscle activity associated with dynamic plantar flexion. *Magn. Reson. Imaging.* 2003 21, 853-61.

Rossiter, H.B., Howe, F.A., Ward, S.A. (2005). Intramuscular phosphate and pulmonary VO_2 kinetics during exercise: Implications for control of skeletal muscle oxygen consumption. In A.M. Jones and D.C. Poole (Eds.), *Oxygen uptake kinetics in sport, exercise and medicine* (pp. 154-184). Oxon, Routledge.

Roussel, M; Bendahan, D; Mattei, JP; Le Fur, Y; Cozzone, PJ. [31]P magnetic resonance spectroscopy study of phosphocreatine recovery kinetics in skeletal muscle: the issue of intersubject variability. *Biochim. Biophys. Acta.* 2000 1457, 18-26.

Rowell, LB. Muscle blood flow in humans: how high can it go? *Med. Sci. Sports Exerc.* 1988 20, S97-103.

Sjogaard, G; Saltin, B. Extra- and intracellular water spaces in muscles of man at rest and with dynamic exercise. *Am. J. Physiol.* 1982 243, R271-80.

Taylor, DJ; Kemp, GJ; Thompson, CH; Radda, GK. Ageing: effects on oxidative function of skeletal muscle in vivo. *Mol. Cell Biochem.* 1997 174, 321-324.

Vandenborne, K; Walter, G; Ploutz-Snyder, L; Staron, R; Fry, A; De Meirleir, K; Dudley, GA; Leigh, JS. Energy-rich phosphates in slow and fast human skeletal muscle. *Am. J. Physiol.* 1995 268, C869-C876.

Weidman, ER; Charles, HC; Negro-Vilar, R; Sullivan, MJ; MacFall, JR. Muscle activity localization with 31P spectroscopy and calculated T2-weighted 1H images. *Invest. Radiol.* 1991 26, 309-16.

Williams, CA; Ratel, S; Armstrong N. Achievement of peak VO_2 during a 90-s maximal intensity cycle sprint in adolescents. *Can. J. Appl. Physiol.* 2005 30, 157-171.

Zanconato, S; Buchthal, S; Barstow, TJ; Cooper, DM. 31P-magnetic resonance spectroscopy of leg muscle metabolism during exercise in children and adults. *J. Appl. Physiol.* 1993 74, 2214-8.

In: Physical Activity and Children: New Research
Editor: N. P. Beaulieu, pp. 137-153

ISBN: 978-1-60456-306-1
© 2008 Nova Science Publishers, Inc.

Chapter 6

MECHANICAL AND METABOLIC WORK DURING LOCOMOTION IN YOUNG CHILDREN

Ann Hallemans[1,2,] and Patricia Van de Walle[2,3,4]*

[1]Research Group of Functional Morphology, University of Antwerp, Belgium
[2]Division of Neuro – and Psychomotor Physiotherapy, Department of Health Care, University College of Antwerp, Belgium
[3]Clinical Motion Analysis Laboratory of the University Hospital Pellenberg, Belgium
[4]Department of Rehabilitation Sciences, KuLeuven, Belgium

ABSTRACT

Gage (1991) defined energy conservation as one of the five major determinants of normal gait. The mechanical cost of walking is dependent on the amount of positive work that must be performed by the muscles to move the whole body, to accelerate body segments and to overcome energy absorption at other joints and because of antagonistic co-contractions. Positive mechanical work production requires muscular (metabolic) work. Adults prefer walking at the speed when the energetic cost is minimal (Winter, 1990). The energetics of walking is quite different in young children as the kinematics, kinetics and muscle activation patterns during gait are still maturing (Cavagna et al., 1983; Hallemans et al., 2004; Ivanenko et al., 2004; Schepens et al., 2004). Also changes in size and morphology during childhood affect the mechanical en metabolic costs of locomotion (De Jaeger et al., 2001). Mechanical work necessary to lift the body against gravity is large at the onset of independent walking, since the energy saving inverted pendulum mechanism is not yet fully mastered (Hallemans et al., 2004; Ivanenko et al., 2004). Also the work necessary to move the limbs relative to the centre of mass is greater in children than in adults (Cavagna et al., 1983; Hallemans et al., 2004; Schepens et al., 2004). Furthermore, standing energy expenditure rate is large in 3 to 4 year old children and decreases with age (De Jaeger et al., 2001). The age related decrease in metabolic

* Contacting author: Ann Hallemans, Research Group of Functional Morphology, Department of Biology, University of Antwerp, Universiteitsplein 1, B-2610 Antwerp, Belgium. Phone: +32/(0)3/ 820.22.60; Fax: +32/ (0)3/ 820.22.71; ann.hallemans@ua.ac.be

energy expenditure is larger than the observed decrease in normalised mechanical work. This suggests that young children have a lower muscular efficiency of (positive) work production than adults (Schepens et al., 2004). Differences in mechanical work, metabolic energy cost and muscular efficiency between children and adults disappear by the age of 10 (Cavagna et al., 1983; De Jaeger et al., 2001; Schepens et al., 2004).

INTRODUCTION

In 1991 Gage added a fifth determinant, namely conservation of energy during walking, to the four determinants of normal gait that were proposed by Perry (1985), i.e. stability in stance, clearance in swing, pre – positioning of the foot for heel contact and adequate step length. Abnormalities in one of the first four determinants of normal gait will result in a higher energy expenditure rate. Already since the 1950's the energetic cost of locomotion is of great interest in gait studies, as it contains information on gait efficiency (Winter, 1990). Energy expenditure can be considered as an objective measure of functional ability since it provides an indication of endurance, fatigue and the ability to accomplish the routine daily task of locomotion (Koop & Stout, 2004). Even during level walking at a constant speed, energy is consumed. Energy is lost at each step and has to be put into the system again. The total amount of mechanical work that has to be performed during walking comprises work to raise the body against gravity, work associated with speed variations during walking and the work necessary for acceleration and deceleration of the limbs (Cavagna, Saibene & Margaria, 1963). Additional metabolic work is performed during walking because of static muscular activity, work for stiffening the limbs and work performed because of antagonistic co - contractions. It seems that there is an optimal speed at which the energetic cost is minimal. For healthy adults, this is at about 3 – 4 km/hr (Margaria, 1938).

The cost of walking might be quite different for children as they largely differ in kinematics, kinetics and muscle activation patterns. At the onset of independent walking, children walk at low speed (0.6 m/s) with short (20 cm), quick (180 steps/min) steps. Other important features of immature gait are the broad base of support, abduction and external rotation of the arms with the elbows flexed (guard position), absence of a consistent heel strike, a flexed position of the hips and knees in stance and simultaneous flexion of the hips and knees in swing. During childhood the immature walking pattern gradually evolves towards a mature and stable state. Researchers have been able to distinguish two different phases in the gait maturation process (Bril & Breniere, 1989; Thelen, 1999; Cheron, Bengoetxea, Bouillot & Lavquaniti, 2001). A first rapid development phase spans the first three to six months after a child started to walk independently. During this period drastic changes are observed in all spatio – temporal and kinematic gait parameters. This first developmental burst is followed by a period of slow maturation. Not all gait parameters reach adult values at the same time. The temporal organisation of the gait cycle is already mature three months after the onset of independent walking. Step- and stride length reach adult values by the age of three (after correction for size differences between adults and children, Clark, Truly & Phillips 1990). A mature ground reaction force profile is seen by the age of five (Endo & Kimura, 1972; Sutherland, Ohlson, Cooper & Woo, 1980; Sutherland, Ohslon, Byden & Wyatt, 1988). At seven years of age muscle activation patterns are mature but it lasts until the age of eight until kinetic parameters reach adult values (Sutherland et al., 1988;

Ounpuu, Gage & Davis, 1991). Considering a walking person as a mechanical system, kinematic and kinetic differences during gait could result in different energy and power requirements of the system.

This paper reviews the literature regarding the energetic cost of walking in children with a normal gait pattern and compares it to the cost of walking in young adults. Although gait maturation has been extensively studied, changes that occur in the mechanical cost of walking due to growth or maturation of gait and the factors that drive these changes are much less understood. It is only recently that more attention has been paid to this topic.

CALCULATING ENERGY EXPENDITURE

During walking, muscles transform chemical energy into mechanical work. Energy expenditure during locomotion can be characterized either by measuring, directly or indirectly, the rate of energy utilization or alternatively by calculating the amount of mechanical work that is performed.

All cellular processes in the body result in the production of heat. It is possible to measure the amount of heat production by the human body. To do so, a person is placed in an airtight room that is thermally insulated and can act as a calorimeter. Despite the fact that these direct measures of energy production are highly sensitive, it is a very impractical method, especially for studies of walking or running (Koop & Stout, 2004). Energy expenditure during walking can also be measured indirectly from oxygen consumption. All energy metabolisms in the body depend on the utilization of oxygen. Oxygen uptake can be measured at rest and during locomotion, providing an indirect estimate of energy expenditure. Measurements of oxygen uptake are based on the principle of conservation of mass. It is assumed that the amount of oxygen that is actually consumed during the energy metabolism equals the difference in oxygen in inhaled and exhaled air and no oxygen is lost. This assumption holds true during steady-state locomotion (Vandewalle, 2004). Oxygen uptake measurements can be performed either by closed- or open-circuit spirometry. In closed-circuit spirometry a subject breathes and re-breathes from a pre-filled container with oxygen. Usually, 100% oxygen is used to prevent that the oxygen level in the container falls beneath critical limits. This method has several disadvantages: it is a stationary set-up, resistance to breathing can be substantial and removal of carbondioxide might not be sufficient (Koop & Stout, 2004; Vandewalle, 2004). During open-circuit spirometry, the subject inhales ambient air. The difference in oxygen and carbondioxide between ambient and exhaled air is investigated. This technique used to be very cumbersome but recently portable devices have been developed, that take breath-by-breath measurements of oxygen uptake, carbondioxide output, heart rate, ventilation volumes and respiratory rate. The systems are lightweight and telemetric so they do not hinder walking (Koop & Stout, 2004; Brehm, Groepenhof & Harlaar, 2004).

When oxygen uptake is used as a measure of the metabolic cost of walking, two different parameters are most often used: oxygen consumption and oxygen cost. Gross oxygen consumption is expressed in millilitre oxygen per minute per kilogram bodyweight. It is actually the rate of oxygen uptake that is directly measured by the equipment. Gross oxygen consumption is dependent on the basal metabolic rate (i.e. the amount of energy expended while at rest), which can differ substantially between subjects of different age and size. This problem can be overcome by calculating the net oxygen consumption (basal metabolic rate is subtracted from gross oxygen consumption to become the net oxygen consumption). On the other hand, net oxygen consumption seems to be more variable within subjects than gross oxygen consumption (Brehm, Becher & Harlaar, 2007.). Variability can be reduced by using careful standardisation (Schwarz, Koop, Bourke & Baker, 2006) and a multiple repetition study design (Brehm et al., 2007). For normalization purposes, standard practice is to divide oxygen consumption by body mass. However, this method is inadequate to eliminate confounding effects that arise from variations in age and size. Schwarz (et al., 2006) proposes a new standardisation scheme that is based on the use of net oxygen consumption and non-dimensional gait variables. Details on the normalisation procedure can be found in table 1. Net non-dimensional oxygen consumption is largely independent of relevant physiological and anatomical factors. Oxygen consumption is an indicator of the intensity of physical effort and is time dependent. It gives a good idea of the perceived exertion of a subject or patient. In turn, oxygen cost describes the amount of energy needed to walk a given distance and is not time dependent. Oxygen cost is calculated by dividing the oxygen rate by walking speed ($ml*m^{-1}*kg^{-1}$). This measure is related to the efficiency of locomotion. More detailed descriptions on the calculation of gross oxygen consumption, net oxygen consumption, oxygen cost and the relationships between these parameters of metabolic energy expenditure and the actual amount of work performed can be found in literature (Brehm et al, 2004; Waters et al., 1999). As a rule of thumb, 1 ml of O_2 consumption equals approximately 5 cal or 20.93 joules (Waters et al., 1999).

Mechanical energy calculations are based on biomechanical models of increasing complexity. They allow insight into at which joints and when during the gait cycle energy is used and possibly provide links to motor control (Winter, 1990). Mechanical work calculations are always an estimation of the total amount of work that has to be performed. The actual amount of work that needs to be performed is underestimated since work resulting from elastic energy storage, isometric muscle contractions or antagonist co – contractions are not taken into account (Winter, 1990). Two primary different methods for calculating mechanical energy are available. The first is based on inverse dynamics, the second on the work energy theorem.

Table 1. Standard (General method GM) and net non-dimensional (NN) normalisation for oxygen consumption parameters

	GM normalization	NN normalisation
Walking speed	v $[m.s^{-1}]$	v x 1/ $\sqrt{g.L_{leg}}$
Oxygen Consumption	O_2^{gross} x 1/m $[J.kg^{-1}.s^{-1}]$	(O_2^{gross} - O_2^{net}) x 1/(mg. $\sqrt{g.L_{leg}}$)
Oxygen Cost	(O_2^{gross} / v) x 1/m $[J.kg^{-1}.m^{-1}]$	(O_2^{gross} - O_2^{net}) / v x 1/mg

m = total body mass; v = walking speed; g = 9.81 $m.s^{-2}$.

When performing inverse dynamical analysis, joint kinematics, ground reaction forces and inertial properties of the body segments are put into a biomechanical model and Newtonian mechanics is used to calculate net joint moments and powers at different joints for the plane of motion being considered. Integration of these power curves over a given amount of time reveals the amount of work that is performed at a particular joint in the plane of movement under consideration. An advantage of this method is that can be determined at which joint most of the work is performed. Disadvantages are that usually only lower extremity joints are taken into consideration in biomechanical models, which will largely underestimate the actual amount of work that is performed. Furthermore, calculation errors can be important, depending on measurement errors and errors in the estimation of segmental inertial properties. This technique will not be discussed further on since it has not yet been used to estimate the amount of mechanical work performed during locomotion in children.

The work-energy theorem says that the work done on an object equals the change in energy of that object. Based on this theorem, work performed during locomotion can be estimated from the mechanical energy changes of the body. Total mechanical work can be divided into external work and internal work. External work is the amount of work necessary to lift and accelerate the body (centre of mass) upward and forward during each step. External work calculations can be obtained from force plate recordings, according to the technique that was first published by Cavagna in 1963. Calculations are easy to perform, lead to small errors and are easy to interpret. For details on the calculation method can be referred to numerous publications in literature (a.o. Cavagna et al., 1963; Cavagna & Margaria, 1966; Cavagna, Thys & Zamboni, 1976; Cavagna, Heglund & Taylor, 1977; Cavagna, Franzetti & Fuchimoto, 1983; Willems, Cavagna & Heglund, 1995). A summary can be found in table 2.

Table 2. Formulas for calculating external mechanical work according to Cavagna (1963)

		Unit	Formula	
CoM acceleration	a_x	m/s²	$= F_x/m$	with F_x = lateral GRF-component
	a_y	m/s²	$= F_y/m$	with F_y = fore-aft GRF-component
	a_z	m/s²	$= F_z/m$	with F_z = vertical GRF-component
CoM velocity	v_x	m/s	$= \sum \Delta a_x \cdot \Delta t + Cte$	**Numerical integration**
	v_y	m/s	$= \sum \Delta a_y \cdot \Delta t + Cte$	Numerical integration
	v_z	m/s	$= \sum \Delta a_z \cdot \Delta t + Cte$	Numerical integration
Gravitational potential energy	E_p	J	$= M_{tot} * 9.81 * height_{CoM}$	
Kinetic energy	E_k	J	$= \frac{1}{2} * M_{tot} * (V_x^2 + V_y^2 + V_z^2)$	
Total mechanical energy	E_t	J	$= E_p + E_k$	
External Work	Wext	J	$= \sum \Delta^+ E_t$	Sum of the positive increments in E_t
Recovery	R	%	$=[\Delta^+ E_p + \Delta^+ E_k - \Delta^+ E_{tot}]/[\Delta^+ E_p + \Delta^+ E_k]$	

Internal work comprises all the work performed by the muscles and tendons that does not directly lead to a displacement of the centre of mass of the body. Classically, only the amount of work to move the limb segments is characterised. Classical internal work is calculated from the kinetic energies of the moving limbs, which appears to be high in that body segment where the work is being done (Fenn, 1930). This method of work calculation is more complex than the method of platform analysis to calculate external work. It is more difficult to interpret and results in more noisy data. Different assumptions have to be made when energy calculations are performed: assumptions regarding the physical properties of the body segments and assumptions on the energy transfers that are allowed between segments (Willems et al., 1995)

THE METABOLIC COST OF WALKING

In healthy adults, oxygen cost is minimal at intermediate speeds (Margaria, 1938; Cavagna et al., 1977). As expected, net energy expenditure is greater in children than in adults (Silverman & Anderson, 1972; Waters, Hislop, Thomas & Campbell, 1983; Rogers, Olson & Wilmore, 1995). In young children (3 – 6 year old) walking at their highest speed, net oxygen cost is 40 to 70% greater than in adults. As children grow older, their gross and net oxygen cost during walking decreases. Age-related changes are also observed in the comfortable walking speed, which is the speed at which energy expenditure during locomotion is minimal. In adult men, this speed is approximately 1.37 m/s. Women prefer walking slightly slower, with a comfortable walking speed of 1.23 m/s. In 6 to 12 year old children this decreases to 1.17 m/s (Waters et al., 1999). At comfortable walking speed, mean oxygen uptake in 6 –12 year old children is 15.3 ml/kg/min. For teenagers (13-19 years old) this decreases to about 12.9 ml/kg/min, which is very close to the value of 12 ml/kg/min that is observed in adults (Waters et al., 1983). In healthy individuals, walking at comfortable walking speed requires little effort. Oxygen consumption amounts 28 to 32% of maximal oxygen consumption capacity (VO_2 max) and the anaerobic metabolism is not activated. This situation changes as walking speed increases. Within a functional range of walking speeds, the energy versus speed relationship is approximately linear. At fast speeds, in adults oxygen consumption increases to 18.4 ml/kg/min. In children this increases to 19.6 ml/kg/min (Waters et al., 1999).

These results all come from descriptive cross-sectional studies that can mask inter-individual differences. In 2002, Morgan and colleagues performed a 5-year follow up study in 23 healthy able-bodied children, measuring oxygen consumption during treadmill walking over a range of speeds. A longitudinal follow-up study can provide more insight into the relation between growth and locomotor oxygen consumption. Their results confirm previous observations that oxygen consumption decreases with age, between the ages of six and eight. At the age of six, on average, oxygen consumption is 27% higher than at the age of ten. Changes observed after the age of eight were only minor and not statistically significant. However, oxygen consumption in 10-year olds was still significantly higher than values reported in literature for healthy young adults. An interaction was also observed between age and speed. Across all ages, oxygen consumption at the fastest speed was significantly larger than at other speeds. But it was only in the 9-year olds that truly a positive linear relationship was observed between oxygen consumption and speed. Apart from looking at average values, inter-individual variability in oxygen consumption was also investigated. Across all ages this was relatively large, between 32% and 41%. In healthy adults, variability in oxygen consumption (measured during overground locomotion) is only 28% (Booyens & Kietinge, 1957 in Morgan et al., 2002).

Different explanations for the higher energy expenditure rate in children have been proposed. An increased net oxygen cost during locomotion can be related either to a greater amount of mechanical work that is performed or to a smaller efficiency of muscular contraction. Both possibilities will be discussed further on. Waters et al (1983) formulated another explanation. They claim that the increase in net oxygen cost can partially be attributed to a higher standing energy expenditure rate. In 3 – 4 year olds, standing oxygen cost amounts 3.42 ± 0.48 W/kg (6.04 ml/kg per min) while in adults it is only 1.95 ± 0.22 W/kg (3.5 ml/kg per min). Basal metabolic rate seems to decrease by 2% every decade throughout childhood and adolescence. The higher basal metabolic rate is a consequence of the lower proportion of lean body mass relative to a higher proportion of fat and skeletal tissue (Waters et al., 1999). Schepens, Bastien, Heglund and Willems (2004) relate this to differences in body size. During growth, there is a 4-fold increase in body mass and a 2-fold increase in leg length. Based on allometric growth, a decrease of 33% is expected in net oxygen cost. A decrease between 0 and 40% is observed. This observation is supported by the data of Rogers et al. (1995) who found an allometric exponential relationship between sub-maximal oxygen consumption and body surface area. Further evidence for the important role of body size is the observation that most differences in energy expenditure between adults and children disappear when differences in body size are accounted for by plotting oxygen cost as a function of dimensionless speed. However, this assumption of dynamic similarity only holds true for children above the age of 4 (De Jaeger, Willems & Heglund, 2001). Morgan et al. (2002) claim that physical immaturity and morphological variation are important factors that are also responsible for the increased inter-individual variability in oxygen consumption during locomotion in children.

EXTERNAL MECHANICAL WORK

As mentioned above, on of the possible explanations for the higher energetic cost of locomotion in children is a higher amount of mechanical work production during locomotion. In healthy adults, the amount of external work that is actually performed is speed dependent and is minimal at intermediate speeds (around 4 km/hr). In figure 1 mass specific external work is plotted as a function of walking speed. External work shows a U – shaped relationship with speed. Energy expenditure during walking is not only due to external work, but results suggest that, in healthy adults with a normal gait pattern, energy expenditure per unit distance is minimal when external work per unit distance is also minimal (Cavagna et al., 1976). External work is mainly performed in two phases: the first phase serves to generate a push forward, the second to complete the vertical lift of the centre of mass. Most work is performed for lifting the body. The forward push can be sustained by the energy recovered from the falling body (Cavagna et al., 1963).

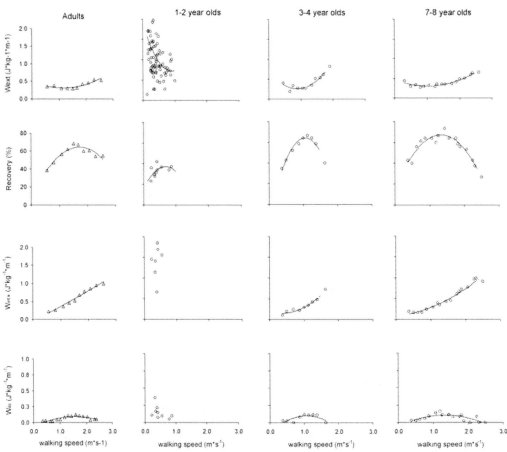

Data from adults are from Willems et al., 1995; Data from 1-2 year old children are from Hallemans et al., 2004; Data from 3 – 8 year old children are from Schepens et al., 2003, Bastien et al., 2004.

Figure 1. Mass specific external work (W_{ext}), recovery, classical internal work ($W_{int,k}$) and work during double contact (W_{dc}) are plotted as a function of walking speed for adults and children of different ages. The average adult regression lines are represented by broken line the on the graphs of the children.

The first to perform mechanical energy calculations in children was Cavagna in 1983. He showed that when two – year old children walk at a speed of 4 km/h (1.11 m/s), external work is 2 – 3 times greater than in adults. Nevertheless, external work showed a U- shaped relationship with speed (figure 1) thus an optimal speed could be identified, even in very young children. The optimal speed increases with age from 2.8 km/hr (~ 0.8 m/s) at the age of two to 5.0 km/hr (~ 1.4 m/s) at the age of twelve. There are abrupt changes in external mechanical work and optimal speed from 1-2 years to 3-4 years. After the age of four there is a more gradual change in external work is observed. The amount of external work that is performed largely increases at speeds above the optimal speed. These changes are more drastic in younger children (figure 1).

Kerrigan (1995) showed that the vertical displacement of the pelvis is strongly correlated with oxygen consumption. Saunders and co – workers, already recognized this idea in 1953. Hip flexion and extension (without flexion of the knees) leads to a compass-type gait with large vertical excursions of the centre of mass and consequently energy expenditure and external work performed during locomotion are large. In normal gait, vertical excursions of the centre of mass are limited to minimize energy expenditure during locomotion by increasing stride length through pelvic rotation (1), the knee flexion – ankle plantar flexion couple (2) and ankle plantar flexion at push-off (3). Anterior pelvic tilt prior to toe-off (4), knee flexion of the stance limb (5) and lateral pelvic displacements (6) also contribute to the smoothening of the path of the centre of mass. These six determinants of Saunders are not present at the onset of independent walking (Statham & Murray, 1971; Hallemans, Otten, De Clercq & Aerts, 2004; Hallemans, De Clercq & Aerts, 2006). Consequently, vertical centre of mass oscillations are large for their small stature, on average 4.6 cm (own observations). In adults vertical centre of mass oscillations amount approximately 4.5 cm (Saunders et al., 1953). Therefore the amount of external work that needs to be performed by toddlers is substantial.

THE INVERTED PENDULUM MECHANISM

To further minimize external work, adults make use of an imperfect inverted pendulum mechanism of energy exchange (figure 2). During a gait cycle the body moves over the supporting leg in an arc. Potential (height) and kinetic (velocity) energy of the body's centre of mass oscillate through maxima and minima as the body raises and falls, accelerates and decelerates. Like in a pendulum, there is the possibility of energy exchange between kinetic and potential energy. In a perfect pendulum, kinetic and potential energy are oscillating exactly 180° out of phase. Kinetic energy can be completely transferred into potential energy and vice versa. All energy can be recovered and no work has to be done to keep the pendulum moving. However, in locomotion there is no complete transformation. Energy is lost from the system and external work must be performed at each step. The amount of work to maintain a constant walking speed if there were no energy exchange can be compared to the amount of work that is actually performed. This value can be expressed as a percentage of recovery and was first defined by Cavagna in 1977. Up to 70% of the required mechanical energy can be recovered from the previous step due to this inverted pendulum mechanism of energy exchange (Cavagna et al., 1977). The muscles must actively supply the other 30% of the mechanical work. In young adults with a normal gait pattern, this inverted pendulum model fits very well when walking at intermediate speeds but no longer holds up at speeds above 7 km/hr.

Is the pendulum mechanism innate or is it learned through walking experience? In 1983 Cavagna also calculated recovery values in children. He found that even in young children external work is minimal when recovery is maximal (figure 1). But in 1 – 2 year old children, recovery only reaches a maximum of 40 – 50%, which is significantly smaller than in adults (Cavagna et al., 1983). Hallemans, Aerts, De Deyn, Otten & De Clercq (2004) and Ivanenko, Dominici, Capellini, Dan, Cheron & Lacquaniti (2004), who were the first to study the energetic cost of locomotion during the first months of independent walking, also found recovery values around 40%. When toddlers perform their first independent steps, recovery values are even smaller (28% on average) and highly variable (Ivanenko et al., 2004; Kimura, Yaguramaki, Fuijita, Ogiue-Ikeda, Nishizawa & Ueda, 2005).

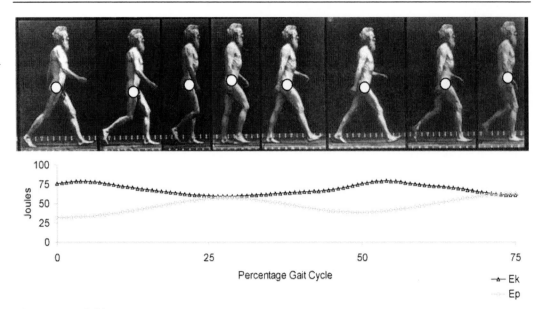

Photo E. Muybridge.

Figure 2. The body's centre of mass (white dot) moves over the supporting limb in an arc. If the leg is considered as a rigid strut this movement represents an inverted pendulum. Kinetic (Ek) and potential (Ep) energy of the centre of mass oscillate out of phase. When the centre of mass is at its highest point Ep is maximal en Ek is minimal. As the height of the centre of mass decreases, the loss in Ep can be used to increase the velocity of the centre of mass both in the vertical and forward directions. Also the kinetic energy of the centre of energy of the centre of mass can be converted into potential energy.

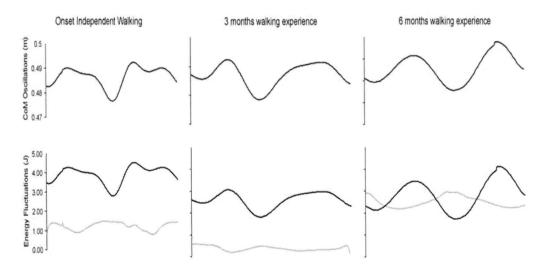

Figure 3. Oscillations of the centre of mass (CoM) and kinetic (in grey) and potential (in black) energy fluctuations are shown for toddlers. Shortly after the onset of independent walking, CoM movements are irregular and the inverted pendulum mechanism of energy exchange is sub optimal. Already a few months after the onset of walking, CoM movements evolve towards a sinusoidal pattern with 2 maxima and 2 minima. A pendular exchange of energy can occur.

Different explanations for the sub-optimal energy exchange can be put forward. In toddlers, trunk and centre of mass oscillations are more variable from step to step than in adults. Also the changes in gravitational potential and kinetic energy of the centre of mass are highly irregular with a variable phase relationship between them. Gravitational potential energy fluctuations are largest in amplitude and almost completely determine the total mechanical energy fluctuations. Kinetic energy fluctuations are small and depend upon walking speed (figure 3). The toddlers' tossing gait in combination with their slow walking speed can explain this large difference in kinetic and potential energy fluctuations. During as much as 25 to 50% of the gait cycle, kinetic and potential energy can be oscillating in phase (Hallemans et al., 2004; Ivanenko et al., 2004; Kimura et al., 2005). Consequently, toddlers fail to demonstrate a prominent energy transfer. A partial energy exchange may occur during some portions of the gait cycle but the classic inverted pendulum behaviour is lacking.

Nevertheless, pendulum – like behaviour rapidly evolves to higher values within a few months of independent walking experience. Already a few weeks after the onset of independent walking, children start to display a clear pendulum – like transfer between kinetic and potential energy of the centre of mass. The vertical centre of mass fluctuations evolve towards a sinusoidal pattern with two maxima and two minima, thanks to improvements in movement coordination (figure 3). Coordinated movements between the hip, knee and ankle joints control the movements of the centre of mass. In turn, improvements in the centre of mass movements affect the potential energy fluctuations. Also the kinetic energy fluctuations increase due to an increase in self – selected walking speed. Recovery values increase and external work decreases (Hallemans et al., 2004; Ivanenko et al., 2004). However, the possibility of energy transfer remains highly variable indicating that toddlers are able to implement the inverted pendulum mechanism of energy exchange but it is not an inherent feature of toddler gait yet.

Not only a slow walking speed and immature movement coordination lead to a sub-optimal exchange of energy, also the small stature of the children might play a role. Figure 4 shows the recovery and the external work expressed as a function of dimensionless speed ($V_f[m*s^{-1}]/\sqrt{9.81[m*s^{-1\,2}]}*leg\_length[m]$) for toddlers, children of different ages and adults. On average, recovery values for children under the age of four (open triangles) are still slightly lower than those of adults. Probably this can be explained by the fact that children under 4 years of age walking at a given speed make steps relatively long for their leg length (Cavagna et al., 1983; Bastien, Heglund & Schepens, 2003). The centre of mass is at its lowest point when the angle between the two legs is the greatest and at its highest when the angle is approximately zero. Thus longer steps increase the vertical excursions of the centre of mass, which results in a higher amount of external work performed. Nevertheless, maximum recovery values are reached at the same dimensionless speed as in adults (i.e. Froude number = 0.4 – 0.5; Cavagna et al., 1963; Hallemans et al., 2004; Kimura et al., 2005). This demonstrates the existence of an efficient speed of human walking that seems to be independent of body size or maturity of walking. Toddlers, on the other hand, at their first unsupported steps, never walked faster than at Froude number = 0.14. Recovery was systematically lower, compared to older children and adults. Both normalised speed and energy recovery increased with age, but 1 – 5 months after the onset of independent walking they were still lower than values observed in older adults and children (Hallemans et al., 2004; Ivanenko et al., 2004; Kimura et al., 2005).

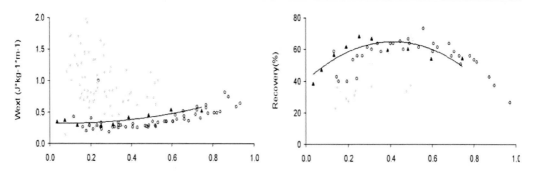

Data from adults are from Willems et al., 1995; Data from 1-2 year old children are from Hallemans et al., 2004; Data from 3 – 8 year old children are from Schepens et al., 2003, Bastien et al., 2004.

Figure 4. External work and recovery are plotted as a function of dimensionless speed. Different age groups are represented by different symbols: ● 1 – 2 year olds, o 3 – 12 year olds, ♦ adults, ♢ 3 – 4 year olds (recovery only).

WORK PERFORMED DURING DOUBLE CONTACT

At the end of each step the body has to be redirected from one pendular arc to the next. At this time in the gait cycle the leading leg is braking. This amount of negative work has to be overcome by the propulsive back leg. Already in 1966 Cavagna and Margaria, as well as Alexander and Jayes in 1978, acknowledged that simultaneous positive and negative work is performed in a step cycle. But until recently this was ignored when mechanical energy calculations were performed. Donelan, Kram & Kuo (2002) were the first to actually calculate the amount of work that is performed during double support when one leg is working against the other to redirect the velocity of the centre of mass. They showed that it is most advantageous when the negative work of the leading leg and the positive work of the trailing leg are performed together. In healthy adults, work during double contact has an inverted U – shaped relationship with speed (figure 1), showing a maximum at intermediate speeds. When this amount of work during double contact is not taken into account, the total amount of external mechanical work during walking can be underestimated substantially (by 33 to 40 % according to Donelan, 2002 & Bastien et al, 2003). Nevertheless, it does not seem to be a major determinant of the cost of walking since optimal speed is not influenced by it.

The double support phase accounts for a substantial portion of the gait cycle in young children. It would be very interesting to find out whether this prolonged phase of double support had an effect on the mechanical work requirements. In very young children work during double contact accounts for 7 to 16% (0.04 – 0.10 J/kg*m) of the work performed on the centre of mass (Hallemans et al., 2004). Contrary to what might be expected, this amount of work is small compared to adults in which it accounts for up to 40% of the work performed on the centre of mass (Bastien et al., 2003). Partially, this might be explained by the fact that the external work performed on the centre of mass is much larger in younger children. Because of the toddlers tossing gait, the most important component of work is the work necessary to lift the centre of mass against gravity. Compared to this, work resulting from the opposite action of the front and the back limb necessary to maintain a (slow) constant walking speed is relatively small. Also the slow walking speed reduces the amount of work performed during double contact. At the age of 3, work during double contact has increased to up to 40% of the total amount of work performed on the centre of mass. Across all ages work during double contact shows an inverted U-shaped relationship with walking speed (figure 1). At slow and intermediate speeds, the back leg generates a forward push at about 20 – 40% of the way through double support. At higher speeds, this forward push shifts to the beginning of double contact, while propulsive forces are generated during the second half of double contact. This reduces the amount work than one leg can perform against the other and therefore work during double contact is lower at higher speeds. At very low speeds work during double contact is also minimised because there is almost no simultaneous work performed by the front and back leg. This is a consequence of passive work transfers between the front and back limb and the velocity of the centre of mass. Nearly all the positive work performed during double contact increases the energy of the centre of mass.

Thus across all ages work during double contact is maximal at intermediate speeds but the maximum occurs at lower speeds in younger subjects. When speed is normalised based on the assumption of dynamic similarity, work during double contact reaches a maximum at the same Froude number (~ 0.35) in adults and children above 5 years of age. Notably at this speed, energy consumption as well as external work is minimal. This shows that also in children work during double contact is not a major determinant of the energetic cost of walking (Bastien et al., 2003). Furthermore, the observed speed - dependent changes in external work and work during double contact are primarily a result of body size.

INTERNAL MECHANICAL WORK

Internal work comprises all the work performed by the muscles and tendons that does not directly lead to a displacement of the centre of mass of the body. It comprises work necessary for acceleration and deceleration of the limbs, static muscular activity, work for stiffening the limbs and work performed because of antagonistic co - contractions. At intermediate speeds, internal work is small in adults but at speeds above and below 4 km/hr the amount of internal work becomes substantial (Cavagna et al., 1963). Internal work done per stride increases with speed, both in children and adults. As walking speed goes up, the velocity of the head and trunk segments relative to the surroundings increases. Consequently, the backward velocity of the supporting limb relative to the centre of mass increases, as does the forward velocity of the swing limb. At a given speed, children above 3 years of age perform the same amount of internal work per unit body mass per stride. However, mass specific internal power is greater in the children because of the higher step frequency (Schepens et al., 2004). A higher step frequency results in higher segmental velocities in children, which increases the cost of accelerating and decelerating the legs. Mechanical work to accelerate the limbs is likely to be 15 to 33% greater in children due to the higher rotational speeds and accelerations that are required when walking with a higher step frequency, even despite the smaller inertias of the body segments (Cavagna et al., 1963). The difference is greater at higher speeds and in younger subjects (Schepens et al., 2004).

In toddlers, internal work per unit distance and per unit mass is significantly higher (0.74 ± 0.09 J/kg*m) than in adults (0.27 ± 0.06 J/kg*m) walking at natural speed (Ivanenko et al., 2004). This can be explained by the fact that step frequency, and consequently the angular velocities of the body segments, are very high in toddlers. If body size is taken into account by expressing speed as the dimensionless Froude number, internal work in toddlers is smaller than in adults. Moreover, internal work in toddlers is almost completely dependent on the work to swing the limb forward because the head, trunk and arms are kept stiff at the onset of walking and therefore their kinetic energy is small (Hallemans et al., 2004).

MUSCULAR EFFICIENCY

Total mechanical work can be calculated by summing external work, work during double contact and classical internal work thereby taking into account possible energy transfers. The efficiency of positive work production can then be calculated as the ratio of total mechanical power to the net energy consumption rate. In adults, efficiency reaches a maximum of 0.30 – 0.35 at 1.25 m/s. In children of all ages total mechanical power and net oxygen consumption increase with walking speed but the increase is greater the younger the subject. The efficiency of positive work production is also speed dependent. Before the age of 7, the increase in net oxygen consumption cannot be fully explained by an increase in total mechanical power. Part of the extra cost could be due to a reduction in muscular efficiency e.g. in 3 – 4 year old children maximal efficiency is only 0.15 – 0.25. This lower efficiency could be due to immature muscular activation patterns below the age of five, such as increased isometric and/or antagonistic co-contractions. Unnithan et al. (1996) showed that muscular co-contractions could explain up to 50% of the metabolic cost of walking. Differences between adults and children disappear after the age of 10 (Schepens et al., 2004).

CONCLUSION

Both metabolic cost and mechanical work are large in children compared to adults, when walking at the same absolute speed. The difference is greater the younger the subject. Different factors, apart from higher mechanical work requirements, contribute to the increased metabolic cost of walking in children. These are their smaller size, the higher basal metabolic rate and lower muscular efficiency. On average, the largest differences between adults and children disappear by the age of ten.

Although extensive research has been performed regarding age-related changes in the oxygen cost during walking, only recently attention has been paid to the mechanical work performed during locomotion in children. Most studies have primarily focussed on the maturation of external work production and the inverted pendulum mechanism of walking. Children perform a greater amount of mass specific external work when walking at the same speed than adults. But above the age of 4 most differences disappear when speed is expressed as the dimensionless Froude number. In very young children however, size differences do not fully account for the increased amount of mechanical work performed during locomotion. In 1 – 2 year old children recovery values remain low and mass specific external work is large, suggesting that the inverted pendulum mechanism of energy exchange during walking is not innate and has to be learned through experience.

The greater amount of mechanical work that is performed when children walk at the same absolute speed than adults is likely to be a very important contributing factor to the higher weight specific oxygen consumption during walking compared to adults. However, to prove this point simultaneous measurements of mechanical and metabolic work during locomotion in children of different ages are required. Until now, no such dataset has ever been published. Researchers have been unable to detect a clear correlation between external work and oxygen cost. Further research is necessary on this topic.

Although the inverted pendulum is a very simple and attractive model, it largely underestimates the cost of walking. Equal and opposite limb movements, isometric muscle contractions or antagonistic co-contractions are not taken into account. In an immature gait pattern these might be substantial and largely increase the energetic cost of locomotion. Alternative methods to calculate mechanical work need to be explored and compared to the measured rate of energy expenditure.

REFERENCES

Alexander R. Mc.N. & Jayes AS. (1978) Optimum walking techniques for idealized animals. *J. Zool. Lond.*, *192*, 97-117.

Bastien GJ., Heglund NC. & Schepens B. (2003) The double contact phase in walking children. *J. Exp. Biol.*, *203*, 2967-78.

Brehm MA., Groepenhof H. & Harlaar J. (2004) Validation of the portable VmaxST system for oxygen uptake measurement. *Gait & Posture, 20*, 67 - 74.

Brehm MA., Becher J. & Harlaar J. (2007) Reproducibility evaluation of gross and net walking efficiency in children with cerebral palsy. *Dev. Med. Child Neurol.*, *49*, 45 - 48.

Bril B & Brenière Y. (1989) Steady State velocity and temporal structure of gait during the first six months of autonomous walking. *Hum Mov Sci.*, *8*, 99-122.

Cavagna GA., Saibene FP. & Margaria R. (1963) External work in walking. *J. Appl. Physiol.*, 18/1, 1-9.

Cavagna GA. & Margaria R. (1966) The mechanics of walking. *J Appl Physiol.*, *21(1)*, 271-8.

Cavagna GA., Thys H. & Zamboni A. (1976) The sources of external work in level walking and running. *J. Physiol.*, *262*, 639-657.

Cavagna GA., Heglund NC. & Taylor CR. (1977) Mechanical work in terrestrial locomotion: two basic mechanisms for minimizing energy expenditure. *Am. J. Physiol.*, *233/5*, R243-R261.

Cavagna GA., Franzetti P. & Fuchimoto T. (1983) The mechanics of walking in children. *J Physiol.*, *343,* 323-39.

Cheron G., Bengoetxea A., Bouillot E., Lacquaniti F & Dan B. (2001) Early emergence of temporal co-ordination of lower limb segments elevation angles in human locomotion. *Neurosci. Lett.*, *308,* 123-27.

Clark JE., Truly S. & Phillips SJ. (1990) A dynamical systems approach to understanding the development of lower limb coordination in locomotion. In: *Sensory-Motor Organizations and Development in Infancy and Early Childhood*. Eds. Bloch, H. & Bertenthal, B. I. The Netherlands: Academic Press; 363-78.

De Jaeger D., Willems PA.& Heglund NC. (2001) The energy cost of walking in children. *Pflügers Arch, 441,* 538-43.

Donelan JM., Kram R. & Kuo A. (2002) Simultaneous positive and negative external mechanical work in human walking. *J. Biomech., 35,* 117-24.

Endo B. & Kimura T. (1972) External force of foot in infant walking. *Journal of the Faculty of Science: Section 5: Antropology (Tokyo), 4,* 103-17.

Fenn, W.O. (1930) Work against gravity and work due to velocity changes in running. *Am. J. Physiol.,* 93, 433-462.

Gage JR (Ed.) (1991) *Gait analysis in Cerebral Palsy.* London: MacKeith Press, 61-95.

Hallemans A., Aerts P., De Deyn PP.,Otten E. & De Clercq D. (2004) Mechanical Energy in toddler gait: A trade-off between economy and stability? *J. Exp. Biol., 207,* 2417-2431.

Hallemans A., Otten E., De Clercq D. & Aerts P. (2005) 3D analysis of toddler gait: A cross-sectional study spanning the first rapid developmental phase *Gait & Posture, 22 (2),* 107-118.

Hallemans A., De Clercq D. & Aerts P. (2006) Changes in 3D joint dynamics during the first 5 months after the onset of independent walking: a longitudinal follow-up study. *Gait & Posture, 24 (3),* 270 – 279.

Ivanenko YP., Dominici N., Cappellini G., Dan B., Cheron G. & Lacquaniti F. (2004) Development of pendulum mechanism and kinematic coordination from the first unsupported steps in toddlers. *J Exp Biol., 207(Pt 21),* 3797-810.

Kerrigan DC., Vibramontes BE., Corcoran BJ. & LaRaia PJ. (1995) Measured versus predicted vertical displacement of the sacrum during gait as a tool to measure biomechanical gait performance. *Am J Phys Med Rehabil.,74(1),* 3-8.

Kimura T., Yaguramaki N., Fuijita M., Ogiue-Ikeda M., Nishizawa S. & Ueda Y. (2005) Development of energy and time parameters in the walking of healthy human infants. *Gait & Posture, 22,* 225-32.

Koop S. & Stout J. (2004) Chapter 10: Energy consumption *In: The treatment of gait problems in cerebral palsy.* Ed. Gage J.; Mac Keith Press.

Margaria, R. (1938) Sulla fisiologia e specialmente sul consuma energetico della Marcia e della corsa a varie velocità ed inclinazioni del terreno. *Atti. Acad. Naz. Lincei Memorie, 7,* 299 – 368.

Morgan DW., Tseh W., Caputo JL., Keefer DJ., Craig IS., Griffith KB., Akins AB., Griffith GE. & Martin PE. (2002) Longitudinal profiles of oxygen uptake during treadmill walking in able-bodied children: the locomotion energy and growth study. *Gait & Posture, 15,* 230-5..

Ounpuu S., Gage JR. & Davis RB. (1991) Three-dimensional lower extremity joint kinetics in normal pediatric gait. *J. Pediatr. Orthop., 11,* 341-9.

Perry J. (Ed.) (1985) *Normal and pathological gait.* Thorofare NJ: Slack Inc.

Rogers DM., Olson BL. & Wilmore JH. (1995) Scaling for the VO2 to body size relationships among children and adults. *J. Appl. Physiol., 79,* 958-967.

Rose J., Gamble JG., Medeiros J., Burgos A. & Haskell WL. (1989) Energy cost of walking in normal children and in those with cerebral palsy. *J. Pediatr. Orthop., 9,* 276-279.

Saunders J., Inman V. & Eberhart H. (1953) The major determinants of normal and pathological gait. *J. Bone Joint Surg., 35,* 543-58..

Schepens B., Bastien GJ., Heglund NC. & Willems PA. (2004) Mechanical work and muscular efficiency in walking children. *J. Exp. Biol., 207,* 587-96.

Silverman M. & Anderson SD. (1972) Metabolic cost for treadmill exercise in children. *J. Appl. Physiol.*, *33*, 696-698.

Sutherland DH., Ohlson R., Cooper L. & Woo S.L-Y. (1980) The development of mature gait. *J. Bone joint Surg.*, *62-A(3)*, 336-353.

Sutherland DH., Olhsen RA., Biden EN. & Wyatt MP. (Eds.) (1988) *The development of mature walking.* Philadelphia: J.B. Lippincott.

Schwarz M., Koop SE., Bourke JL. & Baker R. (2006) A non-dimensional normalization scheme for oxygen utilization data. *Gait & Posture, 24,* 14-22.

Thelen E. (1999) Motor development: a new synthesis. *Am Psychol.*, *50,* 79-95.

Unnithan VB., Dowling JJ., Frost G. & Bar – Or O. (1996) Role of co - contraction in the O2 cost of walking in children with cerebral palsy. *Med. Sci. Sport Exerc., 28,* 1498-1504.

Waters RL., Hislop HJ., Thomas L. & Campbell J. (1983) Energy cost of walking in normal children and teenagers. *Dev. Med. Child Neurol., 25*, 184-188.

Willems PA., Cavagna GA. & Heglund NC. (1995) External, internal and total work in human locomotion. *J. Exp. Biol., 198,* 379-93..

Winter D. (Ed.) (1990) *Biomechanics and Motor Control of Human Movement (2nd. Ed.),* New York: John Wiley & Sons.

In: Physical Activity and Children: New Research
Editor: N. P. Beaulieu, pp. 155-175

ISBN: 978-1-60456-306-1
© 2008 Nova Science Publishers, Inc.

Chapter 7

FIELD-DEPENDENT CHILDREN: A LESS ATHLETICALLY SKILLED AND LESS PHYSICALLY ACTIVE SUBPOPULATION

Wenhao Liu[*]

Physical Education Department, Slippery Rock University,
Slippery Rock, Pennsylvania, USA

ABSTRACT

While children are among the most active segments of our society, their physical activity amounts decrease with age during school years, and a considerable portion of children are physically inactive. Physically inactive children are more likely to remain sedentary in their adulthood years, which will result in a higher rate of prevalence and premature death of lifestyle diseases. Thus, early identification of sedentary children and "untracking" of sedentary living are critical to public health promotion and disease prevention. Accumulative research results, plus the most recent findings, have documented that field-dependent children may be a less athletically skilled and physically inactive subpopulation that needs immediate attention and intervention.

Field-dependent children, which constitute one-quarter of total children and adolescents population, are consistently and constantly documented to be less competent in sport-related settings. Compared with their field-independent counterpart, field-dependent children and adolescents are less athletically skilled, less involved in school varsity sports, and slower or less effective in motor skill acquisition. In addition, in a series of studies comparing field-independent and field-dependent children's learning behaviors in physical education classes, field-dependent children are found to have more problems to understand and remember directions, have more off-task behaviors, and tend

---

[*] Correspondence should be addressed to: Wenhao Liu, Ph. D. Physical Education Department, Slippery Rock University, Slippery Rock, PA 16057-1326, USA. Phone: (724) 738-2819; Fax: (724) 738-2921; e-mail: wenhao.liu@sru.edu

to reduce complex tasks to simpler and easier ones when performing them. As a result, field-dependent children experience much less success academically.

Given the consistent findings regarding field dependence-independence in sport-related settings and the importance of regular physical activity participation to health promotion and disease prevention, the research has recently been extended by investigating the relationship between field dependence-independence and children's physical activity participation. It has been found that, compared with field-independent children, field-dependent children are less likely to participate in organized sports, tend to choose physical activities with less energy expenditure, and have significantly smaller daily physical activity amounts. In addition, new research findings also suggest that African-American children who are less physically active than Caucasian children are significantlly more field-dependent than the latter.

This chapter will introduce the concept and assessment of field dependence-independence first, and then report the accumulated findings regarding the impact of field dependence-independence on sports levels, novel motor skill aquization, and behaviros in phsycial education. Finally, the latest research results with respect to field dependence-independence and children's physical activity participation will be reported. The possible strategies enhancing field-dependent children's sports skill and physical activity level will also be discussed.

INTRODUCTION

Field dependence-independence is a construct that initially came from Witkin and his colleagues' research (Witkin et al., 1954). In the 1940s, when Witkin and his colleagues were seeking to determine how people locate the upright position as quickly and accurately as they ordinarily do, subjects were found, unexpectedly, to be markedly different from one another in their performance on locating the upright position (Witkin & Goodenough, 1981). The Rod-and-Frame Test was used in Witkin's experiments. In administering the Rod-and-Frame Test, the participant sat in a completely darkened room facing a luminous tilted rod surrounded by a luminous tilted square frame, which were the only things the participant could see in the room. The participant was asked to adjust the tilted rod until he or she considered the rod was in a physically vertical position (Figure 1). Some participants were so influenced by the tilted frame that they could not adjust the rod to a position close to the verticality. Other participants, in contrast, apparently relied mainly on their body (the kinesthetic verticality feeling of the body) as a reference and could adjust the rod to a relatively vertical position ignoring the influence of the tilted frame. As a result, individuals relying mainly on self to adjust the tilted rod in the Rod-and-Frame Test were classified as "field-independent" individuals, who could adjust the rod to a relatively vertical position. Those influenced very much by the tilted frame in the Rod-and-Frame Test were classified "field-dependent" individuals, who can not adjust the rod to a vertical position (Witkin & Goodenough, 1981).

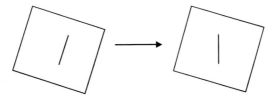

Figure 1. During administration of the Rod-and-Frame Test, the participant is asked to adjust the tilted rod to the vertical position overcoming the misguidance of the tilted square frame.

In 1960s, a portable (table-top size) rod-and-frame apparatus came into being (Oltman, 1968). This small apparatus does not require a completely darkened room for administration, and is small enough to be taken to schools and any other locations where the target participants are conveniently available. The portable rod-and-frame apparatus is the same in construction as Witkin's apparatus, mainly comprising a titled square frame and a rotatable rod, which is surrounded by the frame. With a seated position, the participant puts his/her eyes against an opening at one end of the apparatus and looks into it. The only thing that the participant can see is a tilted rod surrounded by a tilted square frame. During the test the participant is required to adjust the tilted rod to a physically vertical position against the influence of the tilted square frame. Figure 2 and Figure 3 are a version of the portable rod-and-frame apparatus. Because of its enhanced availability and portability, the portable rod-and-frame apparatus has been used widely afterward to operationally define field-dependent individuals and field-independent individuals.

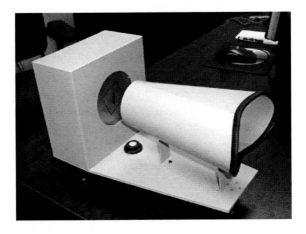

Figure 2.

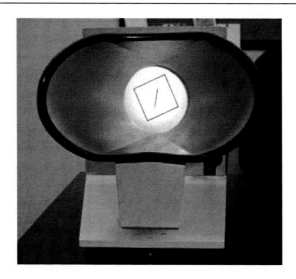

Figure 3.

Another frequently used instrument to assess field dependence-independence is Embedded Figures Test (Oltman, Raskin, & Witkin, 1971). In administering the Imbedded Figures Test the participant is to identify simple figures embedded in more complex patterns within a time frame. It was hypothesized that the individuals who could separate the rod from the tilted frame in the Rod-and-Frame Test (field-independent individuals) could identify simple figures embedded in more complex patterns more easily and faster, and that those who experienced more difficulties in separating the rod from the tilted frame in the Rod-and-frame Test (field-dependent individuals) would feel more difficult in identifying simple figures within more complex patterns (Witkin & Goodenough, 1981). That is, the two instruments share the similarity in separating an item (the rod or a simple figure) from a field (the tilted frame or a complicated figure) by which field-dependent individuals and field-independent individuals can be identified. As a result, both the Rod-and-Frame Test and Embedded Figures Test have been used to operationally define field dependence-independence (Brady, 1995).

However, each of the two instruments measures and emphasizes a different aspect of field dependence-independence. The Rod-and-Frame Test reflects differences mainly in perception of the upright due to reliance on internal versus external cues when the subject is adjusting a rod to a vertical position against influence or disturbance of a tilted square frame. By contrast, the Embedded Figure Test is considered to be more related to cognitive restructuring ability by identifying a simple figure hidden in a more complicated figure (Witkin & Goodenough, 1981). The cognitive restructuring ability is considered to be more related to intelligence and make an important contribution to performance in school, "since the skills required in school tasks are the same as those involved in the tests used to evaluate this dimension of cognitive style; analytical capacity and the ability to develop strategies for organizing and restructuring information." (Páramo & Tinajero, 1990, p. 1084).

In addition, taking the Embedded Figure Test requires a large short-term memory capacity. During the administration of the test, the participants can not see both simple forms and complex figures simultaneously because the simple forms are printed on the back cover of the test booklet and the complex figures are on the booklet pages. Individuals with larger short-term memory do not need to look back at the simple forms too many times thus can identify more simple forms within a time frame. Consequently, field-independent individuals, who can identify relatively more simple forms in the Embedded Figure Test, are considered to have larger short-term memory capacity than field-dependent individuals (Frank, 1983; Witkin & Goodenough, 1981).

Based on many years' research and accumulative findings, Witkin and colleagues summarized and described the construct of field dependence-independence as follows (Witkin & Goodenough, 1977, 1981). Field dependence-independence is the tendency to rely on external frames (given situations, circumstances, and significant or authoritative others) or internal frames (oneself and one's own body) for information processing and behavior. Those who are likely to rely on external referents, or "fields", as guides in information processing are field-dependent individuals. They are more interpersonally oriented and more able to get along with others, but function less autonomously, have less cognitive restructuring ability, and seem likely to adhere to the field. On the other side of the continuum are field-independent individuals, who have the tendency to use internal frames, including body information (kinesthetic feedback and proprioceptive awareness), for their information processing and behaviors. They are more autonomous in decision-making, have stronger cognitive restructuring ability, and are more sensitive to body information. However, they tend to demonstrate lower ability in interpersonal relationship.

Field dependence-independence is considered as a personality trait that is set at a relatively early stage in life (Witkin et al., 1954; Witkin, Goodenough, & Karp, 1967). As with other personality traits, field dependence-independence can affect people in many domains. In fact, the characteristics of field dependence-independence are evident in perceptual, intellectual, educational, vocational, and social domains (Witkin & Goodenough, 1977, 1981; Witkin, Goodenough, & Karp, 1967). That is, relatively field-dependent individuals and relatively field-independent individuals have self-consistent individual differences in diverse domains with regard to characteristics that they bear respectively. One of the most thoroughly investigated areas with regard to field dependence-independence is educational-vocational preferences, choices, and performance (Saracho, 1997; Witkin et al., 1977; Witkin & Goodenough, 1977, 1981). Generally speaking, field-dependent individuals are found to favor and be more competent in careers requiring interpersonal associations such as educational and social work. Field-independent individuals are found to favor and be more competent in careers requiring cognitive restructuring ability with solitary situation such as sciences, engineering, architecture, and art.

FIELD DEPENDENCE-INDEPENDENCE AND SPORT RELATED SETTINGS

Another area that has consistently been found to have consistent relationships with field dependence-independence is sport related settings, which includes sports ability, novel motor skill acquisition, and learning behaviors in physical education classes.

Field Dependence-Independence and Sports Ability

Because field-independent people have a more articulated body concept and tend to rely more on proprioceptive information in detecting their own body position in the Rod-and-Frame test, it was hypothesized that people with higher skills in athletic activities, who must rely on accurate proprioceptive information to make rapid postural adjustments while moving through space, were more field independent than their counterparts who were less athletic skilled (Meek & Skubic, 1971). Along this line several studies were conducted to compare field dependence-independence between national or university athletes and non-athletes.

As early as 1978, Rotella and Bunker made a comparison in dependence-independence between twenty senior male tennis players and a similar aged non-athlete group. As expected, the senior tennis players were found to be significantly more field independent than the non-athlete group. In McLeod's (1985) study, Rod-and-Frame test was administered to 120 subjects who were either participating in varsity sports in swimming, gymnastics, basketball, volleyball and soccer, or non-participants. The comparison indicated that varsity athletes were more field-independent than non-participating subjects. Further, a study by Brady (1995) involved university athletes who were currently participating in Division II of the NCAA and a similarly sized group of non-athletes. Again the resembling results were obtained that highly athletic skilled and physically active individuals are more field independent than the less athletic skilled and less fit ones. The congruent findings also came from Liu (1991), when scores on the Rod-and-Frame Test for elite male high jumpers were compared with those of non-athletes.

The similar comparisons were also made among the public school students, who were obviously much more homogeneous in their sport ability than national or university varsity athletes and non-athletes. Despite this homogeneity, however, the findings were consistent with those discussed above. In their study Meek and Skubic (1971) found the highly skilled high school females were significantly more field independent than the less skilled counterparts. In another study (1972) with junior high school females, Shugart, Souder and Bunker selected 30 girls who got the Rod-and-Frame Test scores at the two extreme ends of the continuum of field dependence-independence (15 field-independent and 15 field-dependent subjects), and a test for dynamic, non-locomotor balancing ability was administered to them. The data analysis revealed that the field-independent group performed significantly better on the stabilometer test of balancing ability. Still with high school students as subjects, Docherty and Boyd (1982) examined the relationship between field dependence-independence and several sport skills via a multiple regression analysis. Results again were consistent with the above-mentioned findings showing that field-independent students demonstrated better performance in volleyball, tennis, and badminton.

In 1990, Raviv and Nabel conducted a study that involved the administration of two instruments, the Rod-and-Frame apparatus and the Embedded Figures Test, to assess field dependence-independence. Ninety-four subjects, boys and girls, again were all high school students. Of these subjects 33 were active in individual sports, 31 were in team sports, and 30 were non-athletes. On both measures, high school student athletes, both in individual sports and in team sports, were characterized by field independence, while non-athletes were relatively field-dependent. Consistent with these findings is McLeod's (1987) study in which public school students were involved. Again student athletes were found more field-independent than their non-athlete counterparts. Further, more recent studies also reported the same direction in the relationship between field dependence-independence and sports ability (Golomer, Cremieux, Dupuis, Isableu, & Ohlmann, 1999; Vuillerme, Teasdale, & Nougier, 2001)

It seems that research on the relationship of field dependence-independence to athletic skills/abilities produced highly consistent results: individuals with highly athletic skills and abilities are more field independent than those with less athletic skills and abilities.

Field Dependence-Independence and Novel Motor Skill Acquisition

If individuals with highly athletic skills and abilities are more field independent than those with poorly athletic skills and abilities, does this mean that field-independent individuals could learn sport skills faster and better than field-dependent individuals?

As discussed in the Instruction section, the Embedded Figure Test is related to cognitive restructuring or analytical ability (Witkin & Goodenough, 1981). Because field-independent people can obtain higher scores on various embedded figures tests than do field-dependent people, the former are considered to have higher analytical ability and will be more successful in learning situation in which the inherent structure is lacking. Conversely, because field-dependent individuals are less competent in analytical and restructuring tasks, therefore, they could be less successful in an unstructured learning situation requiring them to analyze the structure and find the inherent relationship of a new task (Swinnen, 1984). In the physical education area, when students are initially presented with a new sport skill, they are usually unaware of the idea inherent relationship of the parts to the whole skill, experiencing the new skill as a task lacking a clear inherent structure.

In addition, children in physical education class who learn new motor skills rarely have textbooks available. Instead, children depend mainly on physical education teachers for information of new motor skills when teachers give presentation, demonstration, and feedback. This source of information, however, is not always available when students need it, thus making the analytical ability more critical.

Swinnen was one of the most active investigators in this aspect. One of his studies (1984) involved children learning new motor skills on the trampoline. The study was designed so that only some global demonstrations and verbal presentation of the skills were presented, no detailed information of movement parts were given, leaving organization and structuring of the motor skills to the subjects, who were not familiar with the trampoline. The learning aim was to perform the skills as well as possible without external aid after initial global demonstration and presentation. The hypothesis of Swinnen's study was that field-dependent children would show a lower learning rate than field-independent children in an unstructured learning situation. This hypothesis was supported in the study for boys, although not for girls. Two years later, Swinnen and colleagues (Swinnen, Vandenberghe, & Van Assche, 1986) conducted another similar study with more than one hundred 13-year-old boys and girls. Again, the result was in favor of field-independent children.

For their thesis and dissertation, Jorgensen (1972) and MacGillivary (1980) also examined the relationship between field dependence-independence and motor skill learning. In Jorgensen's study, subjects were required to learn a novel movement task - the Alaskan Yo-Yo. The results indicated that the rate of learning for groups was significantly different and in favor of field-independent subjects. In MacGillivary's study, the learning of a ball catching task was used, and field-independent subjects demonstrated a significantly greater rate and amount of learning than the field-dependent subjects. Consistent with the above results is another study by Goulet, Talbot, Drouin, and Trudel (1988) in which it was found again that field-independent subjects tended to learn faster in novel motor skills. Because field independence is concerned with analytic functioning and characterizes a person's problem-solving abilities, and because rapid learning has been associated with similar conceptual elements of differentiation and structuring, it would seem reasonable that rate of motor skill acquisition and field independence are positively related (Jorgensen, 1972).

Swinnen (1983) produced another way to understand the relationship of the rate of motor learning to field dependence-independence. Swinnen argued that, in motor learning, the movement image and the way it was built up were so important that they could be seen as one possible explanation for the better motor performance on the part of field-independent individuals. Based on this argument, the study Swinnen conducted in 1983 involved no actual practice for learning motor tasks. Instead, the subjects were asked to describe the gymnastic skills observed from the video. The results indicated that field-independent subjects tended to give more complete descriptions of observed movements and the difference was statistically significant. Because the field-independent individuals bear the superior analyzing and structuring ability, they can build a more structured visual image of movement in the learning environment lacking a clear inherent structure, and this probably leads them to a better position to learn new motor skills (Swinnen, 1983).

As with the research on the relationship of field dependence-independence to athletic skills/abilities, the research on the relationship of field dependence-independence to novel motor skill acquisition yielded similarly congruent results in favor of field-dependent individuals.

Learning Behaviors of Field-Dependent Children in Physical Education Classes

When it has gradually become unambiguous regarding the relationship of field dependence-independence to athletic skills/ability and motor skill learning, physical educators begins to indicate concerns for field-dependent children, and investigate the learning behaviors of children with different field dependence-independence in the physical education settings.

Field-dependent students, as discussed previously, have less analytical and restructuring ability, view the task as a whole without attempting to discern distinctions. Further, they are also found to have less memory storage capacity and mental energy (Frank, 1983), compared with field-individual students. These limitations, as considered wildly, could make field-dependent students less likely to be successful in a complicated novel motor task learning environment in which analytical and restructuring ability are needed.

Ennis and her colleague (Ennis, Chen, & Fernandez-Balboa 1991; Ennis & Chepyator-Thomson, 1990; Ennis & Lazarus, 1990) carried out a series of studies identifying field-dependent children's specific learning behaviors in physical education classes. In their first two studies (Ennis, Chen, & Fernandez-balboa 1991; Ennis & Chepyator-Thomson, 1990), it was found, compared with field-independent children, field-dependent children indeed had some learning behavior problems within the analytical concept-based curriculum. As a result, they were unable to respond correctly when questions regarding prior directions or the serial order of tasks were asked, and could not work through a set of tasks in a prescribed sequence without watching other classmates working first.

The second salient learning problems observed with field-dependent children in physical education classes was their inability to understand why they had to perform certain tasks. It was especially true when the tasks were related to abstract movement concepts or were repetitive and monotonous, such as hitting the balls with the paddles against walls, or working on a ball-dribbling task. When those tasks were assigned, field-dependent children thought that these tasks were not meaningful and the purpose of practicing them were obscure. This perspective tended to result in off-task behaviors that were disruptive to the educational environment unless the teacher remained close enough providing them with positive and supportive feedback. Field-dependent children's third observed learning problem was that they were uncomfortable with having to work alone. They tried from time to time to diverge from their tasks to join other children when required to work alone and this decreased their on-task time and learning rate.

Consequently, field-dependent children experienced much less success in physical education classes than field-independent children, especially in movement analytical curricula (Ennis, Chen, & Fernandez-Balboa, 1991). It was also found that physical education teachers selected field-dependent children to respond and demonstrate less often than field-independent children (Ennis, Chen, & Fernandez-Balboa, 1991).

Ennis and Lazarus (1990) did the third study in this series to observe and analyze field-dependent children's learning behaviors in the physical education settings. Due to the limitation of memory storage capacity and mental energy on the part of the field-dependent children, it was hypothesized that field-dependent children would choose less effective strategies, which require less memory storage capacity and mental energy, to accomplish a product-oriented motor performance in a complex environment (Ennis & Lazarus, 1990). In their study this complex novel motor task learning environment was intentionally designed. The motor task for the children to accomplish was to intercept a ball that had been rolled down a 3-feet ramp. The children began moving from a marker in front and to the side of the base of the ramp as soon as the ball was released at the top of the ramp, and were encouraged to intercept the ball as quickly as possible.

The results revealed that, compared with field-independent children, field-dependent children consistently chose an angle of approach toward the ball that allowed them to have more time to monitor the speed and the direction of the moving ball and their own moving speed to the ball, reflecting their limited capacity to process multiple information within a short time period. When the action of interception of the ball was analyzed, it was found that field-dependent children reduced a complex open task to a closed task in which they could separate the task and thus complete it more easily. Instead of intercepting the ball while running, the field-dependent children broke down the task into three parts: "(a) running to appropriate location to wait for the ball's arrival, (b) turning to face the ramp, and (c) intercepting the ball" (P. 43). This suggested that field-dependent children found it difficult to integrate running with intercepting, which requires bigger working memory capacity and more mental energy for information processing and decision making.

In summary, Ennis and colleagues' studies suggest less effective learning behaviors in the physical education settings on the part of field-dependent children. These less effective learning behaviors are typically evident when analytical concept-based curriculum is involved requiring highly analytical and restructuring ability, or when a complex motor task learning environment is provided requiring fast information procession. The findings of field-dependent children's less effective learning behaviors is in accordance with and parallels the results discussed in the previous sections that field-dependent individuals are less athletic skilled and slower in novel motor task learning. These results suggest important implications in teaching physical education and research directions of the issue in the future.

CHILDREN'S FIELD DEPENDENCE-INDEPENDENCE AND PHYSICAL ACTIVITY PARTICIPATION

While relationship between the field dependence-independence and sports ability, motor learning, and physical education has become increasingly clear, no attempt was made to understand the association of the field dependence-independence with physical activity participation until after 2002. As with other sport-related settings, physical activity participation involves the use of body information. In addition, sport involvement becomes one of major forms of physical activity in the present day for school children, whose physical activity levels might be closely related to sports participation (Corbin, Pangrazi, & Frank, 2000). Given the fact that field-dependent individuals and children consistently demonstrate less desirable performance in sport, motor learning, and physical education settings, field-dependent children might have lower competence and interest in physical activity participation as well, thus being less physically active than their field-independent peers. The lack of the knowledge in field-dependent children's physical activity levels might keep these children at risk of health problem now and later on in their life.

Based on the concerns mentioned above, Liu and his colleague have conducted several studies investigating the association of field dependence-independence and children's physical activity participation. These studies are either unpublished (Liu, 2002), in press (Liu & Chepyator-Thomson, in press), or just published (Liu, 2007), and will be introduced below, respectively.

Study One

In this study (Liu, 2002) 138 middle school children were involved initially. Of these 138 participants, top one-third scorers ($n = 46$, 22 males and 24 females) on the Rod-and-Frame Test (those with larger deviation from vertical position in adjusting the rod) were classified as field-dependent participants, and bottom one-third scorers ($n = 46$, 24 males and 22 females) with smaller deviation as field-independent participants. These 92 students (46 males and 46 females) were the final participants whose data were analyzed. The remaining participants falling into a neutral group in terms of field dependence-independence were excluded from data analysis.

The participants reported their physical activity levels by completing a physical activity questionnaire, which would produce four physical activity variables after data reduction: (a) minutes of physical activity, (b) minutes of moderate to vigorous physical activity (MVPA), (c) physical activity MET, and (d) moderate to vigorous physical activity MET. MET is metabolic equivalent to express energy expenditure and physical activity intensity. One MET refers to metabolic energy expenditure when sitting quietly (resting metabolic rate), which equals one kcal (kilocalorie) per kilogram of body weight per hour. Energy expenditure in any given sport or activity can be expressed as multiples of the resting MET. That is, an activity with 2 METs requires two times the resting metabolic rate, an activity with 4 METs requires four times the resting metabolic rate, and so on. MET values for various sports and activities are listed in published compendium of physical activity (Ainsworth et al., 2000). In addition, a researcher-developed survey was used for participants to report their current participation in organized sports.

The comparison was made at the percentiles of 10, 25, 50, 75, and 90 for each of the four physical activity variables mentioned above between the field-independent and field-dependent groups. The results are graphically summarized in Figure 4 to Figure 7.

The results provided a vivid contrast in terms of the levels of physical activity between the two groups. The levels of physical activity, as expressed by the four variables, of field-independent group tended to be higher than those of field-dependent group at percentile of 10.

They became almost twice, even triple, as high as those in the field-dependent group at percentiles of 50, 75, and 90 across all the four physical activity variables. For example, the ratios of minutes of physical activity (Figure 4) between the two groups were 29:25 at 10 percentile, 58:25 at 25 percentile, 104:48 at 50 percentile, 140:80 at 75 percentile, and 285:141 at 90 percentile.

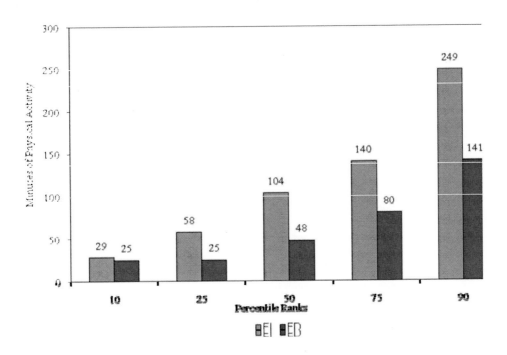

Figure 4. Comparison of Minutes of Physical Activity at Different Percentiles between the Two Groups.

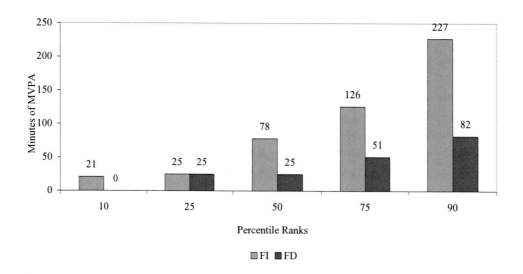

Figure 5. Comparison of Minutes of MVPA at Different Percentiles between the Two Groups.

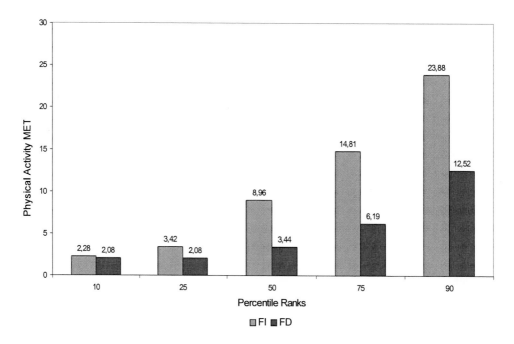

Figure 6. Comparison of Physical Activity MET at Different Percentiles between the Two Groups.

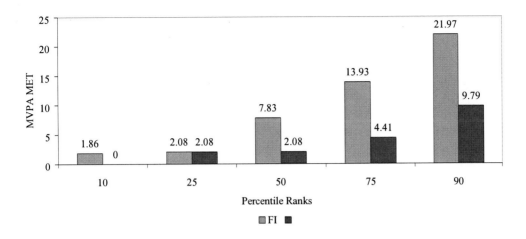

Figure 7. Comparison of MVPA MET at Different Percentiles between the Two Groups.

When a school day was divided into before-school, during-school, and after-school periods, the results indicated significant differences in the patterns of physical activity between the field-independent and the field-dependent children. Specifically, while the field-independent children had almost the same levels of physical activity as did the field-dependent children in before- and during-school periods, the former had a significant higher level of physical activity than did the latter in after-school period. This difference is demonstrated in graphical form in Figure 8 and Figure 9, which suggest that the significant difference in the levels of physical activity between the two groups came mainly from physical activity involvement after school.

Why did the field-independent children demonstrate significantly higher physical activity levels than the field-dependent children in after-school period? A close exam in participation in organized sports revealed the difference in the number of participants who were currently involved in organized sports between the two groups. While there were 20 participants out of 46 involved in organized sports in the field-independent group, the corresponding number in the field-dependent group was 10. Chi-square analysis indicated a significant difference ($\chi^2_{(1, n = 92)}$ = 4.95, p < .05) in numbers of organized-sport participants between the two groups. Most of the organized-sport participants reported the corresponding organized-sport involvement (usually lasted 90 minutes or more) on the physical activity questionnaire. The higher rate of organized sports participation on the part of the field-independent children contributed greatly to their much higher physical activity levels.

Investigation into the physical activity choices would help understand the differences in physical activity participation between the two groups. This investigation was made for the periods of before school and after school only due to the fact that physical activities during school were mainly determined by the contents of physical education classes and did not necessarily reflect the participants' choices. Table 1 provides a summary of the numbers of participants in specific activities and a rank-order list of activity choices for the two groups during the before-school period. Table 2 is the corresponding summary for the after-school period.

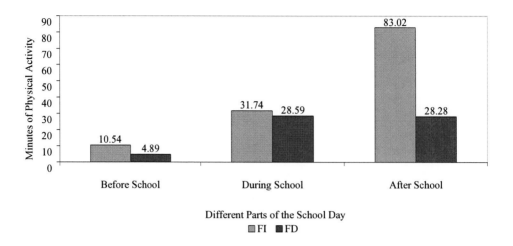

Figure 8. Comparison of Physical Activity Pattern in Mean Minutes of Physical Activity between the Two Groups.

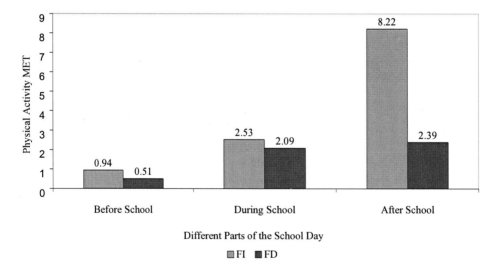

Figure 9. Comparison of Physical Activity Pattern in Mean Energy Expenditure between the Two Groups.

Table 1. Physical Activity Choice before School by Number of Participation and by Rank

Table 1. Physical Activity Choice before School by Number of Participation and by Rank

Physical activity	Field-Independent Group (n = 46)		Field-Dependent Group (n = 46)	
	No.	Rank	No.	Rank
Walking	11	1	8	1
Running	5	2	1	5
Mixed walking/running	4	3	2	2
Weight lifting	4	3	1	5
Exercise (push-ups, sit-ups, etc.)	3	5	1	5
Dance	2	6		
Indoor chores	2	6	2	2
Volleyball	1	8		
Skating	1	8	1	5
Racket sports	1	8		
Ball playing	1	8		
Gymnastics			1	5
Basketball			1	5
Football			1	5
Active games (chase, tag, etc.)			2	2
Outdoor play (hide and seek, etc.)			1	5
Total	35		22	

Note. There were 24 activities reported in the physical activity questionnaire. The activities in which there was no reported participation are not included in this table.

Walking (3.3 METs), running (8.0 METs), mixed walking/running (6.0 METs), and weight lifting (4.5 METs) ranked the first four places for the field-independent group in before-school period. As for the field-dependent group, the top four activities were walking (3.3 METs, mixed walking/running (6.0 METs), indoor chores (3.5 METs), and active games (5.0 METs) (Table 1). There was no much meaningful difference that can be detected except that indoor chores, which involves little athletic skills, was in the top rank (third place) for the field-dependent group. This could be a reflection that the field-dependent children were likely to choose physical activities that were less associated with sport skills. In addition, the energy expenditure related to top four activities was higher in the field-independent group (3.3 + 8.0 + 6.0 + 4.5 = 21.8 METs) than that in the field-dependent group (3.3 + 6.0 + 3.5 + 5.0 = 17.8 METs). In terms of the numbers of the participation in before-school physical activities, the ratio of the field-independent group to the field-dependent group was 35:22, the former was 50% more than the latter.

Table 2. Physical Activity Choice after School by Number of Participation and by Rank

Physical activity	Field-Independent Group (n = 46)		Field-Dependent Group (n = 46)	
	No.	Rank	No.	Rank
Basketball	16	1	2	6
Walking	11	2	9	2
Running	10	3	2	6
Exercise (push-ups, sit-ups, etc.)	8	4	2	6
Skating	5	5	2	6
Mixed walking/running	5	5	6	3
Indoor chores	5	5	14	1
Football	4	8	1	12
Dance	4	8	4	4
Weight lifting	3	10	1	12
Outdoor play (hide and seek, etc.)	2	11	1	12
Combatives (judo, karate, etc.)	2	11	2	6
Outdoor Chores	2	11	1	12
Bicycling	1	12	3	5
Swimming laps	1	12		
Gymnastics	1	12	1	12
Baseball/softball	1	12	1	12
Soccer	1	12	1	12
Racket sports	1	12		
Active games (chase, tag, etc.)	1	12	2	6
Total	84		55	

Note. There were 24 activities reported in the physical activity questionnaire. The activities in which there was no reported participation are not included in this table.

In after-school period, basketball (6.0 METs), walking (3.3 METs), running (8.0 METs), and exercise (8.0 METs) ranked the first four places for the field-independent group, and indoor chores (3.5 METs), walking (3.3 METs), mixed walking/running (6.0 METs), and dance (4.5 METs) for the field-dependent group (Table 2). A remarkable contrast is that indoor chores went up to the first place in the field-dependent group as opposed to basketball in the field-independent group, indicting again that the field-dependent group tended to participate in physical activities with less athletic skills. This tendency was also demonstrated by the fact that, of the top four physical activities for the field-dependent group, only dance was somewhat related to athletic ability. By contrast, there were two physical activities (basketball and exercise) for the field-independent group that were more related to athletic ability.

The contrast of energy expenditure between the two groups became more noticeable in after-school period. While the children in the field-independent group had an energy expenditure of 25.3 METs (6.0 for + 3.3 + 8.0 + 8.0) for the top four activity choices, the corresponding number for the field-dependent group was 17.3 METs (3.5 + 3.3 + 6.0 + 4.5), with a difference of 8 METs (25.3 – 17.3). Again, there were 50% more participation (n = 84) involved in after-school physical activities in the field-independent group than that in the field-dependent group (n =55).

With respect to physical activity choices beyond school time, the field-dependent children, compared with the field-independent children, tended to participate in physical activities that were less related to sports and had less energy expenditure. Further, the field-dependent children also participated less frequently in physical activities beyond school time than did the field-independent children.

In summary, this study indicates that field-dependent children are in a less advantaged position in physical activity participation. Specifically, compared with field-independent children, field-dependent children are much lower in their daily physical activity levels, especially in after-school period, and tend to choose physical activities that are less related to sports and have less energy expenditure. This observation could be largely attributed to their low physical activity level.

Study Two

This study (Liu & Chepyator-Thomson, in press) involved 129 middle school children (62 boys and 67 girls) and used same instruments as those in the first study above, with an addition of two rating sheets for sport ability and interest in physical activity. The rating sheets were five-point Likert scales and participants' physical education teachers evaluated each student's sports ability and interest in physical activity with the rating sheets. The five points of the scales ranged from 1 indicating very poor/low to 5 indicating very strong/high. The four physical activity variables deducted for the physical activity questionnaire were the same as those in the first study: (a) minutes of physical activity, (b) minutes of moderate to vigorous physical activity (MVPA), (c) physical activity MET, and (d) moderate to vigorous physical activity MET.

Different data treatments, however, were used in this second study in an attempt to exam the relationship from another angle. Instead of just using extremely field-dependent children and extremely field-independent children to make comparison and excluding the "neutral" children, this study used all the participants' data, and various correlation analyses were employed to exam the correlation between field dependence-independence and children's physical activity level. The results are reported below.

Correlations between scores on the Rod-and-Frame Test and the four physical activity variables were all significant at the $p < .05$ level for both girls and boys. The correlation coefficients ranged from -.24 to -.28 for girls and -.25 to -.29 for boys, indicating that relatively field-independent children, who had smaller scores on the Rod-and-Frame Test, tended to have higher physical activity levels in both physical activity minutes and energy expenditure.

The correlations between the scores on the Rod-and-Frame Test and participation in organized sports were significant ($r = .30$, $p < .05$) for boys only, indicating that relatively field-independent boys were more likely to participate in organized sports than did relatively field-dependent boys, but not for girls ($r = .20$, $p > .05$). As for the correlations between participation in organized sports and physical activity levels, all the correlation coefficients were medium and large ones, ranging from .37 to .61, and significant at p < .05 level, indicating strong correlations between participation in organized sports and physical activity levels for school girls and boys.

The five-point Likert scales of rating sheets of sport ability and interest in physical activity completed by the physical education teachers were used to determine the correlations of sport ability and interest in physical activity with participation in organized sports and physical activity levels. The ratings in sport ability and interest in physical activity all showed significant correlations (p < .05) with participation in organized sports for both girls and boys, with the coefficients ranging from .47 to .58. The correlations between the ratings in sport ability and the physical activity variables were all significant (p < .05) as well for both girls and boys, with larger correlation coefficients for boys (.45 to .52) than for girls (.32 to .36). The correlations between the ratings in interest in physical activity and the physical activity variables were significant (p < .05) with all the physical activity variables for both genders. Again the coefficients for boys (.42 to .56) were larger than those for girls (.24 to .28).

Finally, the validity of the Rod-and-Frame Test was examined against the rating of sports ability with r values of -.32 (p < .05) for girls and -.45 (p < .05) for boys, and the rating in interest in physical activity with r values of -.23 (p > .05) for girls and -.32 (p < .05) for boys. That is, more field-independent children tended to get higher ratings in sports ability and in interest in physical activity by their physical education teachers.

In summary, this second study again demonstrated the associations between field dependence-independence and physical activity amounts on the part of children. Specifically, field-independent children were found to be more physically active than their field-dependent counterparts, more likely to get involved in organized sports, and got higher ratings in sports ability by their physical education teachers.

Study Three

It has long been reported that black children are less physically active than white children (U.S. Department of Health and Human Service, 1996), and as a result, black children might be in a higher risk of health problem in their future. Some studies have indicated factors that could be related to black children's lower physical activity level. These factors include social and family influences, lower self-efficacy, less access to community-based facilities, and more TV watching (Rate, 1997). Other students have addressed potentially important cultural characteristics that might be related to black children's lower physical activity level, such as different weight loss practices and different body shape-perception (Sallies, Zakarian, Hovell, & Hofstetter, 1996). To understand the relevant factors, Liu (2007) conducted this third study to compare field dependence-independence and physical activity amounts between black children (n = 47) and white children (n = 66). The results indicated a significant difference in minutes of daily physical activity against the black children, with a mean of 77.62 minutes for black children verses a mean of 121.77 minutes for the white children. In addition, a Pearson correlation (r = .35, p < .01) indicated an association of field dependence-independence scores and minutes of physical activity.

CONCLUSION

Accumulative documentations in sports ability, motor skill acquisition, and physical education settings and recent research findings in physical activity levels are consistent in that field-dependent children are a less physically skilled and less physically active subpopulation. From the perspective of theory underlying the Rod-and-Frame Test, field-independent children are less capable of using their body information (kinesthetic feedback and proprioceptive awareness) compared with field-independence children. As a result, field-dependent children have less sports potential or ability, and are less likely to participate in organized sports, which contribute to their lower physical activity levels. From the perspective of theory underlying the Embedded Figure Test, field-dependent children are less competent in analytical and restructuring tasks, thus are less successful in an unstructured learning situation that requires them to analyze the structure and find the inherent relationship of the task for themselves. This condition makes field-dependent children have a less positive experience in learning new sports skills for which they are usually unaware of the inherent relationship at the beginning stage of learning. As a result, they demonstrate less capacity of sports skill, which contribute to their lower physical activity levels.

Immediate attention and physical activity intervention are needed for field-dependent children. Physical educators can make some adaptations in instructional strategies (segmentation, simplification, fractionization, etc.) to facilitate field-dependent children's learning in sports skills, enhancing their competency in physical activity participation. Physical education classes need to be more enjoyable and less competitive for them. Competitive sports that require highly athletic skills are not suitable to field-dependent children given their lower sports ability. More required and organized physical activity in after-school period and integration of lifestyle physical activity (walking to school, taking stairs, doing chores, etc.) are reasonable directions of the intervention. More research investing how to enhance field-dependent children's physical activity level is needed.

REFERENCE

Ainsworth, B., Haskell, W., Whitt, M., Irwin, M., Swartz, A., Strath, S., et al. (2000). Compendium of physical activities: An update of activity codes and MET intensities. *Medicine & Science in Sports & Exercise, 32*(Suppl.), S498-S516.

Brady, F. (1995). Sports skill classification, gender, and perceptual style. *Perceptual and Motor Skills, 81,* 611-620.

Corbin, C., Pangrazi, R., & Frank, B. (March, 2000). Definitions: Health, fitness, and physical activity. *The President's Council on Physical Fitness and Sports Research Digest*, Series 3, No.9.

Docherty, K., & Boyd, D. G. (1982). Relationship of disembedding ability to Performance in volleyball, tennis, and badminton. *Perceptual and Motor Skills, 54,* 1219-1224.

Ennis, C. D., & Chen, A., Fernandez-Balboa, J. M. (1991). Cognitive style differences within an analytical curriculum: Examples of success and nonsuccess. *Early Child Development and Care, 74,* 123-134.

Ennis, C. D., & Chepyator-Thomson, J. R. (1990). Learning characteristics of field-dependent children within an analytical concept-based curriculum. *Journal of Teaching in Physical Education, 10,* 170-187.

Ennis, C. D., & Lazarus, J. C. (1990). Cognitive style and gender differences in children's motor task performance. *Early Child Development and Care, 64,* 33-46.

Frank, B. M. (1983). Flexibility of information processing and the memory of field-independent and field-dependent learners. *Journal of Research in Personality, 17,* 89-96.

Golomer, E., Cremieux, J., Dupuis, P., Isableu, B., & Ohlmann, T. (1999). Visual contribution to self-induced body-sway frequencies and visual perception of male professional dancers. *Neuroscience Letters, 276,* 189-192.

Goulet, C., Talbot, S., Drouin, D., & Trudel, P. (1988). Effect of structured ice hockey training on scores on field dependence-independence. *Perceptual and Motor Skill, 66,* 175-181.

Jorgensen, J. M. (1972). *The relationship between perceptual style and rate of learning a novel movement task.* Unpublished master's thesis, University of Wisconsin.

Liu, W. (1991). A preliminary study of nerve types and field dependence-independence of Chinese male high jump masters of sports. *Acta Psychologica Sinica, 23,* 62-68.

Liu, W. (2002). *Field dependence-independence and physical activity among adolescents.* Unpublished Dissetation, the University of Georgia.

Liu, W. (2007). Field dependence-independence and physical activity of black and white adolescents. *Perceptual and Motor Skills, 104,* 722-724.

Liu, W., & Chepyator-Thomson. (in press). Associations among field dependence-independence, sports participation, and physical activity level among school children.

MacGillivary, W. W. (1980). Perceptual style, critical viewing time, and catching skill. *International Journal of Sport Psychology, 11,* 22-33.

McLeod, B. (1985). Field dependence as a factor in sports with preponderance of open or closed skills. *Perceptual and Motor Skills, 60,* 369-370.

McLeod, B. (1987). Sex, structured sport activity, and measurement of field dependence. *Perceptual and Motor Skills, 64,* 452-454.

Meek, F., & Skubic, V. (1971). Spatial perception of highly skilled and poorly skilled Females. *Perceptual and Motor Skills, 33,* 1309-1310.

Oltman, P. K. (1968). A portable rod-and-frame apparatus. *Perceptual and Motor Skills, 26,* 503-506.

Oltman, P. K., Raskin, E., & Witkin, H. A. (1971). *Group Embedded Figures Tests.* Palo Alto, CA: Consulting Psychologists Press.

Páramo, M. F., & Tinajero, Carolina. (1990). Field dependence/independence and an argument against neutrality of cognitive style. *Perceptual and Motor Skill, 70,* 1078-1087.

Pate, R. R., Trost, S. G., Felton, G. M., Ward, D.S., Dowda, M., & Saunders, R. (1997). Correlates of physical activity behavior in rural youth. *Research Quarterly for Exercise and Sport, 68,* 241-248.

Raviv, S., & Nabel, N. (1990). Relationship between two different measurements of field Dependence and athletic performance of adolescents. *Perceptual & Motor Skills, 70,* 75-81.

Rotella, R. J., & Bunker, L. K. (1978). Field dependence and reaction time in senior tennis players (65 and over). *Perceptual and Motor Skills, 46,* 585-586.

Sallis, J. F., Zakarian, J. M., Hovell, M. F., & Hofstetter, C. D. (1996). Ethnic, socioeconomic, and sex differences in physical activity among adolescents. *Journal of Clinical Epidemiology, 49*, 125-134.

Saracho, O. N. (1997). *Teachers' and students' cognitive styles in early childhood education.* Westport, CT: Bergin& Garvey.

Shugart, B. J., Souder, M. A., & Bunker, L. K. (1972). Relationship between vertical space perception and a dynamic non-locomotor balance task. *Perceptual and Motor Skills, 34*, 43-46.

Swinnen, S. (1983). Role of field dependence in perception of movement. *Perceptual and Motor Skills, 57,* 319-325.

Swinnen, S. (1984). Field dependence-independence as a factor in learning complex motor skills and underlying sex differences. *International Journal of Sport Psychology, 15,* 236-249.

Swinnen, S., Vandenberghe, J., Van Assche, E. (1986). Role of Cognitive style constructs field dependence-independence and reflection-impulsivity in skill acquisition. *Journal of Sport Psychology, 8,* 51-69.

U.S. Department of Health and Human Services. (1996) *Physical activity and health: a report of the Surgeon General.* McLean, VA: International Medical Publ.

Vuillerme, N., Teasdale, N., & Nougier, V. (2001). The effect of expertise in gymnastics on proprioceptive sensory integration in human subjects. *Neuroscience Letter, 311*, 73-76.

Witkin, H. A., & Goodenough, D. R. (1977). Field dependence and interpersonal behavior. *Psychological Bulletin, 84,* 661-689.

Witkin, H. A., & Goodenough, D. R. (1981). *Cognitive styles: Essence and origins.* New York: International Universities Press, Inc.

Witkin, H. A., Goodenough, D. R., & Karp, S. A. (1967). Stability of cognitive style from childhood to young adulthood. *Journal of Personality and Social Psychology, 7,* 291-300.

Witkin, H. A., Lewis, H. B., Hertzman, M., Machover, K., Meissner, P. B., & Wapner, S. (1954). *Personality through perception.* New York: Harper and Brothers.

Witkin, H. A., Moore, C. A., Oltman, P. K., Goodenough, D. R., Friedman, F., Owen, D., & Raskin, E. (1977). Role of the field-dependent and field-independent cognitive styles in academic evolution: A longitudinal study. *Journal of Educational Psychology, 69,* 197-211.

In: Physical Activity and Children: New Research
Editor: N. P. Beaulieu, pp. 177-193

ISBN: 978-1-60456-306-1
© 2008 Nova Science Publishers, Inc.

Chapter 8

CHANGES IN CHILDREN'S MOTIVATION IN PHYSICAL EDUCATION RUNNING PROGRAMS: A THREE-YEAR STUDY

Ping Xiang[1,], Ron E. McBride[1], Jianmin Guan[2] and April Bruene[1]*
[1]Texas A&M University, USA
[2]University of Texas, San Antonio, USA

ABSTRACT

Regular participation in physical activity is considered critical for healthy and active lifestyles among children and adults in the United States. Accordingly, many schools have incorporated running programs into their physical education curricula to maintain and enhance physical activity levels of children. Regular running has been shown to reduce the risk of coronary heart disease, obesity and enhance perceived competence and self-esteem. However, little is known about children's motivation in such programs. Even less is known about how their motivation in such programs might change over time. Inquiry into this area represents a valuable endeavor in the journey to our understanding of how motivational processes might change in children involved in physical activity. Therefore, this longitudinal study examined how children's motivation and performance changed in required running programs conducted during regularly scheduled physical education classes. Specifically, guided by the expectancy-value model of achievement choices, this study examined whether mean levels of children's expectancy beliefs, task values (importance, interest, and usefulness), intention for future running participation, and their running performance changed across grade levels and by gender. Participants (N = 90; 53 boys; 37 girls) completed a timed 1 mile run and questionnaires four times over a three-year period: twice in the fourth grade (September and May) and again at the end of the fifth and sixth grades respectively. During the study, students made the

* *Correspondence should be addressed to:* Ping Xiang. Department of Health and Kinesiology, Texas A & M University, College Station, TX 77843-4243, USA. Phone: 979-845-1668; e-mail: ping@hlkn.tamu.edu; Fax: 979-847-8987

transition from elementary to intermediate school at the beginning of the fifth grade. A 13-item, 5-point Likert scale questionnaire, adapted from previous work with elementary children, assessed children's expectancy beliefs, task values, and intention for future running participation. The 1 mile run assessed the children's running performance. Results revealed no declines in children's expectancy beliefs in running across grades 4-6. But children's task values of running and intention for future running participation decreased as they advanced from elementary to intermediate school. Additionally, children's 1 mile run times consistently improved across all three grades. Lastly, there were no significant gender differences across all variables from fourth to sixth grade. Overall, this study's results are consistent with those of longitudinal classroom research that children's task values of schooling decline over the school years. They also provided empirical evidence that negative effects of school transition on children's motivation observed in the classroom also existed in the physical activity context. Research efforts should be made to help students maintain their motivation for running during the middle school years.

Keywords: The expectancy-value model, longitudinal study, children, running programs

Physical inactivity has been identified as a primary contributing factor of the epidemic of childhood obesity in the United States (Center for Disease Control and Prevention [CDC], 2001). As a result, there is consensus that regular participation in physical activity is critical for children to maintain healthy weight and to live healthy and active lives and that school physical education represents an important avenue to promote and increase physical activity among all children, regardless of their socioeconomic and ethnic backgrounds. Accordingly, many schools have incorporated running programs into their physical education curricula to maintain and enhance physical activity levels of children.

Regular running has been shown to reduce the risk of coronary heart disease, obesity and enhance perceived competence and self-esteem (Sachs & Buffone, 1997). These running programs usually require children to run/walk in their regularly scheduled physical education classes once, twice, or three times a week over the school year. However, knowledge about children's motivation in such programs, particularly the knowledge about how their motivation might change over the school years, is limited.

In earlier studies we found that achievement goals, expectancy beliefs and task values were positive predictors of fourth graders' motivation and performance in a year-long running program (Xiang, McBride, & Bruene, 2004) and that those fourth graders became less motivated about running upon completion of this program (Xiang, McBride, & Bruene, 2006). Inquiry into this area represents a valuable endeavor in the journey to our understanding of how motivational processes might change in children involved in physical activity. Therefore, guided by the expectancy-value model of achievement choices (Eccles et al, 1983; Eccles, Wigfield, & Schiefele, 1998; Wigfield & Eccles, 2000), this longitudinal study examined how children's motivation and performance changed in required running programs conducted during regularly scheduled physical education classes as they progressed from fourth to sixth grade.

A second purpose was to investigate whether boys and girls differed in their running motivation and performance. Research evidence indicates girls are generally less active than boys in school physical education (McKenzie et al., 1995) and the physical activity levels of girls decline much sharper than those of boys (McKenzie, 2003). Therefore, it is important for researchers to take gender differences into account when attempting to assist teachers in maintaining and enhancing boys' and girls' motivation and performance in required physical education running programs. Enhancing motivation and performance may, in turn, lead to increased physical activity levels.

THE EXPECTANCY-VALUE MODEL OF ACHIEVEMENT CHOICES

As developed by Eccles, Wigfield, and their colleagues (Eccles et al., 1983; Eccles et al., 1998; Wigfield & Eccles, 2000), the expectancy-value model of achievement choices addresses that, whether or not children desire to participate in an activity, how much effort they want to put forth into an activity, their level of persistence in the activity, and their performance are all determined by their beliefs about how well they will perform the activity (expectancy beliefs) and the values they attach to the activity (task values). Attainment value (importance), intrinsic value (interest), utility value (usefulness), and cost are the four aspects of task values. Attainment value reflects children's beliefs about the importance of doing well on a given activity. Intrinsic value concerns the enjoyment children get from performing the activity or personal liking of the activity. Utility value refers to children's perceptions of how useful an activity is to them. Children tend to engage in activities if they believe their participation will be of some use to them (Eccles et al. 1998; Wigfield & Eccles, 2000). Finally, cost reflects negative aspects associated with engagement in an activity such as losing time and energy for other activities and experiencing failures. This last value is less researched in both classroom and physical education settings perhaps because of a lack of measures that can reliably and validly assess cost perceived by students. This is particularly true for those students in elementary schools.

Research in physical education reveals expectancy beliefs are positively related to children's timed 1 mile run performance, and task values are positively related to their intention for future participation in physical education as a general subject area and in running as a specific activity (Xiang, McBride, Guan, & Solmon, 2003; Xiang et al., 2004, 2006). These findings are not only consistent with what has been reported in the classroom research (see Eccles et al. 1998, for a review) but also provide empirical evidence that the expectancy-value model can be used to understand and explain children's motivation and performance in the physical activity/physical education domain. In their work on an elementary physical education running program, for example, Xiang et al. (2006) observed that fourth graders' beliefs about how good they were in the running program (expectancy beliefs) and their perceptions of how interesting and fun it was (interest) emerged as the strongest predictors of their motivation for running (intention for future participation in running, persistence, and timed 1 mile run).

Considering that expectancy beliefs and task values are crucial to children's motivation and performance in achievement settings, it is important to understand how these two constructs change as children develop. Consequently, considerable longitudinal work has been undertaken in the domain of academics. Generally, this work reveals children's expectancy beliefs and task values declined over the school years and the extent and rate of such decreases varied by domain (Eccles et al., 1989; Jacbos, Lanza, Osgood, Eccles, & Wigfield, 2002; Wigfield, Eccles, Mac Iver, Reuman, & Midgley, 1991; Wigfield et al., 1997). The Jacbos et al. study (2002) represents exemplary work in this line of inquiry. Over a six year period, they followed children across grades 1 through 12 when examining changes in expectancy beliefs and task values in mathematics, language arts, and sports. They reported that children's expectancy beliefs in all areas declined over time but the extent and rate of such declines differed by domain. For example, children's expectancy beliefs in language arts declined rapidly during the elementary school years, slowed, and finally changed very little after the seventh or eighth grade. In contrast, children's expectancy beliefs in sports changed very little during the first years of elementary school but declined rapidly thereafter. Similar patterns were observed for task values. Children's task values in all subject areas declined across grades 1 to 12. Additionally, children's task values for language arts decreased most rapidly during the elementary school years, while their task values for math decreased most steeply during high school.

Research work has also documented marked declines in children's expectancy beliefs and task values in some domains during transition periods (e.g., transition to middle or junior high school) (see Eccles, Midgley, et al., 1993, for a review). In their longitudinal work on children's achievement-related self-perceptions in math, English, social activities, and sports across the transition from the sixth grade to junior high school, Wigfield et al. (1991) found that children's expectancy beliefs in math, English, and social activities all declined. Similar declines were observed in children's interest in English and social activities. Eccles and Midgley (1989; Eccles, Midgley, et al., 1993) suggested motivational declines during the transition into middle or junior high school could result from a mismatch between the school environments and the developmental needs of students, a perspective known as the stage-environment fit approach.

In the physical activity/physical education domain, few longitudinal studies have been conducted using the expectancy-value model of achievement choices as a theoretical framework. Xiang, McBride, and Guan (2004) examined changes in expectancy beliefs and task values in physical education among children across grades two to five over a two-year period. They reported that second graders' expectancy beliefs declined as they advanced to the third grade but no such decline occurred for fourth graders when they moved to the fifth grade. Children's task values, on the other hand, declined over time. In a more recent investigation of motivational changes among fourth graders in an elementary physical education running program, Xiang et al. (2006) observed no decline in children's expectancy beliefs but reported that children's task values (importance, interest, usefulness) declined across the school year.

The Xiang et al. work provides useful information about how children's expectancy beliefs and task values in physical education and in running changed over the elementary school years, but is a short-term longitudinal project. As a result, long-term changes in children's expectancy beliefs and task values, particularly those of children older than fifth grade, are unknown. Additionally, it is unclear whether the declines observed during the transition to a new grade or new school in the academic settings would occur in physical activity/physical education settings. To this end, future longitudinal work is recommended to go beyond the elementary school years, examine long-term changes, and involve children in the transition from elementary to middle or junior high school.

GENDER DIFFERENCES

Gender differences have long been a focus in the expectancy-value model research conducted in a variety of achievement settings. Generally, boys reported higher levels of expectancy beliefs and task values than girls for "masculine" domains such as math and sports, whereas girls reported higher levels of expectancy beliefs and task values than boys for "feminine" domains such as music and reading (see Eccles et al., 1998, for a review). In their longitudinal study, Wigfield et al. (1997) found that boys had higher expectancy beliefs than girls for math and sports, while girls had higher expectancy beliefs than boys for reading and instrumental music during the elementary school years. Similarly, boys considered sports more important, interesting, and useful than did girls, whereas girls believed reading and instrumental music to be more important, interesting, and useful than did boys. Boys and girls, however, did not differ in their task values for math.

Gender differences have also been observed in physical activity/physical education. In general, boys felt more competent in and placed higher values than girls in most traditional sport and movement activities (Eccles, Wigfield, Harold, & Blumenfeld, 1993; Harter, 1982). Recent findings, however, revealed inconsistencies in gender differences among elementary school children. Xiang et al. (2003), for example, found that boys in grades two and four perceived a higher level of expectancy beliefs in throwing than did girls. However, they did not found that boys and girls differed in their task values for throwing as well as their expectancy beliefs and task values for physical education. Additionally, Xiang et al. (2006) found no gender differences among fourth graders in their expectancy beliefs and task values for running, their 1 mile run performance, and their intention for future participation in running over the course of a year-long running program. Collectively, work conducted in both classroom and physical education reveals the complexity of gender differences in children's expectancy beliefs and task values and suggests gender differences in these two constructs may be specific to activity (task) or children's age.

In sum, the goal of the present longitudinal study is to examine how children's motivation (expectancy beliefs, task values, intention for future running participation) and performance (timed 1 mile run) changed in required physical education running programs as they progressed from the fourth to sixth grade. Specifically, the following research questions were addressed: (a) Are there any mean level changes in children's expectancy beliefs, task values, intention for future running participation, and their 1 mile run performance from fourth to sixth grade? (b) Are there any significant declines in the mean levels of these variables after the transition to a new school from fourth to fifth grade? and (c) Do boys and girls differ in their motivation and performance?

PARTICIPANTS

Participants were part of a longitudinal study examining children's motivation and performance in physical education running programs. A total of 119 fourth graders (67 boys and 52 girls) were initially recruited from an elementary school in a rural community of Texas and were followed until the end of the sixth grade. The community was served by a school district that included four elementary schools, two intermediate schools, two middle schools, and one high school at the time of the study. At the beginning of the fifth grade, the 119 participating fourth graders made the transition to one of two intermediate schools having students in fifth and sixth grades. The final longitudinal sample consisted of 90 children (53 boys and 37 girls), who completed all the measures and tests four times over a three-year period: twice in the fourth grade (September and May) and again at the end of the fifth and sixth grades respectively.

All participants came from lower middle class to middle class families. Their ethnic makeup included: 63.3% Caucasian, 12.2% African American, 10.0% Hispanic, 7.8% Asian American, and 6.7% from other ethnic backgrounds. Participation in the study was voluntary and we obtained institutional, parental, and child permission prior to the study.

RUNNING PROGRAMS

The study was conducted in running programs scheduled during regular physical education classes. During the first year of the study, all children (fourth graders) participated in a year-long running program called Roadrunners. This program was integrated into the physical education curriculum by two physical education specialists (one male and one female) at an elementary school. The school offered children a daily physical education program and each class lasted for 30 minutes. Class size typically ranged from 45 to 70 students.

After completing the fourth grade, the 119 participants made the transition to one of two intermediate schools in the district. The intermediate school had a Run for Your Life running program as part of its required physical education curriculum. Students attended physical education daily for class periods of 45- to 50 minutes taught by three physical education specialists (one male and two females). Class size typically ranged from 27 to 46 students.

"Roadrunners" at the Elementary School

Roadrunners was established to promote cardiovascular health, active lifestyles, and mastery behaviors such as persistence and valuing effort among students. Students were required to run/walk once a week over the course of the school year during their regularly scheduled physical education classes. Children in kindergarten and first grade ran/walked two laps (one lap equals to one third of a mile) each week for the first semester and three laps for the second semester. Second to fourth graders were required to run/walk three laps only for the first two weeks and then could run/walk as many laps as they wished for the remaining 28 weeks. There were four levels of goals for students to achieve: 100 laps, 125 laps, 150 laps, and 175 laps. The two physical education specialists recorded the number of laps children ran/walked every time when they went out for running/walking. Parents or guardians were also welcome to come to class and run with their child.

An awards day occurred at the end of the program awarded children stickers, certificates, trophies, and plaques based on the goal (i.e., the number of laps run/walked) they had achieved in the program. In addition, the number of laps each child ran/walked over the school year was posted on the walls in the gymnasium on the awards day. Children's parents or guardians were also invited to attend the event.

"Run for your Life" at the Intermediate School

The intermediate school incorporated a Run for Your Life running program into the required physical education curriculum. This program aimed to use running as a means for promoting health-related fitness, lifelong physical activity, and goal setting skills among students in physical education classes. It was conducted for approximately 15 consecutive class days during regularly scheduled physical education classes in the spring. During the program students participated in a variety of activities that emphasized the fundamentals (e.g., running form, pacing, mileage/distance, and variety of courses/terrain) of running along with the benefits of running as a lifelong activity. One of the specific goals of the program was to have each student run laps to accumulate enough mileage equivalent to a marathon (i.e., ~26 miles) by the end of the program. Students were encouraged to run as many laps as they could each day when they went out to run. Incentives by the teachers included rewards such as allowing the early finishers their choice of activity for the remainder of the class period and permitting the use of personal stereos while running.

The program posted students' daily accomplishments on the gym wall for the purpose of tracking their progress toward the goals. The postings were not used by the teachers for comparisons among students. Rather, they helped students compare their performances with the goals as they progressed through the program.

VARIABLES AND MEASURES

The students completed questionnaires that included demographic information and self-report measures assessing their expectancy beliefs, task values, and intention for future participation in running. More specifically, while in the fourth grade, students responded to the self-report measures framed in the context of the Roadrunners program; while in the fifth and sixth grades, they responded to those self-report measures framed in the context of the Run for Your Life program.

Demographics

Students responded to questions relating to their age, gender, grade, school, ethnicity, and participation in after-school sports (this last variable was not included in the analysis). Student height and weight measures were recorded but were not analyzed in the present study.

Expectancy Beliefs

Five questions using a five-point Likert scale assessed students' expectancy beliefs about the running programs. Students were asked, "How good at Roadrunners (Run for Your Life) are you?" (1 = very bad to 5 = very good), "If you were to list all the students from the worst to the best in the running program, where would you put yourself?" (1 = one of the worst to 5 = one of the best), "Some kids are better in one subject than in another. For example, you might be better in math than in reading. Compared to your other physical activities in physical education, how good are you at Roadrunners (Run for Your Life)?" (1 = a lot worse in Roadrunners (Run for Your Life) to 5 = a lot better in Roadrunners (Run for Your Life), "How well do you think you will do in Roadrunners (Run for Your Life) this year?" (1 = very bad to 5 = very well), and "How good would you be at Roadrunners (Run for Your Life)?" (1 = very bad to 5 = very well). Responses were averaged to form a score for expectancy beliefs, with a high score indicating a high level of expectancy beliefs and a low score indicating a low level of expectancy beliefs. The Cronbach alpha coefficients of this scale for the fall of the fourth grade, the spring of the fourth grade, the fifth grade, and the sixth grade were .85, .87, 87, and .90, respectively.

Task Values (Importance, Interest, and Usefulness)

Each task value was assessed by two questions using a five-point Likert scale. They were (a) "For me, being good at Roadrunners (Run for Your Life) is?" (1 = not very important to 5 = very important); (b) "Compared to your other physical activities in physical education, how important is it to you to be good at Roadrunners (Run for Your Life)?" (1 = not very important to 5 = very important); (c) "In general, I find Roadrunners (Run for Your Life)" (1 = "way" boring to 5 = "way" fun); (d) "How much do you like Roadrunners (Run for Your Life)?" (1 = don't like it at all to 5 = like it very much); (e) "Some things that you learn in school help you do things better outside of class. We call this being useful. For example, learning about plants might help you grow a garden. In general, how useful is what you learn in Roadrunners (Run for Your Life)?" (1 = not useful at all to 5 = very useful); and (f) "Compared to your other physical activities in physical education, how useful is what you learn in Roadrunners (Run for Your Life)?" (1 = not useful at all to 5 = very useful). Questions (a) and (b) assessed importance; questions (c) and (d) assessed interest; and questions (e) and (f) assessed usefulness. Responses were averaged to form a score for importance, interest, and usefulness, respectively. A high score indicates a high level of these three variables and a low score indicates a low level of the three variables. The Cronbach alpha coefficients for the fall of the fourth grade, the spring of the fourth grade, the fifth grade, and the sixth grade were .85, .86, 85, and .86 for the importance scale, .91, .90, .95, and .94 for the interest scale, and .81, .82, .85, and .87 for the usefulness scale, respectively.

Intention for Future Running Participation

Two questions assessed this construct. They included, "If every Friday in your physical education class is a free activity day, would you choose to do running activities at all?" and

"The Roadrunners (Run for Your Life) program in your physical education class will continue next year. If you have a choice whether you want to participate in it, how much would you like to do it again?" Response scores ranged from 1 = not at all to 5 = very much. Responses were averaged to form a score for the measure, with a high score indicating a high level of intention and a low score indicating a low level of intention. The Cronbach alpha coefficients of this scale for the fall of the fourth grade, the spring of the fourth grade, the fifth grade, and the sixth grade were .77, .78, .68, and .63, respectively.

1 Mile Run Performance

A timed 1 mile run assessed children's performance in running. The 1 mile run test has historically been used as a measure of cardiovascular performance in fitness test programs such as the Presidents' Challenge. Times were recorded in minutes and seconds for each individual student. All students were encouraged to put forth their best effort and run as fast as they could in the test.

The self-report measures on expectancy beliefs, task values (importance, interest, usefulness) and intention for future running participation were adapted from those of the Xiang et al. study (2003)) and were validated through confirmatory factor analysis in an earlier study with students in this sample (Xiang, McBride, & Bruene, 2004). Results of the Xiang et al. study revealed the scores generated by these measures were both valid and reliable. For a more detailed report on the psychometrics of these measures, see the Xiang, McBride and Bruene study (2004).

DATA COLLECTION

Data were collected four times over a three-year period by the researchers: twice in the fourth grade (at the beginning and the end of the Roadrunners program), and again at the end of the fifth and sixth grades. The identical procedure was used across the four data collections. Specifically, the questionnaires were administered to the children during their regularly scheduled physical education classes by the researchers without the physical education teachers' presence. Each item was read aloud to the students. Students were encouraged to ask questions if they had difficulty understanding instructions or questionnaire items. No questions were raised while the students completed the questionnaires that took approximately 30 minutes to administer.

The 1 mile run test was administered by the physical education teachers with assistance of the researchers during the students' regularly scheduled physical education classes after students completed the questionnaires. The children ran a mile as a whole class but were timed individually in minutes and seconds. The test took place on the same tracks where students performed their daily or weekly runs.

Finally, the researchers measured students' height and weight on standard weight scales during their regularly scheduled physical education classes upon completion of the 1 mile run test.

DATA ANALYSIS

After descriptive analyses, a doubly-multivariate analysis of variance (MANOVA) was conducted to examine mean level changes over time in students' expectancy beliefs, task values (importance, interest, and usefulness), intention for future running participation, and performance on the 1 mile run. The doubly-MANOVA consisted of one within-subject factor (year in school: fall of the fourth grade, spring of the fourth grade, the fifth grade, and the sixth grade), and one between-subject factor (gender). Follow-up univariate tests were performed when the doubly-MANOVA yielded significant main effects for year in school and gender. Bonferroni tests were conducted for the post hoc comparisons of mean level changes over four different times in students' expectancy beliefs, task values, intention for future running participation, and performance on the 1 mile run.

RESULTS

Means and standard deviations of expectancy beliefs, task values, intention for future running participation, and 1mile run for the total sample as well as for boys and girls are presented in Table 1. In general, regardless of gender, students reported scores above the midpoint of the scales (i.e., 3) on expectancy beliefs, importance, and usefulness across grades four to six. However, they reported scores slightly below the midpoint of the scales (i.e., 3) on interest and intention for future running participation after the transition from elementary school in the fourth grade to intermediate school in the fifth grade. These data seem to suggest the students in this study developed less positive motivational responses about the Run for Your Life running program at the intermediate school by the end of the sixth grade.

Table 1. Means and Standard Deviations of Variables for Total Sample, Boys, and Girls

Variable	Total sample (N=90)		Boys (n = 53)		Girls (n = 37)	
	M	SD	M	SD	M	SD
Fall of fourth grade						
Expectancy	3.92	0.71	3.87	0.78	3.97	0.62
Importance	4.16	0.78	4.14	0.87	4.18	0.66
Interest	3.71	0.99	3.58	1.07	3.87	0.86
Usefulness	4.07	0.84	4.02	0.86	4.13	0.84
Intention	3.60	1.10	3.67	1.17	3.52	1.02
1 mile run (min.)	12.02	2.77	12.00	2.90	12.05	2.63
Spring of fourth Grade						
Expectancy	3.85	0.79	3.82	0.89	3.88	0.65
Importance	3.76	1.08	3.53	1.24	4.06	0.74
Interest	3.28	1.21	3.30	1.42	3.26	0.89
Usefulness	3.77	1.01	3.67	1.17	3.91	0.74
Intention	3.32	1.12	3.17	1.30	3.51	0.81

Table 1. (Continued)

Variable	Total sample (N=90)		Boys (n = 53)		Girls (n = 37)	
	M	SD	M	SD	M	SD
1 mile run (min.)	11.10	3.00	11.47	3.29	10.61	2.53
Fifth grade						
Expectancy	3.72	0.77	3.73	0.80	3.72	0.74
Importance	3.38	1.13	3.18	1.25	3.64	0.88
Interest	2.88	1.36	2.83	1.51	2.95	1.12
Usefulness	3.51	1.22	3.29	1.38	3.91	0.74
Intention	2.54	1.05	2.45	1.09	2.65	1.00
1 mile run (min.)	9.60	1.81	9.55	1.74	9.66	1.91
Sixth grade						
Expectancy	3.73	0.82	3.73	0.90	3.73	0.72
Importance	3.34	1.09	3.16	1.16	3.59	0.97
Interest	2.89	1.21	2.76	1.27	3.05	1.13
Usefulness	3.24	1.15	3.11	1.28	3.41	0.95
Intention	2.93	1.09	2.91	1.17	2.95	0.98
1 mile run (min.)	9.02	1.92	8.95	1.85	9.11	2.03

Note. Expectancy = expectancy beliefs; Intention = intention for future running participation.

Prior to the MANOVA analysis, the assumption of multivariate normality and of homogeneity of variance-covariance matrices was examined. The values of skewness ranged from -1.20 to 2.24, indicating that the variables were approximately normally distributed. The Box M test, however, revealed the assumption of homogeneity of variance-covariance matrices was not met ($F = 1.21$, $p = .007$). To address the violation of this assumption (Chen & Zhu, 2001; Tabachnick & Fidell, 2001), the alpha level for significance was set at .01 for subsequent analyses.

Results of the MANOVA analysis, reported in Table 2, indicated no significant effect for the interaction between gender and year in school and no significant main effect for gender. The main effect, however, was statistically significant for year in school, Pillai's Trace = .83, $F (18, 71) = 19.04$, $p = .001$, $\eta^2 = .83$. Follow-up univariate tests and post hoc comparisons using Bonferroni tests revealed the results as follows.

Table 2. Results of MANOVA: Effects of Gender and Year in School on Children's Motivation and Performance Variables (N = 90)

Source	Pillai's Trace	F	H_o df	Error df	p	η^2
Between-subject factor						
Gender	.09	1.42	6.0	83.0	.22	.09
Within-subject factor						
Year in school x gender	.315	1.82	18	71	.04	.32
Year in school	.83	19.04	18	71	.00	.83

Expectancy Beliefs

No significant effect of year in school was found on children's expectancy beliefs in running. That is, children's expectancy beliefs did not change as they progressed from the fall of the fourth grade to sixth grade.

Importance

There was a significant main effect for year in school, $F(3, 264) = 16.69$, $p <. 001$, $\eta^2 = .16$. The post hoc tests showed that in the fall, the fourth grade students considered running more important than they did later in the spring, in the fifth grade, and in the sixth grade. Students also perceived higher importance of running in the spring of the fourth grade than in grades five and six, indicating a decline after the transition to the intermediate school. There was no significant difference between grades five and six.

Interest

There was a significant main effect for year in school, $F(3, 264) = 15.50$, $p <. 001$, $\eta^2 = .15$. The post hoc tests showed a similar trend as for importance. While in the fall of the fourth grade, students considered running more interesting than they did in all other school years. Students also perceived higher interest of running in the spring of the fourth grade than in grades five and six, indicating a decline after the transition to the intermediate school. As with importance, there was no significant difference between grades five and six.

Usefulness

There was a significant main effect for year in school, $F(3, 264) = 14.04$, $p <. 001$, $\eta^2 = .14$. The post hoc tests showed that while in the fall of the fourth grade, students believed running was more useful than they did in all other school years. Additionally, students perceived higher usefulness of running in the spring of the fourth grade than in grade six. There was no significant difference between the spring of the fourth grade and grade five and between grades five and six.

Intention for Future Running Participation

A significant effect for year in school was found on children's intention for future running participation, $F(3, 264) = 24.56$, $p = .00$, $\eta^2 = .22$. The post hoc tests showed students expressed similar level of intention within the fourth grade (from fall to spring) and had less desire to participate in running in physical education classes as they advanced from the spring of the fourth grade to the fifth grade. However, students reported stronger intention at the sixth grade than they did at the fifth grade. A significant difference observed between the spring of the fourth grade and fifth grade indicated a decline after the transition to the intermediate school.

1 Mile Run Performance

A significant effect for year in school was also found on children's 1 mile run performance, $F (3, 264) = 72.37, p = .00, \eta^2 = .45$. The post hoc tests revealed an increase in children's 1 mile run performance across all school years, indicating children performed better in the 1 mile run as they advanced from the fall of the fourth grade to the sixth grade.

CONCLUSION

Guided by the expectancy-value model of achievement choices, the present study was designed to examine the mean level changes in children's motivation and performance in required physical education running programs across grades four to six. This study attempts to extend previous longitudinal classroom research (Eccles et al., 1989; Jacbos et al., 2002; Wigfield et al., 1991; Wigfield et al., 1997) to the physical activity/physical education domain. Results of this study revealed a somewhat complex picture of mean level changes in children's motivation and performance in running programs over the school years.

Surprisingly, the mean levels of children's expectancy beliefs in running did not significantly decline over time. That is, children held similar beliefs in their competence in running as they progressed from the fourth to sixth grade. This finding is inconsistent with classroom research that children's expectancy beliefs in math, language arts, and sports declined as they got older (Jacobs et al., 2002; Wigfield et al., 1997). One possible explanation for the disparity might be that children's expectancy beliefs in the present study were assessed within a specific physical activity, running. Children's expectancy beliefs in classroom setting were assessed within a subject domain such as math and language arts.

Perhaps the lack of declines observed in the present study reflected the impact of the physical maturation process. There is potential for children to improve their performance on running with physical maturity (Gallahue, 1989). Our data that children improved their 1 mile run performance across grades four to six seems to lend support to this view. With improved running performance, perhaps children were less likely to feel incompetent in running as they progressed across the grade levels. In their cross-sectional study with students in grades 4, 8, and 11, Xiang and Lee (1998) found no declines in students' perceived competence in running. Taken together, these findings seem to suggest children's ability beliefs (expectancy beliefs and perceived competence) in running remain stable across the school years.

The mean levels of children's task values (importance, interest, usefulness) toward running programs, however, decreased across the fourth and fifth grades with no change in the sixth grade. The mean levels of children's intention for future running participation also decreased across the fourth and fifth grades but increased by the end of the sixth grade. Overall, children in the present study viewed their running programs as being less important, interesting, and useful compared to their responses in the fall of the fourth grade. They also expressed a lower intention to participate in running in the future as they moved from elementary to intermediate school. These findings are in line with previous longitudinal classroom research that documented declines in children's task values in math, language arts, and sports across the school years (Jacobs et al., 2002; Wigfield et al., 1997). They are also consistent with the finding of the Xiang, McBride, and Guan study (2004) that children's task values of physical education decreased across grades two to five.

Research consistently demonstrates that task values are positively related to students' motivated behaviors such as activity choice, effort, and persistence. Students tend to engage in and persist in activities they enjoy and see as important and useful (see Eccles et al., 1998, for a review). Related research within the framework of the theory of planned behavior has indicated intentions are also essential to individuals' achievement behaviors (Ajzen & Fishbein, 1980). Given the importance of task values and intention to students' motivated behaviors, the declines observed in the present study are disturbing. It can be speculated that, if children tend to devalue running programs as they progress through school, they may become less motivated and less engaged in those running programs. This downward trend toward running motivation could eventually run counter to the purpose of running programs in many schools – promoting running as a lifelong activity to maintain and enhance physical activity levels of children.

Longitudinal classroom studies (see Eccles et al., 1993, for a review) have also shown that children's expectancy beliefs and task values decline after they make school transitions, particularly the transition to middle or junior high school. This research finding reveals the possibility that school transition may have a negative impact on children's motivation. No research, however, has been conducted documenting this declining motivational phenomenon with students in the physical activity/physical education domain. The present study represents an initial effort in this line of inquiry. Declines observed during school transitions in academic settings also occurred in our sample population. Task values such as importance and interest and an intention for future running participation after making the transition to an intermediate school at the beginning of the fifth grade mirrored similar declines observed in academic settings.

Eccles and Midgley (1989; Eccles, Midgely, et al., 1993) argued that declines in motivation associated with school transitions, particularly the transition to middle or junior high school, could result from a mismatch between the school environments and the developmental needs of students. They further content that students could become motivated and do well academically if they transitioned to school environments that were responsive to their changing needs and provided opportunities for continued growth and well being. Without this environment, motivational declines could result.

While the present study provides the first documentation that some of children's motivation decreased after they made the transition from the fourth grade in elementary school to the fifth grade in intermediate school, we did not examine the learning environments of the running programs these children participated in across the elementary and intermediate schools. As a result, the contribution of the learning environments of the running programs to the declines observed with the transition to a new school in the present study is unknown. Future research is therefore recommended to identify and determine factors that may contribute to these transition-related declines. Such inquiry may help teachers establish a learning environment in running programs that can better meet the developmental needs of children which, in turn, may sustain motivation for running during the middle school years (grades five to eight).

Contrary to previous research work (Eccles, Wigfield, et al., 1993; Harter, 1982; Wigfield et al., 1997), no significant gender differences were found on the mean levels of expectancy beliefs, task values (importance, interest, usefulness), intention for future running participation, and 1 mile run performance across grades four to six. These results suggest the boys and girls in this study demonstrated similar levels of running motivation and performance. This is encouraging, particularly in light of running being a potential lifelong physical activity for both boys and girls.

Three possible explanations might account for the lack of gender differences revealed in the present study. First, gender differences in children's expectancy beliefs, task values, and motivated behaviors were found most often in gender-role stereotyped activities. For example, boys are likely to report higher levels of expectancy beliefs and task values in masculine-typed activities (e.g., football and basketball), whereas girls tend to feel more competent in and value more of feminine-typed activities (e.g., dance and gymnastics). In this study, however, children's motivation and performance were assessed within running, a physical activity that is not stereotyped as either masculine or feminine. It is possible that students in this study felt that running was appropriate for both genders.

A second explanation is that boys and girls in the present study demonstrated similar performances on the 1-mile run tests across grades four to six. According to the expectancy-value model, children's expectancy beliefs and task values can also be influenced by prior performance experiences. Boys and girls in the present study were tested in 1 mile run four times over a three year time period. This provided opportunities for them to: use previous performances on the 1 mile run tests as a basis for ability judgment, along with other factors such as perception of running as appropriate for both genders, and develop their expectancy beliefs and task values of running across the school years. Because boys and girls in the present study demonstrated the same levels of performance in running from fourth to sixth grade, it is likely that they developed similar belief structures (i.e., expectancy beliefs, task values, intention) of this activity.

A third explanation is that teacher instructional practices may influence how boys and girls perceive, interpret, and respond to learning activities in school. Such influences may contribute to the gender differences observed in achievement-related cognitive, affective, and behavioral responses. Wright (1997), for example, examined how teachers' choice in language during both single sex and co-educational physical education classes contributed to students' stereotypical beliefs about physical activities. She reported that teachers' use of language was not neutral but rather contributed to a gendered learning environment where male students were more enthusiastic about and skilled at traditional team sports than their female counterparts.

Although no data were collected on possible teacher gender differentiation treatment, we observed that the teachers at both the elementary and intermediate schools made the running programs personal or relevant to students in a number of ways. They emphasized cardiovascular health benefits associated with regular running, offered boys and girls equal opportunities for participation, and primarily encouraged all students on their effort and improvement. These practices have been shown to have a positive influence on girls' motivation and achievement (Eccles, 1987; Koehler, 1990). That no gender differences emerged on the mean levels of children's motivation and performance variables over three years in the present study may be attributable to this equitable treatment of boys and girls in the running programs. Additional study, however, is needed to support or refute this postulation.

In summary, the present study adds to the understanding of how children's motivation and performance change in required physical education running programs. Results of the study revealed students' valuing of running declined as they moved from elementary to intermediate school, supporting the view that students' task values generally decline across the school years. This study also revealed declines in some of the students' running motivation (importance, interest, intention for future running participation) as they made the transition to the intermediate school, providing the first empirical evidence that negative effects of school transition on children's motivation observed in the classroom also existed in the physical activity context. We recommend that teachers be cognizant of these negative effects on students' motivation and work with researchers to find ways to help minimize such effects during the transition from elementary to intermediate or middle school. Finally, since boys and girls did not differ significantly in their belief structures of running and performance on the 1 mile run, teachers may expect that both genders are capable of attaining similar levels of accomplishment in running programs during early adolescent years.

REFERENCES

Ajzen, I., & Fishbein, M. (1980). *Understanding attitudes and predicting social behavior.* Englewood Cliffs, NJ: Prentice Hall.

Centers for Disease Control and Prevention (CDC), (2001). Physical activity and good nutrition: Essential elements to prevent chronic diseases and obesity. Retrieved Oct. 24, 2007, from http: www.cdc.gov/nccdphp/dnpa/dnpaaag.htm

Chen, A., & Zhu, W. (2001). Revisiting the assumptions for inferential statistical analyses: A conceptual guide. *Quest, 53,* 418-439.

Eccles, J. S. (1987). Gender roles and women's achievement-related decisions. *Psychology of Women Quarterly, 11,* 135-172.

Eccles, J. S., Adler, T. F., Futterman, R., Goff, S. B., Kaczala, C. M., Meece, J., et al. (1983). Expectancies, values and academic behaviors. In J. T. Spence (Ed.), *Achievement and achievement motives* (pp. 75-146). San Francisco: W. H. Freman.

Eccles, J. S., & Midgley, C. (1989). Stage/environment fit: Developmentally appropriate classrooms for early adolescents. In R. E. Ames & C. Ames (Eds.), *Research on motivation in education* (Vol. 3). New York: Academic Press.

Eccles, J. S., Midgley, C., Wigfield, A., Buchanan, C. M., Reuman, D., Flanagan, C., & Mac Iver, D. (1993). Development during adolescence: The impact of stage/environment fit on young adolescents' experiences in schools and families. *American Psychologist, 48,* 90-101.

Eccles, J. S., Wigfield, A., Flanagan, C. A., Miller, C., Reuman, D. A., & Yee, D. (1989). Self-concepts, domain values, and self-esteem: Relations and changes at early adolescence. *Journal of Personality, 57,* 283-310.

Eccles, J. S., Wigfield, A., Harold, R. D., & Blumenfeld, P. (1993). Age and gender differences in children's self- and task perceptions during elementary school. *Child Development, 64,* 830-847.

Eccles, J. S., Wigfield, A., & Schiefele, U. (1998). Motivation to succeed. In W. Damon (Series Ed.) & N. Eisenberg (Vol. Ed.), *Handbook of child psychology* (5th ed., Vol. 3, pp. 1017-1095). New York: Wiley.

Gallahue, D. (1989). *Understanding motor development: Infants, children, adolescents* (2nd ed.). Indianapolis, IN: Benchmark.

Harter, S. (1982). The perceived competence scale for children. *Child Development, 53,* 87-97.

Jacobs, J. E., Lanza, S., Osgood, D. W., Eccles, J. S., & Wigfield, A. (2002). Changes in children's self-competence and values: Gender and domain differences across grade one through twelve. *Child Development, 73, 509-527.*

Koehler, M. S. (1990). Classrooms, teachers, and gender differences in mathematics. In E. Fennema & G. Leder (Eds.), *Mathematics and gender* (pp. 10-25). New York: Teachers College.

McKenzie, T. L. (2003). Health-related physical education: Physical activity, fitness, and wellness. In S. J. Silverman & C. D. Ennis (Eds.), *Student learning in physical education* (2nd ed., pp. 207-226). Champaign, IL: Human Kinetics.

McKenzie, T. L., Feldman, H., Woods, S., Romero, K., Dahlstrom, V., Stone, E., et al. (1995). Student activity levels and lesson context during third grade physical education. *Research Quarterly for Exercise and Sport, 66,* 184-193.

Sachs, M. L., & Buffone, G. W. (1997). *Running as therapy: An integrated approach.* Lincoln, NE: University of Nebraska Press.

Tabachnick, B. G., & Fidell, L. S. (2001). *Using multivariate statistics* (4th ed.). Needham Heights, MA: Allyn & Bacon.

Wigfield, A., & Eccles, J. C. (2000). Expectancy-value theory of achievement motivation. *Contemporary Educational Psychology, 25,* 68-81.

Wigfield, A., Eccles, J. S., Mac Iver, D., Reuman, D., & Midgley, C. (1991). Transitions at early adolescence: Changes in children's domain-specific self-perceptions and general self-esteem across the transition to junior high school. *Developmental Psychology, 27,* 552-565.

Wigfield, A., Eccles, J. S., Yoon, K. S., Harold, R. D., Arbreton, A. J., Freedman-Doan C., et al. (1997). Change in children's competence beliefs and subjective task values across the elementary school years: A 3-year study. *Journal of Educational Psychology, 89,* 451-469.

Wright, J. (1997). The construction of gendered contexts in single sex and coeducational physical education lessons. *Sport, Education, and Society, 2,* 55-72.

Xiang, P., & Lee, A. (1998). The development of self-perceptions of ability and achievement goals and their relations in physical education. *Research Quarterly for Exercise and Sport, 69,* 231-241.

Xiang, P., McBride, R., & Bruene, A. (2004). Fourth graders' motivation in an elementary physical education running program. *The Elementary School Journal, 104,* 253-266.

Xiang, P., McBride, R., & Bruene, A. (2006). Fourth-grade students' motivational changes in an elementary physical education running program. *Research Quarterly for Exercise and Sport, 77,* 195-207.

Xiang, P., McBride, R., & Guan, J. M. (2004). Children's motivation in Elementary Physical Education: A longitudinal study. *Research Quarterly for Exercise and Sport, 75,* 71-80.

Xiang, P., McBride, R., Guan, J. M., & Solmon, M. (2003). Children's motivation in elementary physical education: An expectancy-value model of achievement choice. *Research Quarterly for Sport and Exercise, 74,* 25-35.

In: Physical Activity and Children: New Research
Editor: N. P. Beaulieu, pp. 195-210

ISBN: 978-1-60456-306-1
© 2008 Nova Science Publishers, Inc.

Chapter 9

DEVELOPMENT OF MOTOR ERROR DETECTION CAPABILITY IN AN UNDERHAND THROWING TASK

Melissa A. Fleischauer and David E. Sherwood[*]
University of Colorado, Boulder, CO, USA

ABSTRACT

The purpose of the study was to determine the rate of development of motor error detection capability in elementary school children. Fifty-five children aged 6 - 11 yrs and 9 adults (mean age 26 yrs) tossed 2 oz and 4 oz beanbags with eyes closed to a floor target located 198 cm away. Participants performed 16 acquisition trials using an underhand toss, 8 trials for each weight bag using both dominant and non-dominant hands. Following each trial, the participant was asked to estimate where the tossed bag landed by placing a second beanbag at the predicted landing point. The actual landing point was then revealed to the participant. Following the acquisition trials, 8 trials were performed without feedback of the actual landing point. The mean absolute difference in distance between the actual landing point and the estimated landing point was the measure of error detection capability. Throwing accuracy was also determined by measuring the absolute distance between the landing point of the toss and the center of the target board. Acquisition accuracy improved significantly with age, from 58 cm error for the 6 yr olds to 21 cm for the adults. Error detection capability also improved significantly with age with estimation errors decreasing from 51 cm in the 6 yrs olds to 20 cm in the adults. Accuracy and estimation errors were reduced on the no feedback trials compared to acquisition. Trial-to-trial variability also improved with age for both accuracy and estimation scores. The results suggest that accuracy in force production and the ability to detect errors based on proprioceptive feedback improves markedly with age. The results imply that teachers, coaches, and clinicians can expect reliable estimations from children about their movements, particularly as they approach 11 and 12 years of age.

---

[*] Address correspondence to: David E. Sherwood, Department of Integrative Physiology, 354 UCB, Boulder, CO 80309-0354, or e-mail: Sherwood@Colorado.edu.

One of the most important processes underlying human motor learning is the capability to self-detect and self-correct movement errors. Learners who can evaluate their own movement errors based on sensory feedback information and correct those errors can continue to improve without the constant need of a teacher or coach (Schmidt, 1987). In fact, the capability to successfully detect and correct movement errors is a milestone that signaled the passage from the verbal-motor stage to the motor stage of learning and allowed the learner to continue to improve without knowledge of results (Adams, 1971).

According to closed-loop control principles, error detection requires the formation of a reference of the intended movement to enable comparisons with the sensory feedback of the current movement. According to Adams theory (1971) or schema theory (Schmidt, 1975), error detection capability is a function of the strength of the recognition memory, which is developed with physical practice and knowledge of results (KR). The recognition memory provides reference information for the intended movement, called the *perceptual trace* by Adams (1971) or *expected sensory consequences* by Schmidt (1975), that are compared with response-produced feedback. Any difference between the expected sensory feedback and the response produced feedback results in an error signal that serves as the basis for correcting the response. The movement correction generated by the error detection process can be applied during the movement if time allows, or if not, on the next practice trial. With practice, the learner becomes consciously aware of the error and can verbalize it via an error labeling process (Schmidt, 1975). The error labeling process is controlled by an error-labeling schema, which is also developed with practice and knowledge of results. The strength of the error detection and error labeling capability is usually indexed by the correlation and/or the mean absolute difference between actual and estimated movement characteristics. As learners are better able to detect and label errors, the correlation between the actual and estimated scores should increase while the difference between the scores should decrease. Interested readers should also see Rubin (1978) for an excellent analysis of current error detection methods and alternative approaches from the perspective of signal detection theory.[1]

Early research by Schmidt and White (1972) using adults provided strong evidence that a temporal error detection capability developed with physical practice. They asked participants to estimate their errors in a timing task with a goal movement time of 150 msec. The correlation between the estimated and actual times reached a maximum of .76 over 170 practice trials. Schmidt and Wrisberg (1973) provided further evidence for the learning of an error detection mechanism in rapid hand movements by showing increases in the correlation between actual and estimated movement times of .13 over 45 practice trials. Other evidence suggests that the reference can be auditory in nature (Newell, 1976; Zelaznik & Spring, 1976; Zelaznik, Shapiro, & Newell, 1978), or based on proprioception (Sherwood & Nishimura, 1999), and can be strengthened by variable practice (Newell & Shaprio, 1976).

However, little research has focused on identifying the rate at which error detection skills develop. For example, Marshall, Elias, and Wright (1985) asked young and older adults to discriminate distance in slow positioning movements of 20-30 cm that varied by 5, 10, 15 or 20%. All participants were poor at discriminating differences of 5% of the movement distance, but discriminability improved as the difference between the criterion and presented

---

[1] Although the methods described by Rubin (1978) are preferred in some cases, the number of practice trials required for a similar analysis of error detection capability were not appropriate for the age groups involved in the current study.

movements increased. The middle aged and older participants tended to have lower detection scores than the younger participants. However, the youngest participants in this study were 18-21 yrs, an age where error detection and corrections capabilities are likely to be fully developed.

Even though there is a lack of research on the error detection process in young children, much work has been done on elements closely related to error detection. For example, in order to detect errors effectively, one must be sensitive to changes in sensory feedback that accompanies movement. Of course, vision provides a rich source of information for movement control (Schmidt & Lee, 2005), but in many cases vision is not available, or is experimentally restricted to study the sensitivity to feedback from proprioceptors (i.e., muscle spindles, Golgi tendon organs). The sensitivity to proprioceptive feedback has been defined by Keogh and Sugden (1985) as kinesthetic acuity and it reflects the capability to detect differences in variables such as location, distance, weight, force, time, speed and acceleration. According to Laszlo and Bairstow (1980) and Bairstow and Laszlo (1981) kinesthetic acuity improves rapidly from age 5 to age 8, and can reach adult performance levels by age 12. In their "runway" task, participants slid blocks up ramps set at different angles and were asked to report which object went higher. Absolute errors decreased from about 20° to about 4° from age 5 to age 8 when active movements were made. Although errors were higher for passive movements, both active and passive movements showed the same trend with age. According to these results, children became better able to determine where their limbs are in space with age, and they were better able to determine differences in limb position when vision is not available. Such improvements in kinesthetic acuity with age would appear to be a necessary element for successful error detection since one must know where their limb is to be able to determine differences with the appropriate reference state. Accordingly, the finding that rapid improvements in kinesthetic acuity are made during childhood, suggest that similar improvements in error detection ability are likely due to the more effective sensitivity to proprioceptive feedback.

Another line of investigation has focused on the capability of young children to use proprioceptive feedback in movement control. Since young children are relatively insensitive to differences in proprioceptive feedback compared to older children, they may not use sensory feedback for the closed-loop control of movement. Rather they may use open-loop or ballistic control at an early age and shift to closed-loop control when they are more confident in their ability to analyze and use sensory feedback. For example, Hay (1978) examined the age progression of kinesthetic acuity by comparing the accuracy of active and passive pointing movements across different age levels in children. The participants consisted of children, ages 4 to 11, who performed two different types of tasks: an active movement-positioning task, and a passive movement-positioning task. In the active task, children pointed to a visual target on a tabletop using movements in the horizontal plane with vision restricted to the target lights. For the passive test, the participant's arm was moved slowly towards the targets by a machine until the participant thought that they were accurately pointing at the target and ordered the movement to stop. In both cases, the absolute distance between the subject's finger and the actual target was measured. Surprisingly, the 4, 5, and 6 year olds were as accurate in the active condition as the 10 and 11 year olds and the adults. The 7, 8, and 9 year olds showed significantly more undershooting of the targets compared to the other age groups. Errors in the passive condition were higher than the active conditions and the 4 and 5 year olds performed better than all other groups. Although kinematic or EMG data was not recorded, the author suggested that the 4 and 5 year olds used an open-loop or ballistic control strategy to reach the targets in both the active and passive conditions rather closed-loop control relying on sensory feedback. According to this notion, the 7, 8 and 9 year olds performed poorer than the 10 and 11 year olds and the adults due to the lack of experience with the appropriate analysis of sensory feedback used in closed-loop control.

More recently, Smyth and Mason (1998) asked 5-8 year olds to make aiming movements to targets that were specified by either vision, proprioception, or both. In this task, targets were placed on the top of a table and participants could either see the target or placed a finger of one hand on the target, or both. They attempted to move an unseen hand located beneath the tabletop to the target position by placing a pin at the estimated target location. All of the age groups were very accurate with average errors typically less than 1 cm, particularly with vision of the target. The 5 year olds performed somewhat better than the other age groups. Participants tended to overshoot the targets with the left hand and undershoot them with the right hand. However, as in earlier studies, kinematic data was not available to help determine whether the movements were controlled by open- or closed-loop processes. Clearly the 5 year olds were not at a disadvantage when relying on proprioception.

Although studies directly focusing on the development of error detection capability in children have not been done, there is considerable evidence that children can improve kinesthetic acuity with age and learn to use proprioceptive feedback in movement control as they age. Given that these two important elements of error detection do improve with age in young children, one would also expect error detection capability to improve in a similar way. Taken together, these two lines of evidence suggest that movement error detection should improve with age between the years of 6 and 10. Beginning with age 11 or 12, error detection should be very similar to young adults. Young children also appear to use open-loop control to a greater extent than older children, who are more adept at closed-loop control. However, in the current study a ballistic throwing task was chosen to equate the type of control used by the participants. Accordingly, any changes in throwing accuracy with age should be due to more efficient motor programming processes rather than the better use of sensory feedback and online corrections.

METHODS

Participants

The participants were 55 normal elementary school students from the same private school between the ages of 6 and 11 years and 9 adults aged 21-47 (mean age 26 years) from the student, faculty and staff university population who volunteered for the study. The participant, or the parent or guardian of each participant gave informed consent. Descriptive data for the participants are shown in Table 1.

Table 1. Age and Gender of the Participants

Age	n	Male	Female	LH	RH
6	8	5	3	1	7
7	5	1	4	0	5
8	12	6	6	2	10
9	14	4	10	3	11
10	11	4	7	2	9
11	5	1	4	0	5
Adults	9	4	5	0	9
Totals	64	25	39	8	56

Note: LH is left-handed and RH is right-handed.

Apparatus and Task

The task required the participant to toss turtle-shaped beanbags to a floor target 198 cm away with an underarm throw with the eyes closed. The beanbags were either 2 oz or 4 oz and were tossed with both the dominant and the nondominant hand. The target was a 30.5 cm x 30.5 cm square at the center of a 91.4 cm x 91.4 cm Styrofoam board that was divided into 9 geometrically identical regions. The target region in the middle of the board was colored blue and it was surrounded by 8 other 30.5 cm x 30.5 cm areas of different colors. The board was placed flat on the floor. Testing was done individually in a quiet part of the gymnasium or the library.

Procedures

Before testing, the participant filled out a brief questionnaire asking them to identify their dominant hand for writing and what kinds of sports and other activities they enjoyed. The experimenter then demonstrated the underhand throwing motion to be used for the task and explained the procedures to be followed. The participant was instructed to stand behind a strip of floor tape indicating the "foul line", positioned 152 cm from the front edge of the target board, hold the bean bag in their hand with their eyes open and look at the target in the center of the target board. The participant was positioned so that their throwing arm was aligned with the center of the target board. When they were ready, the participant closed their eyes and tossed the beanbag toward the target. The experimenter recorded the distance between the landing point of the beanbag and the center of the target with a standard measuring tape, and then picked up the beanbag noting the location of the landing point on a scoring sheet. The participant was then asked to open their eyes, and indicate where they believed the beanbag had landed. They indicated this by placing a second beanbag of the same weight at the estimated landing location. Once the second beanbag had been placed, the experimenter replaced the thrown beanbag at the landing location providing KR of their throwing and error estimation accuracy. The absolute difference in distance between the actual and estimated landing location was the measure of error detection capability. The acquisition phase consisted of 16 KR practice trials, given in four 4-trial blocks combining the dominant and non-dominant hands and the 2 oz and 4 oz beanbags. The order of the test blocks (dominant-2 oz, dominant-4 oz, nondominant-2 oz, nondominant-4oz) was randomly determined for each participant. An 8-trial no KR retention test followed acquisition with 2 trials given for each hand/weight combination. Participants estimated the landing point during acquisition and retention. After the children had completed both acquisition and retention tests they were rewarded with stickers for their participation.

Data Analysis

Throwing accuracy was determined by calculating the mean distance from the nearest edge of the beanbag to the center of the target (i.e., the radial error) for each block of trials for acquisition and retention. Estimation error was determined by measuring the distance from the nearest edges of the beanbags at the actual and estimated landing locations. The mean radial error and estimation error were compared across hands and weights with a 2 (Side: Dominant/Nondominant) x 2 (Weight: 2 oz/4 oz) x 2 (Type: Accuracy/Estimation) x 7 (Age) ANOVA with repeated measures on the first three factors. Separate analyses were done for acquisition and retention.

Trial to trial consistency was determined by calculating the variable error (VE) for each set of four trials in each weight and hand condition. The VE scores were compared across hands and weights with a 2 (Side: Dominant/Nondominant) x 2 (Weight: 2 oz/4 oz) x 2 (Type: Accuracy/Estimation) x 7 (Age) ANOVA with repeated measures on the first three factors. Separate analyses were done for acquisition and retention.

RESULTS

Throwing and Estimation Accuracy

The relation between age and throwing accuracy and estimation error for acquisition is shown in Figure 1, summarized with power functions.[2] Accuracy improved markedly between the ages of 6 and 11 years and reached the minimum score at age 26. The effect of age was significant, $F(6,57) = 15.7$, $p < .001$, $\varepsilon^2 = 0.62$. Estimation errors also improved with age in a similar way as the accuracy scores. In general, errors in estimation were less than errors in throwing accuracy. The main effect of type was also significant, $F(1,57) = 31.9$, $p < .001$, $\varepsilon^2 = 0.36$. The error in estimation appeared to be substantially less than the actual error for the 7 year olds compared to the other age groups, but the Age x Type interaction was not significant ($p > .1$).

---

[2] The use of power functions to depict the age effect was found to account for more of the variance in the data compared to linear, logarithmic, polynomial or exponential functions.

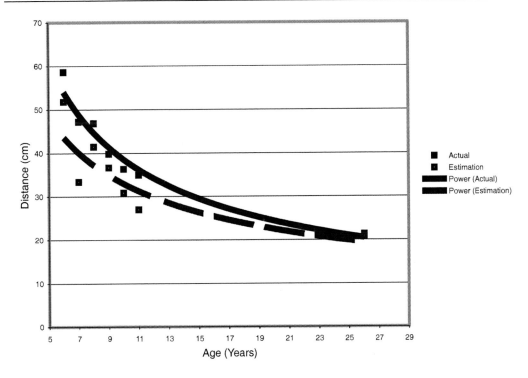

Figure 1. Actual errors in throwing and estimation errors in landing location for all age groups for acquisition. Power functions accounted for 97% and 79% of the variance in the actual and estimated errors, respectively.

The relation between age and throwing accuracy and estimation error for retention is shown in Figure 2. Accuracy again improved markedly between the ages of 6 and 11 years and reached a minimum at age 26. The effect of age was significant, $F(6,57) = 11.3$, $p < .001$, $\varepsilon^2 = 0.54$. Estimation errors also improved with age in a similar way as the accuracy scores. In general, errors in estimation were less than errors in throwing accuracy. The main effect of type was also significant, $F(1,57) = 9.8$, $p < .01$, $\varepsilon^2 = 0.15$. The effects of side and weight were not significant for either analysis. The difference between the error in estimation and the actual error appeared to be greater for the 6-7 year olds compared to the other age groups, but the Age x Type interaction was not significant ($p > .2$).

Since there was no effect of side or weight for acquisition or retention, accuracy and estimation scores were averaged across side and weight for comparisons between acquisition and retention. The 2 (Condition: Acquisition/Retention) x 2 (Type: Accuracy/Estimation) x 7 (Age) ANOVA with repeated measures on the first two factors revealed significant main effects for condition, $F(1,57) = 4.5$, $p < .05$, $\varepsilon^2 = 0.07$, type, $F(1,57) = 23.6$, $p < .001$, $\varepsilon^2 = 0.29$, and age, $F(6,57) = 15.9$, $p < .001$, $\varepsilon^2 = 0.63$. Overall, accuracy was better on retention (34.5 cm) compared to acquisition (40.6 cm) and errors in estimation were lower on retention (37.8 cm) compared to acquisition (42.7 cm) as well.

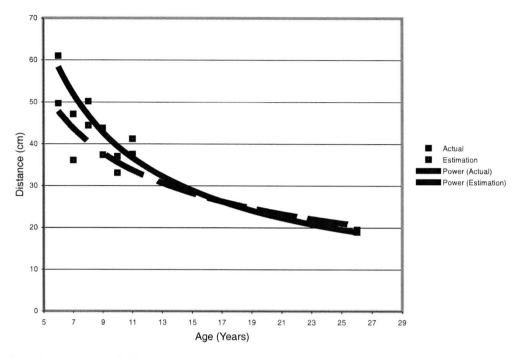

Figure 2. Actual errors in throwing and estimation errors in landing location for all age groups for no KR retention. Power functions accounted for 97% and 83% of the variance in the actual and estimated errors, respectively.

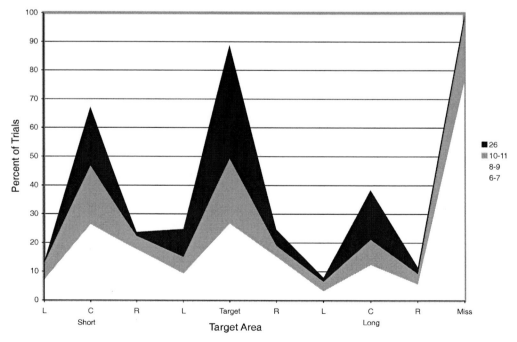

Figure 3. The distribution of throwing errors and correct throws for each age group combined over acquisition and retention. The area represents the number of trials in each category (L is left, R is right, C is center). Short errors are undershoots, and Long errors are overshoots. Miss refers to throws missing the target board.

The distribution of the errors and correct trials in throwing are shown in Figure 3 for the age groups for summed over acquisition and retention. For clarity of presentation, age groups were combined to form four groups. The area on the graph represents the proportion of throws landing in each of the nine areas of the target board. Undershoots and overshoots could have also shown directional errors (L for left and R for right) or been the proper direction (C, center). Throws could have hit the target (Target) or been the proper distance but not the correct direction. The proportion of throws that missed the board is also displayed (Miss). Most of the errors were undershoots rather than overshoots and were errors in distance rather than direction. The same pattern of errors is shown for each age group. As age increased, the proportion of misses decreased and the proportion of target hits increased.

Consistency in Throwing and Estimation

The mean VE scores for movement accuracy and estimation for each age group are shown in Figure 4 for acquisition and Figure 5 for retention. Trial-to-trial consistency improved with age for both movement accuracy and errors in estimation for both acquisition and retention. The effect of age was significant for acquisition, $F(6,57) = 10.02$, $p < .001$, $\varepsilon^2 = 0.51$, and retention, $F(6,57) = 9.12$, $p < .001$, $\varepsilon^2 = 0.49$. Generally, participants were more consistent in their error estimations compared to their actual performance errors. The effect of type was significant for acquisition, $F(1,57) = 10.45$, $p < .01$, $\varepsilon^2 = 0.16$, but did not reach traditional significance levels for retention, $F(1,57) = 3.55$, $p < .07$, $\varepsilon^2 = 0.06$. The Age x Type interaction was not significant for acquisition ($p > .2$) or retention ($p > .3$).

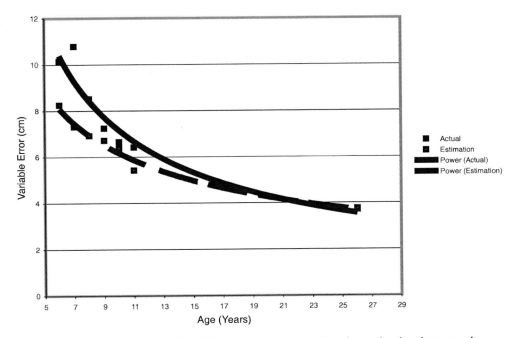

Figure 4. Mean trial to trial variability (VE) for actual errors in throwing and estimation errors in landing location for all age groups for acquisition. Power functions accounted for 95% and 98% of the variance in the VE scores for the actual and estimated scores, respectively.

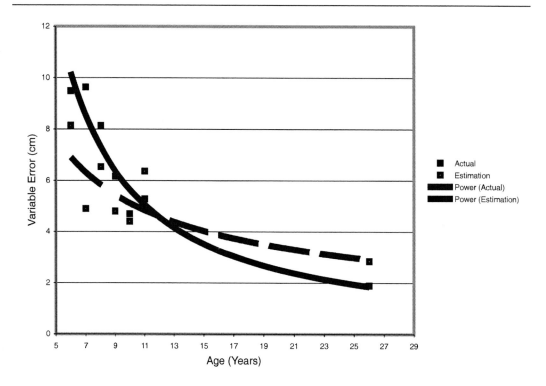

Figure 5. Mean trial to trial variability (VE) actual errors in throwing and estimation errors in landing location for all age groups for no KR retention. Power functions accounted for 96% and 69% of the variance in the VE scores for the actual and estimated scores, respectively.

Since there was no effect of side or weight for acquisition or retention, VE scores for accuracy and estimation were averaged across side and weight for comparisons between acquisition and retention. The 2 (Condition: Acquisition/Retention) x 2 (Type: Accuracy/Estimation) x 7 (Age) ANOVA with repeated measures on the first two factors revealed significant main effects for condition, $F(1,57) = 11.6$, $p < .01$, $\varepsilon^2 = 0.17$, type, $F(1,57) = 8.6$, $p < .01$, $\varepsilon^2 = 0.13$, and age, $F(6,57) = 14.8$, $p < .001$, $\varepsilon^2 = 0.61$. Overall, trial-to-trial variability in accuracy was lower on retention (15.0 cm) compared to acquisition (17.8 cm) and variability in estimation was lower on retention (15.0 cm) compared to acquisition (17.8 cm) as well.

DISCUSSION

The major goal for the current study was to determine how error detection capability develops with age. Participants tossed beanbags attempting to hit a target 198 cm away without vision, but with KR provided during acquisition. The main procedural departure from earlier studies involving adults (e.g., Schmidt & White, 1972) was that error detection capability was determined by having the participants place a second beanbag where they thought the thrown beanbag had landed. The absolute distance between the two beanbags was the estimate of error detection capability. Based on previous research, one expected improvements in both throwing accuracy and error detection capability with age.

Throwing Accuracy and Age

As expected, throwing accuracy improved with age (Figures 1 and 2). The youngest age group missed the target board on almost half their throws, and when they did hit the target board, they missed the target square by nearly 60 cm (2 target zones). Clearly, tossing beanbags without vision was challenging for the 6-year-old group. However, as age increased marked improvements were noted in throwing accuracy. By ages 10 and 11, throwing errors were less than 38 cm on average, and the target board was missed only 20% of the time. By adulthood, throwing errors were less than 25 cm, and the target board was missed less than 2% of the time. The current pattern of results replicates earlier work by Gardner (1979) who had children toss tennis balls into a basket with a 13.5 in (34.3 cm) diameter from either 6 feet (183 cm) or 9 feet (274 cm) with vision available. In this study throwing accuracy improved from 26% to 53% successful tosses as age increased from 5 to 8 years of age. Older children tossing to the 9-foot (274 cm) target showed improvements from 32% to 53% successes between the ages of 9 and 15 years. Of course, the advantage of the current study was that errors were measured precisely, rather than the hit/miss dichotomy used by Gardner (1979). Nevertheless, the study supports the notion that as children mature they become better able to produce accurate movements without vision by adjusting the amount of force used (Whiting & Cockerill, 1972, 1974).

According to motor programming theory, movements of different distance are accomplished by selecting a force or amplitude parameter to be used with the generalized motor program for throwing (Schmidt, 1975; Schmidt & Lee, 2005). The youngest children in the current study had difficulty selecting the proper force parameter and producing effective throws relative to the other children and the adults. However, as age increased, children were more successful in choosing the correct force parameter and improving throwing accuracy. According to schema theory (Schmidt, 1975), the older children had formed a strong recall schema, which allowed them to appropriately vary the force parameter to reduce throwing errors in the absence of visual feedback. The youngest children were still in the process of developing recall schemas for force parameterization.

For acquisition and retention, the errors in throwing were about 30% of the goal distance in the 6 year olds compared to about 10% for the adults. The relative errors here are very similar to errors reported by Whiting and Cockerill (1972) in a task where children had to push a trolley up a ramp different target distances without vision. For the trolley task, relative errors for the 5 and 6 year olds were about 29% for the shortest distance target (i.e., 60 cm) and between 22% and 24% for target distances ranging from 119 cm to 169 cm. Relative errors for the adults ranged from 13% to 11% as distance increased. With vision relative errors were reduced markedly in the trolley task to about 15% in the 5 and 6 year olds and to 10% in the adults. With age, it is clear that children can also improve their relative errors in throwing as well as the absolute errors as the force production processes become more efficient.

Despite the high absolute and relative errors in the 6 year olds, performance of the group on the retention trials was very good. In fact, the actual errors and the errors in estimation for all groups were smaller on retention compared to acquisition. This finding suggests that all groups had acquired the task well enough to perform the task without extrinsic feedback.

The analysis of errors indicated that all participants tended to undershoot the target rather than overshoot (Figure 3). In fact the proportion of target hits and undershoots was about equal for the children. By adulthood, the target square was hit a majority of the time, with errors equally distributed between over- and undershoots. The preponderance of distance errors, rather than directional errors, suggests that the errors were due to differences in the amount of force produced or to the timing of the release point instead of variations in the path of the hand.

One surprising result was the lack of difference between the dominant and nondominant hands in terms of accuracy or trial-to-trial variability, particularly for the older children. Prior work had demonstrated a greater throwing accuracy advantage for the dominant hand compared to the nondominant hand in 10-13 year olds compared to 6-9 year olds (Burge, 1952). More recently, Rigal (1992) has shown a dominant hand advantage for a number of basic motor abilities involving the hand including visually-based aiming and arm-hand steadiness in 6-9 year olds. However, nearly all the comparisons between dominant and nondominant hands in young children have used motor tasks where vision was available. In the current study throwing was done without vision suggesting that differences in dominant and nondominant hand for ballistic tasks may not emerge until later in childhood. However, lateral asymmetries have been established in more complicated throwing actions (i.e., the overarm throw) in 4-10 year olds when vision is available (Teixeira & Gasparetto, 2002). But, it is possible that the high trial-to-trial variability in throwing under non-visual conditions masked any between-hand differences in throwing accuracy. Clearly further work is needed in this area.

Error Estimation and Age

As noted above, the main goal of the current study was to determine how error detection capability develops with age. As shown in Figure 1, errors in estimation decreased with age from about 51 cm of error in the 6 year olds to just over 25 cm in the 11 year olds. Adult participants estimation errors were less than 25 cm. The same general pattern was shown on retention (Figure 2) but the age effect was somewhat weaker, probably due to the small number of retention trials provided. The results suggest that the 6-year-old group was relatively poor at error detection compared to the other age groups. In term of schema theory (Schmidt, 1975), the youngest participants had not yet developed a strong recognition schema for the evaluation of proprioceptive and/or auditory feedback. As age increased errors in detection decreased suggesting that recognition schema strength had improved with age. As expected, the adults had the lowest estimation error suggesting they had developed the most effective error detection capability and the strongest recognition schema.

The improvement in the error detection process with age could have been due to several factors. Older children could have had better kinesthetic acuity (Bairstow & Laszlo, 1981; Laszlo & Bairstow, 1980), which would have allowed them to discriminate short and long throws more effectively, for example. The older children could also have been better at translating proprioceptive feedback into locations in extrapersonal space. That is, they could translate differences in sensory feedback to locations on the target board more effectively than the younger children. The current work, together with research with older adults (Marshall et al., 1985), suggests that error detection capability improves rapidly over childhood, is optimal throughout young adulthood and middle age, and then declines in the elderly.

Interestingly, work has also shown that children can be trained to observe and detect errors in the movements of others. For example, Liang (2001) demonstrated that fifth graders were better able to observe and detect movement errors in manipulative motor skills compared to third graders. The current work has shown that children can also learn to detect their own movement errors, and this capability improves with age. Taken together, such results imply that teachers and coaches can expect older children to reliably estimate their own movement errors, paving the way for continued improvements without the constant help of an instructor.

Performance Consistency

As age increased, participants reduced trial-to-trial variability in throwing accuracy and estimated error (Figures 4 and 5). Trial-to trial variability was the greatest in the 6 and 7 year olds relative to the 8-11 year olds. The adult group was the most consistent. The high VE in the youngest age groups suggests that they had difficulty producing a consistent force from trial to trial. It was common for participants in the 6 and 7 year old groups to show differences as much as 89 cm between consecutive throws with the same weight and the same hand. In contrast, adult participants rarely showed trial-to-trial variations in performance more than 25 cm. The relatively high trial-to-trial variability in the youngest children could have been caused by variability in the force production processes resulting in variable throwing patterns. Work by Smits-Engelsman, Westenberg, and Duysens (2003) and Lazarus, Whitall and Franks (1995) have shown that the variation in isometric force production improves dramatically from age 6 to age 9. Forssberg, Eliasson, Kinoshita, Johansson, and Westling (1991) showed that trial-to-trial variability in grip force production decreases with age, particularly between the ages of 1 to 8 years. Other work has shown that young children show more variable and less smooth aiming movements than older children and adults (Smits-Engelsman, Sugden, & Duysens, 2006; Yan, Thomas, Stelmach, & Thomas, 2000, 2003). Based on the work cited here, the improved trial to trial variability in throwing accuracy with age was likely due to the reduction in variability of force production processes resulting in smoother and less variable kinematic movement patterns. Clearly one important aspect of motor development is the capability of producing consistent motor output with regards to force production.

A second finding of interest was that participants were generally more consistent in their error estimations compared to their accuracy scores. Although the Type x Age interactions were not significant, there was a tendency for the younger participants to be more consistent in their estimated errors compared to their actual errors relative to the older age groups. The younger age groups tended to select a specific part of the target board for their estimated landing locations, rather than vary them appropriately with the actual landing point. The reduced variation in the estimated landing locations could be due to a so-called centering tendency (Cain, 1973; Stevens & Greenbaum, 1966) whereby subjects reduce the range of the variable under their control.

In summary, the current work has demonstrated that error detection capability develops rapidly between 6 and 11 years of age. The pattern of the age effect was similar for both throwing accuracy and errors in estimation, and the pattern of change with age was similar to the change in kinesthetic acuity (Bairstow & Lazlo, 1981; Lazlo & Bairstow, 1980), and accuracy in related tasks (Gardner, 1979; Whiting & Cockerill, 1972). The results imply that teachers, coaches, and clinicians can expect reliable estimations from children about their movements, particularly as they approach 11 and 12 years of age.

ACKNOWLEDGEMENTS

The authors wish to thank James Hill for his help in data collection and analysis. Melissa Fleischauer is currently with the Leadership in Healthcare Organizations program at the University of California, San Diego. Support by the Undergraduate Research Opportunities Program at the University of Colorado is also appreciated.

REFERENCES

Adams, J. A. (1971) A closed-loop theory of motor learning. *Journal of Motor Behavior*, 3, 111-150.

Bairstow, P. J., & Lazlo, J. I. (1981). Kinaesthetic sensitivity to passive movements and its relationship to motor development and motor control. *Developmental Medicine and Child Neurology*, 23, 606-616.

Burge, I. C. (1952). Some aspects of handedness in primary school children. *British Journal of Educational Psychology*, 22, 45-51.

Cain, W. S. (1973) Nature of perceived effort and fatigue: roles of strength and blood flow in muscle contractions. *Journal of Motor Behavior*, 5, 33-47.

Forssberg, H., Eliasson, A. C., Kinoshita, H., Johansson, R. S., & Westling, G. (1991). Development of human precision grip I: Basic coordination of force. *Experimental Brain Research*, 85, 451-457.

Gardner, R. A. (1979). Throwing balls in a basket as a test of motor coordination: Normative data on 1350 school children. *Journal of Clinical Child Psychology*, 8, 152-155.

Hay, L. (1978). Accuracy of children on an open-loop pointing task. *Perceptual and Motor Skills*, 47, 1079-1082.

Keogh, J., & Sugden, D. (1985). *Movement skill development*. New York: MacMillan.

Lazarus, J-A. C., Whitall, J., & Franks, C. A. (1995). Isometric force regulation in children. *Journal of Experimental Child Psychology*, 60, 245-260.

Lazlo, J. I., & Bairstow, P. J. (1980). The measurement of kinaesthetic sensitivity in children and adults. *Developmental Medicine and Child Neurology*, 22, 454-464.

Liang, G. (2001). Teaching children qualitative analysis of fundamental motor skill (Doctoral dissertation, West Virginia University, 2001). Dissertation Abstracts International, 62 (5A), 1794.

Marshall, P. H., Elias, J. W., & Wright, J. (1985). Age related factors in motor error detection and correction. *Experimental Aging Research*, 11, 201-206.

Newell, K. M. (1976) Motor learning without knowledge of results through the development of a response recognition mechanism. *Journal of Motor Behavior*, 8, 209-217.

Newell, K. M., Shapiro, D. C. (1976) Variability of practice and transfer of training: some evidence toward a schema view of motor learning. *Journal of Motor Behavior*, 8, 233-243.

Rigal, R. A. (1992). Which handedness: Preference or performance? *Perceptual and Motor Skills*, 75, 851-966.

Rubin, W. M. (1978). Application of signal detection theory to error detection in ballistic motor skills. *Journal of Experimental Psychology: Human Perception and Performance*, 4, 311-320.

Schmidt, R. A. (1975) A schema theory of discrete motor skill learning. *Psychological Reviews*, 82, 225-260.

Schmidt, R. A. (1987) The acquisition of skill: some modifications to the perception-action relationship through practice. In H. Heuer & A. F. Sanders (Eds.), *Perspectives On Perception and Action* (pp. 77-103). Hillsdale, NJ: Erlbaum.

Schmidt, R. A., & Lee, T. D. (2005) *Motor control and learning*. Champaign, IL: Human Kinetics.

Schmidt, R. A., & White, J. L. (1972) Evidence for an error detection mechanism in motor skills: a test of Adams' closed-loop theory. *Journal of Motor Behavior*, 4, 143-153.

Schmidt, R. A., & Wrisberg, C. A. (1973) Further tests of the Adams' closed-loop theory: response-produced feedback and the error detection mechanism. *Journal of Motor Behavior*, 3, 155-164.

Sherwood, D. E., & Nishimura, K. M. (1999) Spatial error detection and assimilation effects in rapid single and bimanual aiming movements. *Journal of Motor Behavior*, 31, 381-393.

Smits-Engelsman, B. C. M., Sugden, D., & Duysens, J. (2006). Developmental trends in speed accuracy trade-off in 6-10-year-old children performing rapid reciprocal and discrete aiming movements. *Human Movement Science*, 25, 37-49.

Smits-Engelsman, B. C. M., Westenberg, Y., & Duysens, J. (2003). Development of isometric force and force control in children. *Cognitive Brain Research*, 17, 68-74.

Smyth, M. M, & Mason, U. C. (1998). Direction of response in aiming to visual and proprioceptive targets in children with and without Developmental Coordination Disorder. *Human Movement Science*, 17, 515-539.

Stevens, S. S., & Greenbaum, H. B. (1966) Regression effect in psychophysical judgment. *Perception & Psychophysics*, 1, 439-446.

Teixeira, L. A., & Gasparetto, E. R. (2002). Lateral asymmetries in the development of the overarm throw. *Journal of Motor Behavior*, 34, 151-160.

Whiting, H. T. A., Cockerill, I. M. (1972). The development of a simple ballistic skill with and without visual control. *Journal of Motor Behavior*, 4, 155-162.

Whiting, H. T. A., Cockerill, I. M. (1972). Eyes on hand-eyes on target? *Journal of Motor Behavior*, 6, 27-32..

Yan, J. H., Thomas, J. R., Stelmach, G. E., & Thomas, K. T. (2003). Developmental features of rapid aiming movements across the lifespan. *Journal of Motor Behavior*, 32, 121-140.

Yan, J. H., Thomas, K. T., Stelmach, G. E., & Thomas, J. R. (2003). Developmental differences in children's ballistic aiming movements of the arm. *Perceptual and Motor Skills*, 96, 589-598.

Zelaznik, H. N., Shaprio, D. C., & Newell, K. M. (1978) On the structure of motor recognition memory. *Journal of Motor Behavior*, 10, 313-323.

Zelaznik, H. N., & Spring, J. (1976) Feedback in response recognition and production. *Journal of Motor Behavior*, 8, 309-312.

In: Physical Activity and Children: New Research
Editor: N. P. Beaulieu, pp. 211-223

ISBN: 978-1-60456-306-1
© 2008 Nova Science Publishers, Inc.

Chapter 10

ANAEROBIC CRITICAL VELOCITY: A NEW TOOL FOR YOUNG SWIMMERS TRAINING ADVICE

Ricardo Fernandes[*], Inês Aleixo, Susana Soares, J. Paulo Vilas-Boas

University of Porto. Faculty of Sport. Porto, Portugal

ABSTRACT

The regression line equation obtained through the relationship between swimming distances and respective time durations has been used to provide the estimation of the critical velocity value. This value is considered a good indirect indicator of the anaerobic threshold and, consequently, a measure of the functional aerobic capacity of swimmers. However, even in young swimmers, the majority of swimming events last less than 2.30 minutes, which reflects the importance of the anaerobic energy production as a major contributor during competition.

The purpose of this study was to assess, in young swimmers, an "anaerobic" critical velocity (AnCV), assessed with shorter test distances that could allow scientists and coaches to possess a new tool for anaerobic training control. The existence of a relationship between the AnCV and the performance during a 100 m front crawl event (first and second 50 m splits, and total time), being accepted as a good example of an anaerobic swimming effort, was tested.

A group of 32 competitive swimmers of the North of Portugal regional swimming team, 15 girls (12.3±0.7 years old, 160.5±4.7 cm, 45.6±6.6 kg and 6.3±0.5 training sessions/week) and 17 boys (13.2±0.7 years old, 169.8±9.0 cm, 54.5±7.6 kg and 6.6±0.9 training sessions/week) were included in the study. To obtain the AnCV values through the distance/duration regression line, the swimmers swam three distances in front crawl (12.5, 25 and 50 m) at maximum velocity, separated by a 30-minute rest interval. This

---

[*] ricfer@fade.up.pt

methodology is a mode-specific non-invasive method, hypothesised to estimate parameters normally obtained from blood lactate analysis. The 100 m front crawl performance values were obtained in real competition events. Mean plus SD values for AnCV and 100 m front crawl were 1.48 ± 0.06 m/s and 68.3 ± 2.0 s, and 1.62 ± 0.06 m/s and 62.4 ± 2.6 s, respectively for female and male swimmers (differences between genders were observed for both parameters for a $p < 0.001$). It was found a strong inverse relationship between the AnCV and the 100 m front crawl time ($r = -0.84$), the first 50 m partial ($r = -0.87$) and the second 50 m partial ($r = -0.79$), all for a $p < 0.001$ ($n = 32$). The value of the AnCV converted in 100 m time was not different from the 100 m front crawl event duration for each gender group ($p > 0.05$).

To our knowledge, it was the first time that the anaerobic critical velocity concept was presented for front crawl, suggesting that AnCV can be used as a control parameter for the training development of anaerobic capacities.

Keywords: Swimming, anaerobic exercise, testing, critical velocity

INTRODUCTION

With the increasing participation of children in sports (Bar-Or, 1995; Baxter-Jones and Mundt, 2007), young swimmers, like adults, strive to achieve higher performances through more developed and specific training processes. This is particularly true in swimming, since it is a sport that encourages children to begin their participation in competitive events at very young ages. Platonov and Fessenko (1994) emphasized that the ages corresponding to the beginning of systematic swimming practice, and to the involvement in the specialized training, are major determinants for achieving high-level performances.

The training control and evaluation of swimmers is considered a fundamental tool for increasing the efficiency of training processes (Mujika et al., 1995; Maglischo, 2003) and to the prediction of performance (Wright and Smith, 1994). From the several determinants of swimming performance presented in Figure 1, the bioenergetical factor seems to be one of the most important and, consequently, one of the most studied by coaches and scientists (Costill et al., 1992). Clarys (1996) observed that the studies of bioenergetics accounted for 18% of the total amount of 685 publications related to swimming. The bioenergetical studies are based upon the characterization of the capacity and power of the two larger body energy systems (the aerobic and the anaerobic ones) through the assessment of well-known physiological parameters, like the anaerobic threshold, the maximum oxygen uptake and the maximum blood lactate concentrations.

The main purpose of the bioenergetical training control and evaluation of swimmers is to determine their bioenergetical profile, and to observe the corresponding physiological changes due to the training process. In this sense, there are some valid and well accepted tests that allow swimming coaches and scientists to dispose objective and pertinent data related to the aerobic energy system. From this, it is possible to assess the anaerobic threshold through the 30-minute continuous test (Olbrecht et al., 1985), the Mader's two-speed test (Mader et al., 1978) and the critical velocity test (Wakayoshi et al., 1992a), as well as to assess the velocity corresponding to the maximum oxygen uptake using the 7 x 200 m front crawl protocol (Pyne et al., 2000; Fernandes et al., 2003).

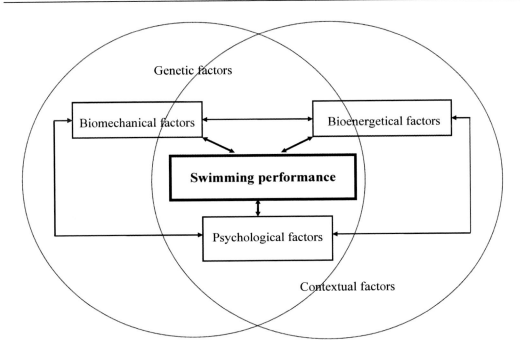

Figure 1. Determinant factors of swimming performance (adapted from Fernandes, 1999). Bioenergetic, biomechanic and psychological factors assume a direct influence, and genetic and contextual factors an indirect influence in swimming performance.

Nonetheless the importance of aerobic capacity in swimming performance (Olbrescht, 2000; Maglischo, 2003), the majority of the swimming competitive events lasting less than 2.30 minutes, even when performed by young swimmers, reflects the importance of the anaerobic energy system as a major contributor during competition. Holmér (1983) referred that for the 50 and 100 m events the anaerobic contribution is about 80%, or even more. Thus, a large anaerobic capacity, with high rates of glycogen breakdown and glycolytic enzyme activities in the muscles, may be a prerequisite for fast swimming (Trappe, 1996). However, quantitative assessments of anaerobic metabolism are difficult to achieve, since invasive measures (e.g. muscle biopsies, blood samples and magnetic resonance) are costly and unavailable in a field test setting, since it demands knowledgeable technicians and require a considerable amount of sophisticated equipment (Rohrs et al., 1990).

The purpose of this study was to implement a simple and non-invasive test that could allow coaches and scientists to have a new tool for anaerobic training control and evaluation of swimmers. This test is called "anaerobic" critical velocity (AnCV) and was based upon the concept of critical velocity. The AnCV assessment method uses the regression line equation obtained through the relationship between sprint swimming distances and the respective time durations, to provide a hypothetical measure of the functional anaerobic capacity of swimmers. As it will be more detailed in the discussion section, the literature related to critical velocity allows us to understand that the longer the testing distances used in its assessment, the stronger the relationships found with aerobic threshold and with long distance performances, allowing one to suppose that the shorter the testing distance, the stronger the relationship with short distance events, and with anaerobic potential. Thus, it was assessed the AnCV in young trained swimmers and tested the existence of a relationship between the

AnCV and the performance during a 100 m front crawl event (first and second 50 m splits, and total time), once it is accepted as a good example of an anaerobic swimming effort for age-group swimmers.

MATERIAL AND METHODS

A group of 32 young trained swimmers of the North of Portugal regional swimming team volunteered for this study. The eight top ranked swimmers from the season 2006/2007 according to FINA ranking tables born in 1994 and 1995 (girls) and in 1993 and 1994 (boys) were included in the study. One girl was excluded of the study, reducing the girls group to a total of 15 subjects. Two boys born in 1993 were matched identically in 8th and 9th position of the ranking and both were included in the boys group (n = 17). The testing protocol was included in a training campus with two days of duration and each subject had an informed consent form signed by their parents authorizing their participation. A medical examination at the beginning of the training season revealed that all subjects were in good general health. The physical characteristics and weekly frequency of training of the female and male groups of swimmers are shown in Table 1.

The test sessions took place on a short course (25 m) indoor swimming-pool with a mean depth of 2 m. Water temperature was 27.5° C (81.5° F). AnCV was assessed through the slope of the regression equation established between the 12.5, 25 and 50 m test distances and the corresponding test times (Figure 2). Each test distance was performed in front crawl, at a maximal velocity. In-water starts and flip turns were used. AnCv (represented as a and expressed in m/s) was calculated from the slope of the distance (y) versus time (x) relationship, and b is y-interception value, according to this equation:

$$y = ax + b \tag{1}$$

A rest interval of, at least 30 min, was administered between the three trials. Furthermore, the 100 m front crawl time values were obtained in a real competition event that took place close to the date of the AnCV assessments. The times of the tests were registered by stopwatches (Seiko®) and the competition times through official electronic timing. AnCV was also converted in 100 m time ($AnCV_{100time}$) throughout the ratio obtained between the distance (100 m) and the corresponding swimming velocity (AnCV).

Table 1. Mean ± SD values for the physical characteristics and weekly training frequencies of the subjects

Parameters	Female swimmers (n = 15)	Male swimmers (n = 17)
Age (years) *	12.3 ± 0.7	13.2 ± 0.7
Body mass (kg) *	45.6 ± 6.6	54.5 ± 7.6
Height (cm) *	160.5 ± 4.7	169.8 ± 9.0
Training frequency (sessions.wk[-1])	6.3 ± 0.5	6.6 ± 0.9

n, number of subjects.

* Represents a significant difference between the two gender groups ($p \leq 0.005$).

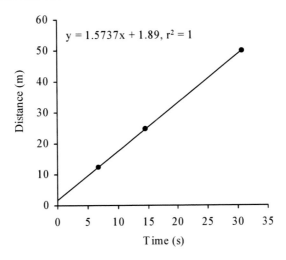

Figure 2. Example of a regression line established between the tests distances of 12.5, 25 and 50 m and the times spent in its achievement at maximum swimming velocity.

Statistical treatment included comparison of group mean values using t-test for independent samples, as well as t-test when comparing tests. The normality of all distributions was verified using a Shapiro-Wilk test before means were compared. Additionally, for estimating the relationships between the AnCV and 100 m front crawl competition values, the Pearson product moment correlation coefficient was used. A statistical significance level of 5% was accepted.

RESULTS

The mean ± SD values of the different variables obtained for both genders and for the total sample are reported in Table 2 (statistical significant differences between gender groups are signed). The value of the AnCV converted in 100 m time was not different from the 100 m front crawl event duration, for each gender group and for the entire group ($p > 0.05$).

Table 2. Mean ± SD values for AnCV, AnCV$_{100time}$, time duration of the 100 m front crawl event, 1st 50 m partial of the 100 m front crawl event, and 2nd 50 m partial of the 100 m front crawl event, in female, male and total group of swimmers

Parameters	Female swimmers (n = 15)	Male swimmers (n = 17)	Entire group (n = 32)
AnCV (m/s) *	1.48 ± 0.06	1.62 ± 0.06	1.56 ± 0.09
AnCV$_{100time}$ (s) *	67.5 ± 2.6	61.7 ± 2.3	64.4 ± 3.8
100 m front crawl (s) *	68.3 ± 2.0	62.4 ± 2.6	65.2 ± 3.8
1st 50 m partial (s) *	33.0 ± 1.1	30.2 ± 1.2	31.5 ± 1.8
2nd 50 m partial (s) *	35.4 ± 1.0	32.3 ± 1.6	33.7 ± 2.1

n, number of subjects
* Represents a significant difference between the two gender groups ($p \leq 0.001$).

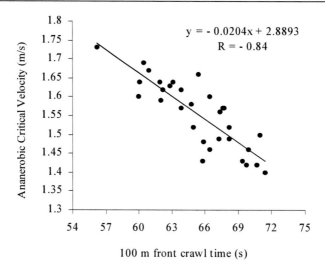

y = - 0.0204x + 2.8893
R = - 0.84

Figure 3. Relationshisp between AnCV and the 100 m front crawl time for the total sample of swimmers (n = 32).

Through the values of the determination coefficient (r^2), and the tests of regression, it was possible to verify a very strong linearity that characterizes the relationship between the distance of the tests and their respective duration, as it is possible to observe in the example of Figure 1 (in the total sample, the mean value of r^2 was higher than 0.99, for a $p < 0.01$).

It was found a high inverse relationship between the AnCV and the 100 m front crawl time duration ($r^2 = 0.72$, $p < 0.0001$) (Figure 3). This relationship was also observed for each gender group: female (r = - 0.47, $p \le 0.05$) and male swimmers (r = - 0.68, $p \le 0.01$).

For the entire group of subjects, a high inverse correlation between AnCV and the first 50 m ($r^2 = 0.76$) and the second 50 m time partials ($r^2 = 0.63$) were found ($p < 0.001$) (Figure 4). Specifically in the male group, these relationships are also observed for AnCV and the first 50 m partial (r = - 0.73, p = 0.001) and for AnCV and the second 50 m partial (r = - 0.60, p < 0.05).

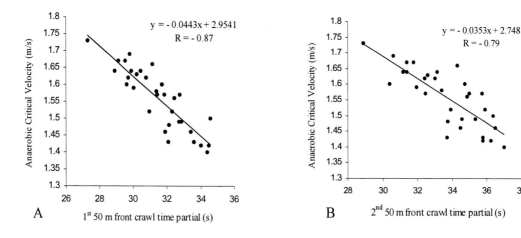

A

B

Figure 4. Relationshisp between AnCV and the first 50 m split time of the 100 m front crawl event (left panel) and the second 50 m partial (right panel) for the total sample of swimmers (n = 32).

DISCUSSION

Monod and Scherrer (1965) have found a linear relationship between total work done by one muscle, or one synergistic muscle group, at several work intensities and time to exhaustion during high intensities exercise. These authors had already observed the existence of a hyperbolic relationship between power output and time to exhaustion, which possesses a curvature constant with an asymptote (Scherrer and Monod, 1960). This asymptote was designated by "critical power" and accepted as a "threshold of local fatigue". The linear relationship was obtained changing the "power" by the "work done" until exhaustion. The slope of the regression line was then considered the critical power value and the y-intercept, accepted as the anaerobic work capacity. When applied to cyclic sports, as running, cycling or swimming, critical power is designated as "critical velocity", which is being considered as a useful tool for estimating aerobic performance (di Prampero et al., 2007).

The critical power concept was specifically developed and adapted for swimming by Wakayoshi et al. (1992a), being defined as the theoretic maximal swimming speed that could be maintained without exhaustion for a long period of time. Wakayoshi and co-authors named this concept "critical swimming velocity" and expressed it as the slope of a regression line established between swimming distance at each corresponding velocity and the duration of exercise, i.e., between the test distances and the time needed to cover them at maximum intensity.

After the pioneer study of Wakayoshi and co-workers, several researchers assessed the critical front crawl swimming velocity as an indicator of the swimmer's functional aerobic capacity as measured through the anaerobic threshold, or equivalent measurement (e.g. Wakayoshi et al., 1992b; Ginn, 1993; Wakayoshi et al., 1993; Wright and Smith, 1994; Vilas-Boas et al., 1997; Dekerle et al., 1999; Fernandes and Vilas-Boas, 1999; Fernandes et al., 2001; Martin and Whyte, 2000; Hill and Smart, 2001; Dekerle et al., 2002; Soares et al., 2003; Greco et al., 2007). These studies allow understanding that the longer the testing (or competition) distances used in critical velocity assessment, the higher the correlation values found with anaerobic threshold and with long distances performances.

Once "critical velocity" was the original expression used to define the velocity sustainable on the basis of maximal oxygen consumption during running exercise (Lloyd, 1966), it is normal that some authors have tried to relate the critical velocity with the velocity corresponding to maximal oxygen consumption. This was accomplished for running and cycling performances (cf. Billat et al., 1999; Morton and Billat, 2000; Berthoin et al., 2003), and more recently also for swimming performance (di Prampero et al., 2007).

Combining the results of these two trends of papers, it is possible to conclude that critical velocity seems to be strongly related both to the velocities corresponding with anaerobic threshold and with the maximum oxygen consumption, suggesting a kind of inconsistency of the critical velocity parameter and/or concept. This is even more noticeable if we consider that Abe et al. (2006) found a strong relationship between the critical velocity determined over 75, 100 and 150 m distances performed in breaststroke by low level swimmers, and a 50 m swimming performance (r = 0.85, p < 0.05), despite the 50 m velocity was about 25% higher than the CV.

This apparent inconsistency, however, may be explained through the methodology used for the assessment of critical velocity. Abe et al. (2006) used, as stated, distances between 75 and 150 m and found relationships with anaerobic performances, despite underestimating their velocities. Di Prampero et al. (2007) found significant relationships between CV and aerobic power, but they used swimming distances between 50 and 200 yards. Moreover, a number of studies concluded about the overestimation of anaerobic threshold by the use of critical velocity, but they selected mostly distances of 200 and 400 m (Wakayoshi et al., 1992b; Wakayoshi et al., 1993; Ginn, 1993; Hill et al., 1995; Ikuta et al., 1996; Fernandes et al., 2001; Greco et al., 2007). Meanwhile, the higher relationships between critical velocity and anaerobic threshold were obtained in studies involving longer distances for the assessment of critical velocity (Wakayoshi et al., 1992a; Wright and Smith, 1994; Vilas-Boas et al., 1997; Dekerle et al., 1999; Fernandes et al., 1999; Brickley et al., 2004). As a consequence, we hypothesize that the longer the distances used for critical velocity assessment, the higher its relationship with lower bioenergetic power regimens, and the shorter those distances, the higher its relationship with more powerful exertions. At this purpose, Wright and Smith (1994) stated some time ago that a long swimming distance, of approximately 15 min duration, should be included as one of the distances used to compute critical velocity, in order to avoid overestimation of these parameter. Dekerle et al. (1999) also stated that swimming critical velocity should be calculated from performances ranging from 200 to 2000 m, i.e., from exhaustion times ranging from 2 to 30 min.

The late reasoning conducted us to explore extreme short distances to assess an AnCV parameter relevant for anaerobic training assessment and advice; a parameter that may replace the controversial b value of the regression line equation. This parameter is assumed, by some authors, to be the swimming distance covered at the expense of the anaerobic capacity (Biggerstaff et al., 1992; Dekerle et al., 2005; di Prampero et al., 2007), although other studies found this value, at least, controversial (Hill et al., 1995; Toussaint et al., 1998; Dekerle et al., 2002; Soares et al., 2003; Almeida e Kokubun, 2004; Soares et al., 2004; Vilar et al., 2004; Thanopoulos et al., 2004; Dekerle and Carter, 2006).

To our knowledge, the present study was the first one to assess the "anaerobic critical swimming velocity" in front crawl swimmers. The present study had also the advantage of being conducted in the best early-teen swimmers of the North of Portugal. The new results found in the present chapter could bring new insights that allow better understanding of the anaerobic bioenergetic system during swimming exercise of short duration and of performance limitations that may be unique to children (Klika and Thorland, 1994).

The high linearity observed in the relationship between distance and time was also verified in the critical velocity related studies that assessed its "aerobic" component (e.g. Wakayoshi et al., 1992a; Wakayoshi et al., 1992b; Wrigth and Smith, 1994; Fernandes et al., 1999; di Prampero et al., 2007). This high linearity shows that it is possible to assess AnCV through simplified calculations, namely using a linear relationship between 3 test distances and its corresponding times.

Both male and female early-teen swimmers presented mean time values of 100 m front crawl similar to those found in other publications for swimmers of the same age and level (e.g. Troup, 1991; Cazorla, 1993; Bar-Or et al., 1994), and higher than swimmers of the same age but of low level of swimming proficiency (Pelayo et al., 1997). The significant differences between genders are easily explained because of the gap in performance levels after puberty, as stated specifically for swimming (Bar-Or et al., 1994) and for sports in general (Van Praagh, 1998). No comparison is made relating the front crawl AnCV values obtained in the present study with the literature, because no other study is available.

Furthermore, a strong inverse relationship between the AnCV and the 100 m front crawl time was found, meaning that 72% of the variability of 100 m front crawl performance is explained by the AnCV. This inverse relationship was also observed for the two 50 m partials of the 100 m event, being 76% and 63% of the variability of the first and the second 50 m time partials, respectively explained by the variability of the AnCV values.

In addition, the value of the AnCV converted in 100 m time was not different of the 100 m front crawl event duration, for each gender group ($p > 0.05$). It occurred precisely the opposite, i.e., the differences in time between the conversion of AnCV and the 100 m event were lower than 1 s, which corroborates the fact that AnCV could be adopted as an index of anaerobic performance in competitive young swimmers. In fact, the 100 m performance at a velocity correspondent to the AnCV exclude the starting action, that will allow to save between 1 and 2 s to the finish time. So, it is possible to conclude that the AnCV overestimates the 100 m swimming velocity, which is coherent with the expectation of relevant aerobic energy participation upon the 100 m event. In future studies, the analysis of the relationship of velocities, and similitude of event times, between the AnCV and the 50 m competition time should be explored. The effect of turning actions is concurrent with the late discussed effect. The effect of the turn during the 50 m test reduce the test time, and increase the slope of the line and, consequently, the AnCV value (that is expectedly lower if no turns are included in the calculations, consequently closer to the 100 m competition time); meanwhile, the 100 m event was performed in a short course swimming pool, including 3 turning actions, and consequently overestimating even more the event velocity. As a conclusion, if the AnCV and the 100 m event were calculated / evaluated without turns, it should be expected a larger difference than the observed one, which will agree even more with a larger participation of the aerobic system in the event, as stated by Gastin (2001), for instance.

AnCV is a mode-specific non-invasive method, which can estimate parameters normally obtained from blood lactate analysis. The method is appropriate for use on subjects of younger ages. Additionally, this methodology is an inexpensive method that allows coaches to estimate anaerobic swimming potential, using minimal equipment (a stopwatch and a PC) and occupying a short time space during training practice. However, this was a preliminary study, which needs future developments, namely in older trained swimmers as well as in other swimming techniques than front crawl.

CONCLUSION

To our knowledge, it was the first time that anaerobic critical velocity concept is presented. The results suggest that AnCV can be used as measure of the anaerobic swimming potential, although future assessments in high level swimmers performing in the four swimming techniques are needed. So, we hope that the AnCV test can be well accepted and applied by coaches in their training control programmes, as well as widely studied by sport scientists.

REFERENCES

Abe, D.; Tokumaru, H.; Niihata, S.; Muraki, S.; Fukuoka, Y.; Usui, S.; Yoshida, T. (2006). Assessment of short-distance breaststroke swimming performance with critical velocity. *J Sports Sci Med* 5, 340-348.

Almeida, A. G. and Kokubun, E. (2004). Validity of y-intercept in tethered and free swimming as anaerobic capacity index. In *CD of Proceedings of the 9th Annual Congress of the European College of Sport Science*. Clermond-Ferrand, France.

Bar-Or, O. (1995). The young athlete: some physiological considerations. *Journal of Sports Sciences, 13,* 31-33.

Bar-Or, O.; Unnithan, V.; Illescas, C. (1994). Physiologic considerations in age-group swimming. In M. Miyashita, Y. Mutoh, A.B. Richardson (Eds.), *Medicine and Science in Aquatic Sports* (39, pp. 199-205. Basel: Karger.

Baxter-Jones, A. G.; Mundt, C. (2007). The young athlete. In N. Armstrong (Edt.), *Paediatric exercise physiology – Advances in sport and exercise science* (pp. 299-324). Philadelphia: Churchill Livingston Elsevier.

Berthoin, S.; Baquet, G.; Dupont, G.; Blondel, N.; Mucci, P. (2003). Critical velocity and anaerobic distance capacity in prepubertal children. *Can J Appl Physiol*, 28 (4), 561-575.

Biggerstaff, K. D.; Hill, D. W.; Jackson, S. L.; Sams, B. R. (1992). Use of the critical power concept to evaluate anaerobic capacity in swimmers. *Med Sci Sports Exerc, 24,* S75.

Billat, V.; Koralsztein, J.P.; Morton, R. (1999). Time in human endurance models. From empirical models to physiological models. *Sports Med*, 27 (6), 359-379.

Brickley, G., Carter H., Dekerle, J., Clark S. (2004). Physiological responses to exercise at critical swimming velocity. In *CD of Proceedings of the 9th Annual Congress of the European College of Sport Science*. Clermond-Ferrand, France.

Cazorla, G. (1993). *Tests specifiques d'evaluation du nageur*. Cestas: Association pour la resherche et l'evaluation en activité physique et en sport.

Clarys, J. (1996). The historical perspective of swimming science. In J. P. Troup, A. P. Hollander, D. Strasse, S. W. Trappe, J. M. Cappaert, T. A. Trappe (Eds.), *Biomechanics and medicine in swimming VII* (pp. xi-xxiv). London: E & FN Spon.

Costill, D. L.; Maglischo, E.W.; Richardson, A. (1992). *Swimming*. London: Blackwell Scientific Publications.

Di Prampero, P. E.; Dekerle, J.; Capella, C.; Zamparo, P. (2007). The critical velocity in swimming. *Eur J Appl Physiol*, 28. DOI 10.1007/s00421-007-0569-6

Dekerle, J.; Carter, H. (2006). The D-T relationship over a century of swimming Olympic performances. A limit of the critical velocity concept. In P. Hellard, M. Sidney, C. Fauquet, D. Lehénaff (Eds.), *Proceedings of the First International Symposium Sciences and Practices in Swimming* (pp. 123-126). Biarritz, France: Atlantica.

Dekerle, J.; Pelayo, P.; Sydney, M.; Marais, G. (1999). Determination of critical speed in relation to front crawl swimming performances. In P. Parisi, F. Pigozzi, G. Prinzi (Eds), *Proceedings of the 4ᵗʰ Annual Congress of the European Colleague of Sport Science* (pp. 127). Rome, Italy: Rome University Institute of Motor Sciences.

Dekerle, J.; Sidney, M.; Hespel, J.M.; Pelayo, P. (2002). Validity and reliability of critical speed, critical stroke rate, and anaerobic capacity in relation to front crawl swimming performances. *Int J Sports Med*, 23 (2), 93-98.

Dekerle, J.; Brickley, G.; Hammond, A.J.; Pringle, J.S.; Carter, H. (2005). Validity of the two-parameter model in estimating the anaerobic work capacity. *Eur J Appl Physiol*, 96 (3), 257-264.

Fernandes, R.J. (1999). Perfil Cinenatropométrico, Fisiológico, Técnico e Psicológico do Nadador Pré-Júnior. Master of Sciences Thesis. Faculty of Sport Sciences and Physical Education of Porto University. Porto, Portugal.

Fernandes, R. and Vilas-Boas, J.P. (1999). Critical velocity as a criterion for estimating aerobic training pace in juvenile swimmers. In K. Keskinen, P. Komi, P. Hollander (Eds.), *Proceedings of the VIII International Symposium of Biomechanics and Medicine in Swimming* (pp. 233-238). Jyvaskyla, Finland: University of Jyvaskyla.

Fernandes, R.; Barbosa, T.; Vilas-Boas, J.P. (2001). Relatioships between some well known indicators of aerobic resistance of swimmers. In J. Mester, G. King, H. Struder, E. Tsolakidis, A. Osterburg (Eds.), *Book of Abstracts of the 6th Annual Congress of the European College of Sport Science* (pp. 1181). Cologne: German Sport University.

Fernandes, R. J.; Cardoso, C. S.; Soares, S. M.; Ascensão, A. A.; Colaço, P. J.; Vilas-Boas, J. P. (2003). Time limit and VO2 slow component at intensities corresponding to VO2max in swimmers. *Int. J. Sports Med.*, 24, 576-581.

Gastin, P. B. (2001). Energy system interaction and relative contribution during maximal exercise. *Sports Med.*, 31 (10), 725-41.

Ginn, E. (1993). *Critical speed and training intensities for swimming: coaches repport.* Belconnen: National Sport Research Center. Australian Sports Comission.

Greco, C. C.; Pelarigo, J. G.; Figueira, T. R.; Denadai, B. S. (2007). Effects of gender on stroke rates, critical speed and velocity of a 30-min swim in young swimmers. *J. Sport Science Med.*, 6, 441-447.

Hill, D. W.; Steward Jr., R. P.; Lane, C. J. (1995). Application of the critical power concept to young swimmers. *Pediatric Exercise Science*, 7, 281-293.

Hill, D. W. and Smart, C. L. (2001). Maximal lactate steady-state velocity and critical velocity in young swimmers. In J. Mester, G. King, H. Struder, E. Tsolakidis, A. Osterburg (Eds.), *Book of Abstracts of the 6th Annual Congress of the European College of Sport Science* (pp. 41). Cologne: German Sport University,

Holmér (1983). Energetics and mechanical work in swimming. In: A. P. Hollander, P. Huijing and G. de Groot (Eds.), *Biomechanics and Medicine in Swimming* (pp. 154-164). Champaign, Illinois: Human Kinetics.

Ikuta, Y.; Wakayoshi, K.; Nomura, T. (1996). Determination and validity of critical swimming force as performance index in tethered swimming. In J. P. Troup, A. P. Hollander, D. Strass, S. W. Trappe, J. M. Cappaert, T. A. Trappe (Eds.), *Biomechanics and Medicine in Swimming VII* (pp. 146-151). London: E& FN Spon.

Klika, R.J.; Thorland, W.G. (1994). Physiological Determinants of Sprint Swimming Performance in Children and Young Adults. *Pediatric Exercise Science*, 6, 59-68.

Lloyd, B.B. (1966). The energetics of running: an analysis of world records. *Adv Science*, 22, 515-530.

Mader, A.; Heck, H.; Hollman, W. (1978). Evaluation of latic acid anaerobic energy contribution by determination of postexercise latic acid concentration of ear capillary blood in middle-distance runners and swimmers. In F. Landry, W. Orban (Eds.), *Exercise physiology* (pp. 187-200). Miami: Symposia Specialists.

Maglischo, E.W. (2003). Swimming Fastest. Champaign, Illinois: Human Kinetics.

Martin, L., Whyte, G.P. (2000). Comparison of critical swimming velocity and velocity at lactate threshold in elite triathletes. *Int J Sports Med* 21, 366-368.

Monod, H.; Scherrer, J. (1965). The work capacity of synergic muscular group. *Ergonomics*, 8, 329-338.

Morton, R., Billat, V. (2000). Maximal endurance time at VO2max. *Med Sci Sports Exerc*, 32 (8), 1496-1504.

Mujika, I.; Chatard, J.-C.; Busso, T.; Geyssant, A.; Barale, F.; Lacoste, L. (1995). Effects of training on performance in competitive swimming. *Can. J. Appl. Physiol.* 20 (4), 395-406.

Olbrecht, J.; Madsen, O.; Mader, A.; Liesel, H.; Hullman, W. (1985). Relationship between swimming velocity and latic acid concentration during continuous and intermittent training exercise. *Int. J. Sports Med.*, 6 (2), 74-77.

Olbrecht, J. (2000). The science of winning. Planning, periodizing and optimizing swim training. Luton, England: Swimshop.

Pelayo, P.; Wille, F.; Sidney, M.; Berthoin, S.; Lavoie, J.M. (1997). Swimming performances and stroking parameters in non skilled grammar school pupils: relation with age, gender and some anthropometric characteristics. *J Sports Med Phys Fitness*, 37 (3), 187-193.

Platonov, V.N. e Fessenko, S.L. (s.d.). *Los sistemas de entrenamineto de los mejores nadadores del mundo. Teoria y prática.* Barcelona: Editorial Paidotribo.

Pyne, D.; Maw, G.; Goldsmith, W. (2000). Protocols for the physiological assessment of swimmers. In C. J. Gore (Edt.), *Physiological tests for elite athletes* (pp. 372-382). Australia: Australian Sports Commission.

Rohrs, D. M.; Mayhew, J. L.; Arabas, C.; Shelton, M. (1990). The relationship between seven anaerobic tests and swim performance. *J. Swimming Research* 6 (4), 15-19.

Scherrer, J.; Monod, H. (1960). Le travail musculaire local et la fatigue chez l'homme. *J. Physiol.*, 52, 419-501.

Soares, S.; Fernandes, R.; Vilas-Boas, J.P. (2003). Analysis of critical velocity regression line informations for different ages: from infant to junior swimmers. In J.-C. Chatard (Edt.), *Proceedings of the IXth World Symposium on Biomechanics and Medicine in Swimming* (pp. 397-401). Saint-Etienne, France.

Soares, S.; Fernandes, R.; Marinho, D.; Vilas-Boas, J. P. (2004). Are the critical velocity and y-intercept values similar when determined with different regression distances? In *CD of Proceedings of the 9th Annual Congress of the European College of Sport Science.* Clermond-Ferrand, France.

Thanopoulos, V.; Bogdanis, G.C.; Maridaki, M. (2004). Evaluation of aerobic and anaerobic fitness of competitive and non-competitive swimmers using the critical speed concept. In V. Klisouras; S. Kellis; I. Mouratidis (Eds.), *Proceedings of Pre-Olympic Congress* (pp. 86-87). Thessaloniki, Hellas.

Toussaint, H. M.; Wakayoshi, K.; Hollander, A. P.; Ogita, F. (1998). Simulated front crawl swimming performance related to critical speed and critical power. *Med Sci Sports Exerc*, 30 (1), 144-151.

Trappe, S.W. (1996) Metabolic demands for swimming. In J. P. Troup, A. P. Hollander, D. Strasse, S. W. Trappe, J. M. Cappaert e T. A. Trappe (eds), *Biomechanics and Medicine in Swimming* – Swimming Science VII (pp. 127-134). London: E & FN Spon.

Troup, J. P. (1991). Developmental changes of age-group swimmers. In J. Troup (Edt.), *International center for aquatic research annual, studies by the International Center for Aquatic Research 1990-91* (pp. 33-41). Colorado Springs: United States Swimming Press.

Van Praagh, E. (1998). *Pediatric anaerobic performance*. Champaign, Illinois: Human Kinetics.

Vilar, S., Fernandes, R.; Campos, A.; Marinho, D.; Vilas-Boas, J. P. (2004). Relationship between the y-interception value obtained by the distance/time regression and b[La]. A study made in age group and junior/senior swimmers. In E. V. Praagh; J. Coudert; N. Fellmann; P. Duché (Eds.), *CD of Proceedings of the 9th Annual Congress of the European College of Sport Science*. Cleremond-Ferrand, France.

Vilas-Boas, J. P.; Lamares, J.P:; Fernandes, R.; Duarte, J.A. (1997). Relationship between anaerobic threshold and swimming critical speed determined with competition times. In *Abstract book of the FIMS's 9th European Congress of Sports Medicine*. Porto, Portugal.

Wakayoshi, K.; Ikuta, K.; Yoshida, T.; Udo, M.; Moritani, T.; Mutoh, Y.; Miyashita, M.; (1992a). Determination and validity of critical velocity as an index of swimming performance in the competitive swimmer. *Eur J Appl Physiol* 64, 153-157.

Wakayoshi, K.; Yoshida, T.; Udo, M.; Kasai, T.; Moritani, T.; Mutoh, Y.; Miyashita, M. (1992b). A simple method for determining critical speed as swimming fatigue threshold in competitive swimming. *Int. J. Sports Med.*, 13, 367-371.

Wakayoshi, K.; Ikut, K.; Yoshida, T.; Udo, M.; Moritani, T.; Mutoh, Y.; Miyashita, M. (1993). Does critical swimming velocity represent exercise intensity at maximal lactate steady state? *Eur. J. Appl. Physiol.*, 66, 90-95.

Wright, B.; Smith, D. J. (1994). A protocol for the determination of critical speed as an index of swimming endurance performance. In M. Miyashita, Y. Mutoh, A. B. Richardson (Eds.), *Medicine and Science in Aquatic Sports, Med. Sport Science* (39, pp 55-59). Karger, Basel.

In: Physical Activity and Children: New Research
Editor: N. P. Beaulieu, pp. 225-239

ISBN: 978-1-60456-306-1
© 2008 Nova Science Publishers, Inc.

Chapter 11

GROWTH RATES BY CHILDREN GRADES 4-8 ON SELECTED FITNESSGRAM TEST ITEMS

Stephen A. Butterfield[1,], Rose M. Angell[2]*
Robert A. Lehnhard[1] and Craig A. Mason[1]
[1]University of Maine, Orono, ME,
[2]Jefferson Village School

ABSTRACT

Children's fitness, once taken for granted, is now the centerpiece of a national effort to improve the health of all Americans (e.g., Healthy People 2010). A critical focus of this effort is the role of school physical education (PE). Recently, concern has shifted to time/space/budgetary constraints and the efficacy of PE to meaningfully impact children's fitness. The purpose of this study was to examine growth rates (i.e., change) in fitness performance by children in grades 4-8 during two consecutive school years (i.e., yr.1 =grades 4-7; yr. 2=grades 5-8). The study's design was multi-cohort sequential (i.e., grades 4-8) with eight repeated measures over 21 months. We used the FITNESSGRAM to test each child's aerobic capacity, muscular endurance, and flexibility. Hierarchical linear modeling (HLM) analyzed the data. HLM is a multi-level form of regression that models intercept and slope for each participant and permits hypothesis testing about rate of change over time, and factors associated with change. In addition to overall growth-rates on selected fitness subtests, we examined the association of age, sex, body mass index (BMI) and participation in organized sports. Our results varied considerably across the three areas of fitness, but four principal findings emerged: a) Very substantial gains occurred in aerobic performance (i.e., PACER score), ($p < .001$); b) we found small but significant gains in muscular endurance (pushups & curl ups) and flexibility; c) high levels of BMI (+1.5 SD) exerted a negative pull on aerobic performance, pushups and curl-ups ($p<.05$); and d) participation in after school sports was positively associated ($p<$

* Contact: Stephen A. Butterfield, Ph. D., 5740 Lengyel Hall, University of Maine, Orono, ME 04469-5740. (O) 207 581 2469; (H) 207 945 3684; (Fax) 207 581 1206; Steve.Butterfield@umit.maine.edu

.05) with better performance, especially PACER score. These results suggest that PE—especially in combination with sports—might foster physical fitness.

INTRODUCTION

The notion that all children should achieve appropriate levels of physical fitness has gained considerable popular support. However, the best means of reaching this important national goal remains elusive. The public, through their elected local school boards often seems reluctant to make youth fitness a priority—at least within the context of physical education (PE) and the traditional 6-hour school day. In some instances, school officials question the efficacy of PE to meaningfully impact children's physical fitness.

Less than a generation ago, children participated in reasonably high levels of vigorous physical activity. Most notably, Ross and Gilbert (1985), employing a large national sample, found that 80.3 % of boys and girls in grades 5-12 participated in PE (Ave.=3.6 classes/week @ 47.6 min./class). They further reported that 45% of boys and 37% of girls participated in vigorous physical activity outside of PE. However, ten years later, data indicated that children were increasingly less physically active (Riddoch & Boreham, 1995). Recently, Sherar, Esliger, Baxter-Jones, and Tremblay (2007) confirmed this trend toward reduced physical activity among boys and girls ages 8-14. Specifically, they found that both moderate and vigorous physical activity by children diminished with chronological and biological age. What seems apparent is a generation long pattern of lower physical activity by children and adolescents.

This disconcerting trend coincides with less time for PE time in the nation's public schools. For instance, contemporary data show an 80% participation rate in PE by 9th graders, which drops to 45% by grade 12. It appears that many schools are reducing PE time to permit greater emphasis on so-called academics. Regrettably, such policy has eluded evidence that time assigned to PE does not limit academic performance, even when PE time is increased relative to other subjects (Faircloth & Stratton, 2005; Morrow, Jackson, & Payne, 1999; Pate, et al., 2006). Furthermore, physically fit children tend to be more involved in community activities, receive PE from a specialist, and participate in regular school-based physical fitness testing (Ross & Pate, 1987).

A number of manageable factors are believed to impact children's physical fitness. The degree to which children participate in year round physical activity is certainly one. Data from a large national study revealed substantial variation in physical activity during the calendar year, with most activity occurring during summer. However, high scoring children on fitness tests (>75th percentile) reported considerably more physical activity during non-summer months than did lower achieving children (<40th percentile). In fact, lower scoring children reported much less vigorous (i.e., high intensity aerobic) activity during the 9-month school year than did their higher scoring peers. This trend is important because most children participate in more than 80 percent of their physical activity outside of PE. According to this data, activity time peaks in the summer, falls off precipitously in the fall and winter, and then rebounds in the spring (Ross & Gilbert, 1985). However, this more than 20-yr-old data does not reflect the substantial increase in 'screen time' experienced by today's youth.

If children's physical activity varies predictably during the year, are their performances on physical fitness tests a reflection of seasonal physical activity? Data reported by Christodoulos, Flouris, and Tokmakidis (2006) indicated improved aerobic performance throughout the school year followed by little or no improvement during the summer break—a time when children are reportedly more physically active. This finding was confirmed by Butterfield, Lehnhard, Mason, and Mc Cormick (2007) who observed improved aerobic capacity by children (grades 4-8) during the course of a school year with a decline in aerobic performance during the summer break.

Another factor related to children's physical fitness is participation in PE. Understandably, PE programs offering a wide array of units produce better test scores than programs with more limited curricula. In addition to more eclectic PE, total time in PE class-- up to a point-- is positively associated with improved fitness. Nevertheless, it is important for children to be physically active in 'other settings' (Ross & Gilbert, 1985). For instance, Butterfield, Lehnhard, Mason, and McCormick, (2007) reported significantly better aerobic performances by children enrolled in organized after school sports than children who did not participate. However, sports participants and non-participants increased their aerobic performances at similar rates. It appears from this limited data that PE and organized sports combine to produce reasonably high levels of aerobic performance during the 9-month school year, but these gains do not necessarily continue during extended times away from school.

Although children's physical fitness remains a matter of national concern (Ross & Gilbert, 1985) there is limited continuous data on seasonal fluctuations in health-related physical fitness. Such information would likely be of interest to professionals as well as those responsible for affecting policy and allocating resources. The purpose of this study was to examine changes in selected items of health-related physical fitness by children in grades 4-7 (ages 8-14) over two school years (yr.1=grades 4-7, yr. 2=grades 5-8; total time= 21 months). We addressed the following specific questions: 1) What is the nature of change in health-related physical fitness by boys and girls in grades 4-8? 2) Are changes in health-related physical fitness associated with age, sex, body mass index (BMI), or organized sports participation?

METHOD

Design

A multi-cohort, sequential design was used in which 3 measurements were collected during year one and 5 measurements in year two. The sample consisted of 91 children in grades 4 through 7 at the start of the project. Permission was obtained from school officials to test more frequently in year two in order to more precisely examine the effect of time on fitness performances. Measurements were taken at approximately equidistant time points, September/January/May in Year 1, and at 8-week intervals throughout Year 2 (September/ November/January/March/May). In addition to being tested at regular intervals, all children participated in regular PE (45min/class by 2 classes/week. The PE program, taught by a state certified PE teacher, with over 20 years experience, consisted of a balanced curriculum aligned with state and national standards (National Association for Sport and Physical

Education NASPE). Moreover, children regularly performed FITNESSGRAM (Cooper Institute for Aerobics Research, 1999) test items (push-ups, curl-ups, and PACER (modified) in PE class. The PE instructor taught children these fitness items and regularly monitored their performance to assure adherence to FITNESSGRAM standards. Prior to data collection, we obtained the University's IRB approval, and all project activities were carried out under their auspices. Because of the repeated measurements nature of this study, children's consent was obtained at each measurement time.

Procedure

The FITNESSGRAM (Cooper Institute for Aerobic Research, 1999) was used to test each child's aerobic performance, muscular endurance, and flexibility. All testing was done during regularly scheduled physical education class. The school's PE teacher (and her assistant) conducted height and weight measurements while the children were in stocking feet. BMI was computed for each child at each test time. School officials verified children's participation in organized sports (school and/or community) at each test time.

Data Analysis

We used Hierarchical Linear Modeling (HLM) to analyze the data. HLM is a powerful tool for examining repeated measures growth-related data. For example, rather than examine growth over time as residualized change or as a simple difference score, HLM allows one to model and test the actual growth curves for children over time. Furthermore, HLM readily incorporates missing measurements at different time periods for different participants.

In an HLM repeated measures design, the overall model is split into two (or more) levels of analysis. Level One essentially describes the individual growth curves that a child experiences over time, such as the level of a given child's aerobic performance at the start of the study, and then how his or her performance increases or decreases over time. Level Two describes how child characteristics influence those individual growth curves, such as how participation in sports at the start of the study may be associated with a higher initial level of aerobic performance or greater increases in aerobic performance over time.

In the present study, a child's eight fitness measurements assessed over two academic years constituted the Level One variables. Student characteristics (e.g., age, sex, & sports participation at the start of the study) constituted the Level Two variables. The present analysis consisted of a four series of HLM models predicting Pacer scores, push-ups, curl-ups, back-right and back-left sit and reach.

RESULTS

Means and standard deviations for participant characteristics and all performance variables appear in Table 1. Information for Level One variables corresponds to all assessments (up to 8) across all participants, while information for the Level Two variables correspond to characteristics of the 91 participants.

A series of HLM analyses were performed predicting Pacer scores, push-ups, curl-ups, back-right and back-left sit and reach. For all analyses, the Level One model predicted a student's performance based on the time of the assessment (months since baseline). The following additional potential Level One effects were examined and included if statistically significant: a 'summer effect' between the end of Year One and the start of Year Two (e.g., an additional drop in performance over the summer months), a differential Year Two time effect (i.e., an increase or decrease in the growth function during the second year, in addition to the overall time effect), and a BMI effect related to the student's BMI measurement at each assessment. The summer effect was assessed through a dummy variable coded as 0 for the three Year One assessments and 1 for the five Year Two assessments. The differential Year Two slope was assessed by a variable coded 0 for the three Year One assessments and the first Year Two assessment, and set equal to the number of months since the start of Year Two for the final four assessments in Year 2.

Table 1. Descriptive Statistics

Level One					
Variable	*N*	*mean*	*SD*	*Min*	*Max*
TIME	662	11.63	6.90	0.00	21.00
PACER	654	28.76	15.90	4.00	89.00
PUSH	475	5.17	5.98	0.00	35.00
CURL	481	34.64	20.94	0.00	75.00
BACK-L	485	9.11	2.71	1.50	12.00
BACK-R	485	9.21	2.64	1.00	12.00
BMI-ASMT	660	21.59	5.07	13.00	40.00
Level Two					
Variable	*N*	*Mean*	*SD*	*Min*	*Max*
GRADE	91	5.52	1.08	4.00	7.00
SEX	91	0.38	0.49	0.00	1.00
SPORT	91	0.78	0.42	0.00	1.00
BMI-BASE	91	21.55	5.28	13.90	39.00

Note: Time = Months since baseline; Pacer = Pacer laps completed; Push = Number of push-ups; Curl = Number of curl-ups; Back-L = Flexibility-left (Back-saver sit and reach); Back-R = Flexibility-right (Back-saver sit and reach); BMI-ASMT = BMI at each assessment; Grade = Year in school; Sex = Child sex (0=Male, 1=Female); Sport = Sport participation at baseline (0=No, 1=Yes); BMI-Base = BMI at baseline.

Level Two predictors included the student's sex (boy=0, girl=1), participation in organized sports at baseline (no=0, yes=1), the child's grade in school at baseline, and the child's BMI at baseline. Grade and BMI were grand mean centered. A preliminary model included these Level Two variables as predictors of the Level One intercept and all significant Level One effects. Non-significant effects were systematically removed resulting in the following final models. For clarity and brevity, only the final models predicting each performance measure are presented.

Aerobic Capacity (Pacer Score)

Analyses resulted in the following Level One and Level Two models predicting Pacer scores:

Level One

$$\text{Pacer}_{ij} = \beta_{oj} + \beta_{1j}\,\text{TIME} + \beta_{2j}\,\text{BMI} \qquad\qquad \text{(Eq. 1)}$$

Where (Level Two)…

$$\beta_{oj} = 21.38 - 6.32*\text{SEX} + 4.67*\text{GRADE} + 2.84*\text{SPORT} - 0.05*\text{BMI} \qquad \text{(Eq. 2)}$$

$$\beta_{1j} = 0.39 + 0.33*\text{SPORT} - 0.02*\text{BMI} \qquad\qquad \text{(Eq. 3)}$$

$$\beta_{2j} = -1.04 - 0.46*\text{GRADE} \qquad\qquad \text{(Eq. 4)}$$

The Level Two model predicting the Level One intercept term (Eq. 2) provides information as to baseline differences between children (e.g., are there sex differences in performance at baseline?). Controlling for other effects, Pacer scores for girls were 6.32 points lower than scores for boys (γ=-6.32, t(86)=-3.533, p<. 01). In addition, older children completed more laps than younger children—equal to approximately 4.67 additional laps with each additional grade in school (γ=4.67, t(86)=4.586, p<.001). Neither baseline sport participation (γ=2.84, t(86)=1.425, p>.10) nor baseline BMI (γ=-0.05, t(86)=-.192, p>.50) had a significant impact on the Level One intercept; however, as these were significant predictors of the Level One Time effect, both were included for model specification.

The Level Two model predicting the Level One Time effect (Eq. 3) provides information as to why children varied in the degree to which their Pacer scores increased (or decreased) over time. For example, youth at the mean baseline BMI who were not involved in sports saw an average slope of .39 over time. However, involvement in sports at baseline was associated with a .33 increase in the Time slope (γ=0.33, t(88)=2.748, p<. 01), for a net effect or slope of .72. Note that because this .33 effect is a difference in the slope, it indicates a cumulative effect that increased monthly, resulting in a steadily increasing difference between these youth over time (see Figure 1). In addition, baseline BMI negatively impacted the Pacer slope over time, corresponding to a .02 reduction in the slope for each one-point increase in baseline BMI (γ=-0.02, t(88)=-2.059, p<. 05).

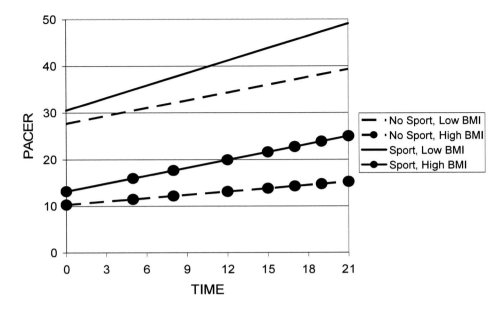

Figure 1. Pacer Score (Completed laps) by Sport Participation and Baseline BMI.

Finally, the Level Two model predicting the Level One BMI effect (Eq. 4) provides information as to the degree that BMI at each assessment influenced a student's performance at that assessment. Specifically, analyses found that having a high BMI at a given assessment negatively impacted older youth more than younger youth. Consequently, with each additional grade in school, the negative effect that BMI had on performance became steadily stronger ($\gamma=-0.46$, $t(89)=-4.688$, $p<.001$).

When predicting Pacer scores, there was no significant Level One Summer effect between the end of Year One and the start of Year Two, nor was there a significant differential time effect for Year Two, and so these Level One effects were not included.

Muscular Endurance (Push-ups)

Analyses resulted in the following Level One and Level Two models predicting Push-up scores:

Level One

$$\text{Push-up}_{ij} = \beta_{0j} + \beta_{1j}\text{TIME} + \beta_{2J}\text{SUMMER} + \beta_{3j}\text{Y2DIFF} + \beta_{4j}\text{BMI} \qquad \text{(Eq. 5)}$$

Where (Level Two)…

$$\beta_{0j} = 2.28 - 2.61*\text{SEX} - 0.79*\text{GRADE} + 2.28*\text{SPORT} \qquad \text{(Eq. 6)}$$

$$\beta_{1J} = 0.07 - 0.10*\text{SEX} + 0.30*\text{SPORT} \qquad \text{(Eq. 7)}$$

$$\beta_{2J} = 1.04 - 2.69*\text{SPORT} \qquad \text{(Eq. 8)}$$

$$\beta_{3J} = -0.03 - 0.26 * SPORT \qquad (Eq.\ 9)$$

$$\beta_{4J} = -0.27 \qquad (Eq.\ 10)$$

The Level Two model predicting the Level One intercept term (Eq. 6) again provides information as to baseline differences between children. Controlling for other effects, girls averaged 2.61 fewer push-ups than boys ($\gamma=-2.61$, $t(87)=-4.750$, $p<.001$). In addition, children performed .79 fewer push-ups at each additional grade level ($\gamma=-0.79$, $t(87)=-2.311$, $p<.05$). Finally, sport participation at baseline was associated with an increase of 2.28 push-ups ($\gamma=2.28$, $t(87)=2.689$, $p<.01$).

The Level Two model predicting the Level One Time effect (Eq. 7) again indicates why youth varied in the degree to which the number of push-ups they performed increased or decreased over time. For males who were not involved in sports at baseline, the overall time effect was not statistically significant ($\gamma=0.07$, $t(88)=0.916$, $p>.10$). In contrast, sport participation at baseline was associated with a significant .30 increase in the slope ($\gamma=0.30$, $t(88)=3.141$, $p<.01$), while being a girl lowered the slope by .10 ($\gamma=-0.10$, $t(88)=-4.653$, $p<.001$).

However, the overall effect for baseline sport participation on push-up performance was more complex than this alone suggests. As reflected in the Summer effect (Eq. 8), youth who were not involved in sports at baseline saw an additional 1.04 gain in the number of push-ups they performed over the course of the summer, although this effect was not statistically significant ($\gamma=-1.04$, $t(89)=1.345$, $p>.10$). However for those involved in sports at baseline, this summer-gain was reduced by 2.69 ($\gamma=-2.69$, $t(89)=-3.023$, $p<.01$), resulting in a net reduction of 1.65 push-ups over the course of the summer. Furthermore, the Year 2 differential time effect (Eq. 9) indicates that the beneficial effect of baseline sports participation upon the slope over time was no longer observed by Year 2 ($\gamma=-.26$, $t(89)=-2.237$, $p<.05$). This complex relationship over time is presented in see Figure 2.

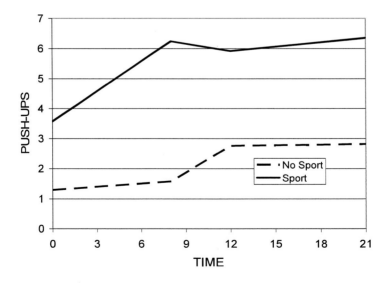

Figure 2. Completed Push-Ups by Sport Participation.

Finally, as reflected in Equation 10, a student's BMI at each assessment significantly impacted his or her performance. Specifically, each additional one-point increase in BMI was associated with a decreased performance of .27 push-ups at that assessment ($\gamma = -.27$ t(90)=-4.761, p<.001). This effect was not influenced by the child's sex, baseline sport participation, grade in school, or baseline BMI.

Muscular Endurance (Curl-ups)

Analyses resulted in the following Level One and Level Two models predicting Curl-up scores:

Level One

$$\text{Curl-up}_{ij} = \beta_{0j} + \beta_{1j}\text{TIME} + \beta_{2J}\text{Y2DIFF} + \beta_{3j}\text{BMI} \qquad \text{(Eq. 11)}$$

Where (Level Two)…

$$\beta_{0j} = 29.18 + 4.50*\text{GRADE} \qquad \text{(Eq. 12)}$$

$$\beta_{1J} = 0.74 \qquad \text{(Eq. 13)}$$

$$\beta_{2J} = -1.21 \qquad \text{(Eq. 14)}$$

$$\beta_{2J} = -0.90 \qquad \text{(Eq. 15)}$$

As reflected in Equation 12, children performed 4.50 additional curl-ups with each additional grade level ($\gamma = 4.50$, t(89)=2.799, p<. 01). In addition, BMI at each assessment negatively impacted the number of curl-ups a child performed, with .90 fewer curl-ups for each one-point increase in BMI at a given assessment (Eq. 15). The existence of a significant time effect and differential Year 2 effect resulted in a more complex association with time. Specifically, the overall time effect indicated an increase of .74 curl-ups per month ($\gamma = 0.74$, t(90)=5.725, p<.001); however, the differential Year 2 effect reduced the slope an additional 1.21 curl-ups per month ($\gamma = -1.21$, t(90)=-4.388, p<.001), for a net reduction of .47 curl-ups per month during Year 2.

Flexibility-Left (Back-saver Sit and Reach)

Analyses resulted in the following Level One and Level Two models predicting Flexibility-Left scores:

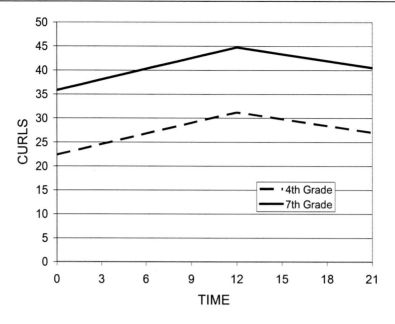

Figure 3. Completed Curl-Ups by Grade in School.

Level One

$$\text{Flex-Left}_{ij} = \beta_{oj} + \beta_{1j}\text{TIME} + \beta_{2J}\text{Y2DIFF} \qquad \text{(Eq. 16)}$$

Where (Level Two)…

$$\beta_{0j} = 7.52 + 1.61*\text{SEX} - 0.18*\text{GRADE} + 0.91*\text{SPORT} \qquad \text{(Eq. 17)}$$

$$\beta_{1J} = 0.02 + 0.05*\text{SPORT} \qquad \text{(Eq. 18)}$$

$$\beta_{2J} = -0.14 + 0.03*\text{GRADE} \qquad \text{(Eq. 19)}$$

As reflected in Equation 17, controlling for all other effects, Flex-Left scores for girls at baseline were 1.61 points higher than boys ($\gamma=1.61$, $t(87)=3.514$, $p<.01$). Neither baseline sport participation ($\gamma=0.91$, $t(87)=1.560$, $p>.10$) nor grade in school ($\gamma=-0.18$, $t(87)=-0.751$, $p>.10$) had a significant impact on the Level One intercept; however, as these were significant predictors of the Level One Time and Year Two differential effects, respectively, both were included for model specification.

Changes over time continued to be complex. Specifically, the overall time effect varied based on whether youth were involved in sports at baseline. The overall time effect for youth involved in sports at baseline was .05 greater than youth not involved in sports at baseline ($\gamma=0.05$, $t(89)=2.955$, $p<.01$). In fact, the overall time effect for youth not involved with sports at baseline was not statistically significant ($\gamma=0.02$, $t(89)=1.163$, $p>.10$). During Year 2, this pattern changed. On average, the existing time-slope decreased by .14 during Year 2 ($\gamma=-0.14$, $t(89)=-7.331$, $p<.001$); however, the degree of this drop in the time-slope varied by the grade-level of the child ($\gamma=0.03$, $t(89)=2.303$, $p<.05$).

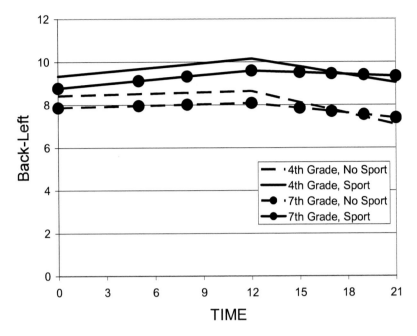

Figure 4. Flexibility-Left (Inches) by Grade in School.

Flexibility-Right (Back-saver Sit and Reach)

Analyses resulted in the following Level One and Level Two models predicting Flexibility-Right scores:

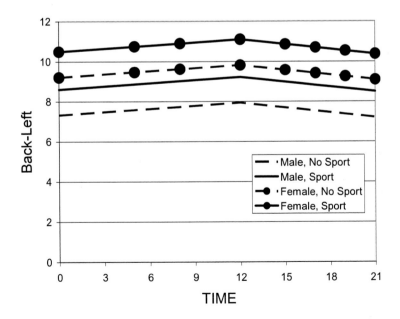

Figure 5. Flexibility-Right (Inches) by Grade in School.

Level One

$$\text{Flex-Right}_{ij} = \beta_{oj} + \beta_{1j}\,\text{TIME} + \beta_{2J}\text{Y2DIFF} + \beta_{3J}\text{BMI} \qquad \text{(Eq. 20)}$$

Where (Level Two)…

$$\beta_{0j} = 7.32 + 1.88*\text{SEX} + 1.29*\text{SPORT} \qquad \text{(Eq. 21)}$$

$$\beta_{1J} = 0.05 \qquad \text{(Eq. 22)}$$

$$\beta_{2J} = -0.13 \qquad \text{(Eq. 23)}$$

$$\beta_{2J} = -0.02 + 0.15*\text{SEX} \qquad \text{(Eq. 24)}$$

As reflected in Equation 21, controlling for all other effects, Flex-Right scores for girls at baseline were 1.88 points higher than boys ($\gamma=1.88$, $t(88)=4.287$, $p<.001$), while baseline sport participation was associated with a 1.29 increase in Flex-Right scores ($\gamma=1.29$, $t(88)=2.439$, $p<.05$). Surprisingly, BMI at each assessment had a positive association for girls, with a .15 increase in Flex-Right scores at that assessment, relative to boys, for each one-point increase in BMI ($\gamma=0.15$, $t(89)=2.938$, $p<.01$). In fact, BMI effect at each assessment was not statistically significant for boys ($\gamma=-0.02$, $t(89)=-0.770$, $p>.10$). Once more, changes over time continued to be complex. The overall time effect was a .05 increase in Flex-Right scores each month post-baseline ($\gamma=0.05$, $t(90)=4.609$, $p<.001$); however, this value was reduced by -.13 during Year 2 ($\gamma=-0.13$, $t(90)=-5.973$, $p<.001$).

CONCLUSION

We found improvement in aerobic performance among all groups over the 21 months of this study. As anticipated, boys performed better at baseline by averaging over 6 laps more than girls. However, boys and girls increased their aerobic performance at equal rates, suggesting similar responses to environmental factors such as physical education and sports. Also noted was a chronological age effect as each additional grade level performed nearly 5 laps more than the preceding grade. These effects are likely attributable to biological events associated with normal growth (i.e., leg length) and maturation in early adolescence. For instance, boys ages 10-14 reach Vo_2 max values of approximately 52 ml/kg/min while 12-yr-old girls consume about 45 ml/kg/min, which by age 16 drops to 40 ml/kg/min. Also, during adolescence, boys increase their muscle mass, and cardiorespiratory organ size, while girls experience more body fat with concomitant reductions in O_2 transport (Krahenbuhl, Skinner & Kohrt, 1985).

Aerobic performance was no doubt related to environmental factors. This finding was most evident when examining the association of sport participation and BMI. Children at mean BMI, who participated in sports, had slopes that were nearly twice that of non-participating children. The result was a cumulative effect whereby after 21 months the performance gap between participants and non-participants—at mean BMI—expanded considerably. Furthermore, this effect was much greater for children at higher levels of BMI (+1.5 SD). At the final measurement time (month 21), children with low BMI (-1.5 SD) who participated in after school sports performed nearly 35 more laps than non-participants in the high BMI group. However, notwithstanding sport participation or BMI status, all groups increased the number of completed laps over the 21 months of the study. These findings are consistent with those reported by Butterfield, Lehnhard, McCormick and Mason (2007), with was one noteworthy difference: In the latter investigation, there was a significant drop-off in aerobic performance over the summer; no such pattern was found in the present study. This summer effect suggests that the nature of opportunities for physical activity varies among communities. Also possible is that opportunities for vigorous activity may be present but less accessible for some children,

The improved performance across time for the entire sample may be due to a learning effect. Possibly, the graded protocol of the PACER systematically shaped performance in such a way that children internalized the concept of pacing as they were being tested. It was apparent that over the 21 months of the study, children adjusted their performance according to the progressive demands of the PACER. In fact, the limited time for PE (40min/class, 2 classes/week) and the broad scope of the PE curriculum (skill development, etc.) negates a physiological training effect as the source of improved children's aerobic performance. Empirical observations made during the test sessions, indicate that improved PACER scores follow more efficient pacing strategy, an observation put forth by Pate & Shepard (1989). This apparent learning effect might be best likened to a 'tortoise and hare' phenomenon. That is, at baseline, many children "took it out too fast' in the early stages of the test.

Although children were instructed to keep pace with the audible 'beep', in many cases they accelerated too quickly, covering the 20 meters well in advance of the next timed cue. Needlessly high speed in the early PACER stages no doubt produced high levels of lactic acid leading to premature fatigue. However, with each test session, the number of children adopting this 'hurry and wait' approach declined as children learned to pace more economically. By the final test session (8th measurement) nearly every child had acquired a reasonably efficient pattern of acceleration. In other words, the slower they were able to go in the early stages, the more laps they completed. Physiologically, this would lead to a more favorable step-wise increase in oxygen consumption from stage to stage. Therefore by effective pacing, children experience a shorter and less steep period of oxygen deficit. Efficient means less reliance on anaerobic metabolism thus delaying a critical (i.e., fatiguing) level of circulating lactic acid.

The increase in aerobic performance we found held true whether a child participated in organized sport or not. However, the rate of improvement among sports participants was greater than their non-participating peers. The reason for this gap cannot be stated with certainty at this time. However, there is a strong likelihood that time spent in practice and competition produced at least minimal physiological adaptation leading to a greater rate of improvement.

Another consideration: Is the PACER inherently motivating? While performing the PACER, children received immediate feedback in terms of laps completed. Therefore it is very easy for children to monitor their progress in easily recognizable steps. Self-monitoring might encourage goal directed behavior. In the final analysis, performance on the PACER appears to be related mainly to normal growth (i.e., leg length), biological maturation and 'learning to pace', findings similar to those reported by Pate and Shepard (1989). Also, after school sports that contain an aerobic component contribute substantially and may partially offset the impact of higher BMI's. Intervening early on behalf of children with high BMI's seems particularly important, as the performance differential between children with high BMI's and their low BMI peers increased with age. Further investigation is needed regarding the cognitive and affective dimensions of aerobic testing and performance. In the meantime, it may be expedient for PE teachers to incorporate the PACER as a teaching as well as an assessment tool. Every effort should be made to provide--and encourage participation in safe, developmentally appropriate, after school sports.

The limited upper body strength and endurance (Pushups) of this group was anticipated, as was the negative association between BMI and number of pushups. Until the proper hormonal profile is in place—especially among boys—large gains in muscular strength would be the exception. Over the first 12 months of this study, children did increase the number of pushups completed followed by a plateau in performance. The initial gain (first 12 months) was probably due to improved muscle fiber recruitment. It must be pointed out that although children at this school worked on pushups as part of their daily routine, they still hit a plateau in year 2.

Abdominal strength/endurance (Curl-ups) scores revealed improved performance during year one only. Again, physiologically, this may have been due to better fiber recruitment with the muscle groups used to perform curl-ups. However, as is the case with any such parameter, motivation can account for some of the unexplained variance. As curl-ups were part of the daily PE routine, we have no ready explanation—other than decreased motivation-- for the decline in curl-up scores in year two.

Growth rates for flexibility (Sit & reach) were likewise marginal. While we found meaningful gains in year one, scores slightly declined (less than an inch) in year two. It is reasonable to argue that a child's range of motion, at any particular joint, may vary from day to day and indeed within any given day itself. And these changes may reflect activity patterns immediately prior to testing thus clouding interpretation. Nonetheless, these results approximate those reported in the FITNESSGRAM (Cooper Institute for Aerobic Research, 1999) as being in the healthy range.

Further research should extend the observation period beyond the middle school years. Given decreased physical activity (and PE) among high school age children continuous data is needed on their fitness status as well. In the meantime, physical educators should be cautious about interpreting a single cardiovascular endurance test as indicative of children's true aerobic capacity. It appears to us that much of the variance in such tests is attributable to a learning effect that may take several test sessions to eliminate. Physical educators should consider the PACER as a powerful teaching tool and as an assessment instrument. We cannot, at this time, make similar recommendations for the pushup, curl-up, and sit and reach test, even when these items are practiced on a regular basis.

REFERENCES

Butterfield, S.A., Lehnhard, R.A., Mason, C., & McCormick, R. (2007). *Aerobic performance by children in grades 4-8: A multiple time point study.* Poster session presented at the American Alliance for Health, Physical Education, Recreation, and Dance Annual Conference, Salt Lake City, Utah.

Christodoulos, A.D., Flouris, A., & Tokmakidis, S.P. (2006). Obesity and physical fitness of preadolescent children during the academic year and summer period: Effects of organized physical activity. *Journal of Child Health Care,* 10, 199-212.

Cooper Institute for Aerobics Research (1999). FITNESSGRAM *test administration manual.* 2nd ed. Dallas, TX: Cooper Institute for Aerobics Research.

Fairclough, S.,& Stratton, G. (2005). Physical activity levels in middle and high school physical education: A review. *Pediatric Exercise Science,* 17, 217-236.

Krahenbuhl, G.S., Skinner, J.S., & Kohrt, W.M. (1985). Developmental aspects of maximal aerobic power in children, *Exercise and Sports Science Reviews,* 13, 503-538.

Morrow, J.R., Jackson, A.W., & Payne, V.G. (1999). Physical Activity promotion and school physical education. *President's Council on Physical Fitness and Sport Research Digest,* 3, 1-8.

Pate, R.R., Davis, M.G., Robinson, T.N., Stone, E.J., McKenzie, T.L., & Young, J.C. (2006). Promoting physical activity in children and youth: A leadership role for schools. *Circulation,* 114, http//www.circ.ahajournals/doi: 10.1161.

Riddoch, C.J., & Boreham, C.A.G. (1995). Health-related physical activity of children. *Sports Medicine*, 19, 86-99.

Pate, R.R., & Shepard, R.J. (1989). Characteristics of physical fitness in youth. In C.V. Gisolfi & D.R. Lamb (Eds.) *Perspectives in exercise science and sport medicine: Youth, exercise and sport.* Indianapolis, IN: Benchmark.

Ross, J.G., & Gilbert, G.G. (1985). The national children and youth fitness study: A summary of findings. *Journal of Physical Education, Recreation, and Dance,* 56, 45-50.

Ross, J.G., & Pate, R.R. (1987). The national children and youth fitness study II: A summary of findings. *Journal of Physical Education, Recreation, and Dance*, 58, 51-56.

Sherar, L.B., Eslinger, D.W., Baxter-Jones, A.D., & Tremblay, M.S. (2007). Age and gender differences in youth physical activity: Does physical maturity matter? *Medicine & Science in Sports & Exercise,* 39, 830-835.

In: Physical Activity and Children: New Research
Editor: N. P. Beaulieu, pp. 241-252

ISBN: 978-1-60456-306-1
© 2008 Nova Science Publishers, Inc.

Chapter 12

PRESCRIBED AEROBIC EXERCISE AND THE RECOVERY FROM TRAUMATIC BRAIN INJURIES (TBI) AMONG CHILDREN AND ADOLESCENTS: A RANDOMISED CONTROLLED TRAIL PROTOCOL

Lawrence T. Lam[*]

Centre for Trauma Care, Prevention, Education, and Research,
The Royal Alexandra Hospital for Children, Sydney, Australia
Discipline of Paediatric and Child Health, the Faculty of Medicine,
The Sydney University, Australia

ABSTRACT

Children with moderate and severe traumatic brain injuries often have associated physical impairments such as muscle weakness, incoordination, and spasticity as long term sequelae of their injury. The current practice is to provide an individualised therapy program consisting of retraining of motor tasks, specific muscle strengthening and coordination exercises, and fitness and balance activities. However the use of an aerobic exercise program specifically prescribed to the needs of patients as part of the therapy regimen has not been used consistently or evaluated formally. This proposed randomised controlled trial aims to evaluate the benefits of including prescribed aerobic exercises as part of the therapy program in this patient population. Eligible subjects for this study will include children and adolescents aged between 6 and 16 years who have sustained moderate and severe traumatic head injuries as determined by their initial Glasgow Coma Scores (GCS) at least 12 months prior to enrolment. Patients who suffer head injuries with a GCS of 13 or higher are classified as a having mild brain injury, 9 to 12 a moderate injury and 8 or less a severe brain injury. Patients satisfying the selection

---

[*] Correspondence to: Lawrence T Lam. CTCPER, The Royal Alexandra Hospital for Children, Locked Bag 4001, Westmead NSW 2145, Australia. Telephone No: +612 9845 3055; Fax. No.: +612 9845 3082; E-mail: lawrencl@chw.edu.au

criteria will be randomly allocated to the control or the intervention groups. Patients in the control group will receive standard rehabilitation therapy as per their conditions. Patients in the intervention group will receive the standard rehabilitation treatment deemed appropriate to their needs, with an extra treatment of a prescribed aerobic exercise program specified by a specialist in sports medicine. The program will last for 12 weeks with 2 sessions per week according to the requirement for significant effects which have been reported in the literature. The primary outcomes of the study are cognition/attention, functional status, mobility, general quality of life, and parental evaluation of the program. Outcome measures have been selected to assess impairment, activity and participation according to the WHO international classification of Functioning, Disability and Health. Data will be collected on each subject at baseline, and 3 months after the intervention. All outcome assessments are measured using standardised and validated clinical assessment tools, or by using calibrated electronic instruments. A standard data analytical approach for randomised controlled trails will be employed for analysing data, taking into consideration multiple outcomes and repeated measurements.

INTRODUCTION

Traumatic head injuries are defined as any non-penetrating injuries to the head in which patients can have extensive skull injuries from collision, impact, or blunt trauma. The severity of brain injury sustained by an individual is classified by the Glasgow Coma Scores (GCS). An individual who suffers head injuries with a GCS of 13 or higher is classified as a having mild brain injury, 9 to 12 is a moderate injury and 8 or less a severe brain injury.

Behavioural and cognitive problems are long-term sequelae of moderate to severe traumatic brain injury (TBI) in children (Levin et al., 1982, Winogron et al., 1984). Conduct disorder, hyperactivity, and cognitive deficits in terms of inattention, initiation, and information processing and memory loss have been identified as major problems (Bijur et al., 1990). A positive correlation has been demonstrated for markers of injury severity such as duration of coma and post-traumatic amnesia, with the neurological, behavioural, and intellectual sequelae at two years post trauma (Ruijs et al., 1993). Longer-term sequelae of TBI such as the ability to maintain employment, psychological/psychiatric problems, and poor relationships with family members have been demonstrated at 20 years post trauma (Klonoff et al., 1993).

The long term physical health of children following TBI has also been shown to be at risk. Results of a recent study have suggested children and adolescents who suffered an acquired brain injury are more likely to be obese as compared with the national population in Australia (Patradoon-Ho et al., 2005). Childhood obesity has been demonstrated to be significantly associated with a multitude of morbidity and mortality among children, and has long term consequences later in adulthood (Must et al, 1992, Must, 1996). The implication for children with TBI is that they might carry an additional burden of disease and ill health as a direct result of their brain injury, as well as the outcome of obesity/overweight which is resultant from TBI.

The current focus of brain injury rehabilitation is often centred on improving the patient's function in day to day activities. This includes reintegration to school and social activities, self-care such as toileting, dressing and food preparation, and vocational planning. Because the focus is on these areas, other aspects of patients' health, such as physical fitness and maintenance of a healthy body weight may be neglected. Other reasons for a lack of focus on physical fitness in rehabilitation programs include the patients' impaired cognition (ie the ability of the patients to participate in the program) and lack of resources (each patient requires an individualised program). Physical fatigue is a common problem noted by clinicians working with children with TBI, and may interfere with their daily activities. Apart from physical fatigue, children with TBI may also experience cognitive fatigue. Anecdotal evidence suggests that cognitive fatigue may be exacerbated by physical fatigue.

The positive effect of physical exercise, particularly aerobic exercise, on the reduction of overweight and obesity among children has been well documented (Sothern et al, 2000, Miller & Dunstan, 2004). In terms of the effect of prescribed aerobic exercise on the health of chronically ill children, there is a growing volume of work (Stranghelle et al., 1988; Shore, & Shepard, 1999; McBurney et al., 2003). However, to the present, there have been no published reports on the effect of prescribed aerobic exercise on the recovery of traumatic brain injury among children. The rationale for prescribing aerobic exercise to children with TBI is to improve cardiorespiratory fitness and thereby potentially reduce the commonly reported physical fatigue. This, in turn, is hypothesised to enhance the overall recovery, including the improvement of cognitive fatigue, of these children.

The aim of this study is to evaluate the effectiveness of an individualised prescribed aerobic exercise program on the recovery from traumatic brain injuries among children and young adolescents. This study will be conducted at the Royal Alexandra Hospital for Children, Sydney, Australia. The hospital is a level one trauma centre for paediatric trauma as well as a tertiary Children's Hospital located in the Western areas of Sydney servicing a child and adolescent population of approximately 3.5 million. Members of the research team of the study include specialists in Rehabilitation, Sports, and Trauma Medicine, a senior Physiotherapist specialised in TBI, a senior Exercise Physiologist, and a senior Epidemiologist and Biostatistician.

METHODS

Study Design

This is a single blind randomised controlled trail of an aerobic exercise program specifically designed and prescribed to individual children or young adolescents who have suffered from traumatic brain injuries. Patients who satisfy the selection criteria will be recruited and entered into the trail prospectively. These patients will be randomly allocated into either the treatment group or the control group. Details of the randomisation are further described in the following section. The treatment or intervention is an aerobic exercise program specifically tailor-made for individual patients. Details are presented in the Intervention section below. Assessments will be conducted at baseline (before implementation of the aerobic exercise program), and at the end of the intervention (i.e. 12 weeks after baseline). A follow up measure on the general quality of life and daily physical activities will also be carried out 6 months post intervention (i.e. 9 months after baseline). All outcomes of the study will be assessed by experts in the field who are blinded to the allocation of groups.

Patients Eligibility and Exclusion Criteria

Eligible subjects of this study will include children and adolescents aged between 6 and 16 years who have sustained moderate and severe traumatic head injuries (as determined by their initial GCS) at least 12 months prior to enrolment. In most cases, these patients have been admitted as inpatients to the Children's Hospital. Moderate and severe TBI patients who have been admitted to the hospital and subsequently discharged are registered on the Brain Injury Rehabilitation Registry of the hospital and are followed as outpatients by the Brain Injury Rehabilitation Team. Subjects who are unable to participate in a prescribed exercise program due to severe physical limitations or severe cognitive disability, such as an inability to walk on a treadmill or sit on an exercise bike, will be excluded.

Recruitment of Patients

Patients with traumatic head injuries who satisfy the eligibility criteria will be selected from the patient list of the Brain Injury Rehabilitation Registry. Suitable patients will be enlisted by the Brain Injury Co-ordinator of the hospital. Parents or caregivers of these enlisted patients will be approached and be informed of the study by research staff. Consent will be sought from parents or caregivers for their children's participation in the trail. Due to the need of information on the effect of prescribed aerobic exercise on different subgroups of traumatic brain injury patients, a mix of different age, sex, and degree of physical disability subjects will be enrolled. In order not to interfere with the on-going rehabilitation that these patients receive, the study is co-ordinated via the Brian Injury Co-ordinator who is also a member of the research team.

Randomisation

Randomisation and treatment allocation will be centralised at the study management centre and will be conducted by the Epidemiologist/Biostatistician who will have no patient contact. In order to avoid the difficulty of having imbalanced allocations to the treatment and control groups, simple randomisation is not recommended. Instead, the permuted block randomisation method will be employed for the allocation of patients. Stratification in randomisation is the method used to avoid imbalance in subject allocation such that certain subgroups of subjects with characteristics more associated with the endpoint are unequally assigned to a particular treatment group. In this study, one particular factor requiring special attention is the sex ratio. It is well established that males have a higher propensity of injury, particularly traumatic brain injuries, than females. The ratio of male to female trauma patients admitted to the hospital is about 2:1. Hence, the randomisation will be stratified according to the sex ratio. Patients will be allocated to either the intervention or control groups prospectively as they are recruited to the study.

Intervention

Consented patients who are randomised to the intervention group will continue to receive the standard rehabilitation treatment deemed appropriate to their needs, with an extra treatment of a prescribed aerobic exercise program specified by a specialist in Sports Medicine and a senior Physiotherapist. The program will last for 12 weeks with 2 sessions per week according to the requirement for significant effects which have been reported in the literature (Takken et al., 2003).

The prescribed aerobic exercise program consists of circuit training. This involves a variety of short activities including cycling, running on a treadmill, stepping on a stepper, rowing, jumping on a mini-trampoline and activities with hoops and balls. Prescription is to be based on the subject's baseline measurement of their physical fitness assessed by peak Oxygen Volume (VO2 max). The aim of the prescribed exercise is for the subject to work at 60-70% of VO2 max for 30-40 minutes 2 sessions per week for 12 weeks. The physical fitness of each patient will be assessed using a standardised protocol, (details are presented in the next section). The heart rate at VO2 max will be recorded as the indicator for measuring the amount of work that the patient achieves during an exercise session. During an exercise session, the patient will wear a Heart Rate Monitor to monitor the intensity of exercise as well as to determine the corresponding VO2 max level. A typical session of aerobic exercise designed for a 14 year old girl who suffered a severe TBI is presented in Table 1. At baseline, the heart rate at VO2 max for this patient was 178 bpm, the exercise aimed to achieve a maintainable heart rate of about 125 bpm. A session will normally last for 50 minutes with 5 minutes for warm-up and warm-down before and after the exercise routine.

The individually-designed program will be carried out in a human movement and exercise laboratory at the hospital. The program will be conducted by a Senior Physiotherapist of the Rehabilitation Department who is specialised in TBI. Throughout the program, children will be under the strict supervision of the Physiotherapist.

Measuring Instruments

The primary outcomes of the study are cognition/attention, functional status, mobility, and parental perception on the general quality of life of the child. Outcome measures have been selected to assess impairment, activity and participation according to the WHO international classification of Functioning, Disability and Health (WHO, 2001). Instruments used in these assessments are all validated and standardised clinical tools that are commonly used in clinical practice.

Changes to cognition, behaviour and attention will be assessed by the Behaviour Rating Inventory of Executive Function (BRIEF, Gioia et al, 2000). The BRIEF inventory is a multidimensional questionnaire specifically designed for assessing the behaviour and cognitive status, particularly executive functions, of children and adolescents aged between 5 and 18 years. This is a fully validated and standardised instrument, and is used as standard practice for the assessment of children with TBI in the hospital's Department of Rehabilitation Medicine.

Table 1. A prescribed aerobic exercise session for a 14 year old girl who has suffered from a Traumatic Brain Injury

Type of activity	Brief description of the activity	Duration	Rating*
1) Treadmill	Walking on a uninclined mini-treadmill with 4.1-4.2 kph	5 mins	3
2) Step-ups	Big steps on stepper at about 60 rpm	5 mins	3
3) Throwing and catching	Bouncing a basket ball off a net to herself and catching it	5 mins	3
4) Hula hoops	Big hula hoop around waist and a small hula hoop around arm. First started with big and then both	3 mins	4
5) Exercise bike	Riding on an exercise bike with resistance level 4 40 rpm	5 mins	4
6) Mini trampoline	Combination of jumping and running	5 mins	4
7) Ball activities	Steeping/ galloping sideways while catching and throwing balls	5 mins	5
8) Skipping	Running step and skipping	4 mins	4
9) Treadmill	Walking on a uninclined mini-treadmill with 4.4-4.5 kph	5 mins	4
10) Step ups	Big steps at 60 rpm and then small steps at 60 rpm	5 mins	5

* Rating on self-perceived exertion: 0=Nothing at all; 1=very weak; 2=weak; 3=moderate; 4=somewhat strong; 5/6=strong; 7-10= very strong.

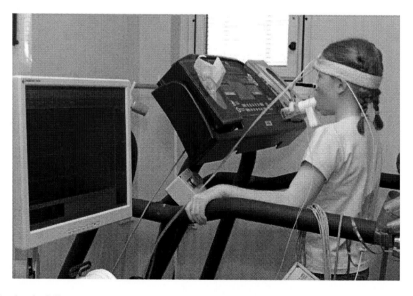

Figure 1. A physical fitness stress test on a Bruce Treadmill with gas analysis using a Medgraphics metabolic cart.

Daily Physical Activities Record

There are different types of activities that your child may do every day. The following is a list that summarises these activities.

Activity Types	Example of activities
1	Sleeping, Resting in bed
2	Sitting, eating, listening, writing, etc.
3	Light activity: standing, washing, combing, etc.
4	Slow walk (<4 km/h), dressing oneself, taking a shower, etc.
5	Light manual work: several house chores, walking at 4 to 6 km/h, etc.
6	Recreational sports and leisure activities: cycling, playing football, trampolining, roller blade, roller skating, skateboarding, scootering, playing, etc.
7	Manual work: lifting, carrying light loads, etc.
8	Higher intensity of sports and leisure activities: swimming, dancing, ice skiing, gymnastics, tennis, horse riding, etc.
9	Intense manual work: competitive sports, carrying heavy loads, jogging and running, training for sports, etc.

To fill in the record, write down the number corresponding to the type of activities that you child has involved at each time slot.

Hour	Min.	Activity	Hour	Min.	Activity
6 am	00		3 pm	00	
	30			30	
7 am	00		4 pm	00	
	30			30	
8 am	00		5 pm	00	
	30			30	
9 am	00		6 pm	00	
	30			30	
10 am	00		7 pm	00	
	30			30	
11 am	00		8 pm	00	
	30			30	
12 noon	00		9 pm	00	
	30			30	
1 pm	00		10 pm	00	
	30			30	
2 pm	00		11 pm	00	
	30			30	

Figure 2. A modified Bouchard activity diary.

Functional status (ie the ability to complete activities of daily living such as dressing, toileting, and feeding) will be measured using the WeeFIM II System (UDS MR, 2004), which is designed as a functional assessment for children and adolescents with acquired and congenital disability (UDS MR. 2004). The WeeFIM II is designed to assess the functional status of children with acquired or congenital disabilities mainly in three domains: self-care, mobility, and cognition.

Mobility will be assessed using a 6-minute walk and the 10 metre velocity tests which are current practice in the Rehab Department. The health specific (but not condition specific) quality of life of patients will also be assessed by using the Child Health Questionnaire–Parent Report (CHQ-PF50, Landgraf, & Ware, 1996).

Secondary outcomes include physical fitness improvement, improvements to physical activities, and body weight. Physical fitness will be assessed using a Bruce treadmill protocol or a fixed bike riding protocol, and gas analysis using a Medgraphics metabolic cart. Values for Heart Rate max, VO2 max and Anaerobic Threshold will be obtained using the build-in computerised gas analyser. (Figure 1) The assessment will be conducted at the human movement and exercise laboratory located at the hospital with a constant environmental control for room temperature. Physical fitness assessments will be carried out by a qualified Exercise Physiologist.

Physical activity will be measured using a modified Bouchard activity diary (Bouchard et al., 1983). Parents or primary caregivers will be asked to conduct physical activity monitoring on their children for one week using the daily physical activity diary. Parents will be asked to nominated three days within a normal school week with one day being a non-school day (i.e. either Saturday or Sunday). They will be instructed on how to fill in the diary using the ratings scale on activity types, to record all activities that their children are involved in at 30 minutes intervals for the full 24 hours of the day. An example of the diary is depicted in Figure 2.

Overweight/obesity will be measured by means of age-specific Body Mass Index (BMI-for-age) according to the international standard (Hammer et al., 1991; Pietrobelli et al., 1998), as well as skin fold measures. Assessments on BMI of patients will also be carried out pre and post intervention.

Other information such as age, sex, cause of injury, time since injury, GCS at admission, physical impairment (hemiplegia, quadriplegia, spasticity, dystonia, ataxia), walking equipment (frames, walking sticks) and splint usage will also be collected.

Procedures

After randomisation, each patient will follow the same procedure for baseline assessments. These include:

- A physical fitness assessment using the Bruce treadmill protocol or a fixed bike riding protocol will be performed (Exercise Physiologist)
- The anthropological measures will be taken to obtain the body weight and height for the calculation of the BMI (Exercise Physiologist)

- Functional status and mobility assessment will be carried out by the senior Physiotherapist based on observation and parental reports (Research assistant)
- Parents or primary caregivers will be asked to complete the BRIEF and CHQ-PD50 (Research Assistant)
- Parents or primary caregivers will be asked to carried out physical activity monitoring on their children for one week using the daily physical activity diary (Research Assistant)

Patients who are allocated to the intervention group will begin the prescribed exercise program in conjunction to the standard rehabilitation treatment. Patients in the control group will receive standard rehabilitation deemed to be appropriate for their condition.

Assessment procedures will be repeated for both groups after 12 weeks. A follow up measure on the general quality of life and daily physical activities will also be carried out 9 months after baseline assessment.

Power Analysis

Due to the lack of available published information on the effect of prescribed aerobic exercise on primary outcomes in this population, a precise power calculation for sample size is not possible. However, a pilot study is currently being conducted aiming to derive this information. The pilot study aims to recruit 10 patients of different age, sex and levels of disability to the intervention group only. The results obtained from these patients will provide information on the effect size of the program for the primary outcomes. This will allow a formal power analysis on all primary outcome measures.

Data Collection and Analysis

Data will be collected on each subject at baseline, and at 3 months (immediately after the intervention). All outcome assessments will be measured using standardised and validated clinical assessment tools, or by using calibrated electronic instruments. Assessments will be conducted by either the qualified Exercise Physiologist or a research assistant employed to the study. Both the Exercise Physiologist and the research assistant are blinded to the allocation of patients. All assessment and clinical data will be collected at the time of assessment, and other clinical information will be extracted from the medical records.

The standard statistical analytical approach for analysing data of randomised controlled trials will be employed. The focus of the study is on the changes in all outcome measures between baseline and the repeated assessment. Since this is a multiple outcome study and all outcome variables are measured as continuous variables, comparisons on the changes in all outcome measures between the intervention and control groups will be conducted using Multivariate Analyses of Variance (MANOVA) to accommodate for the multiple comparisons and to avoid any unnecessary type I errors.

RESEARCH PLAN AND ETHICAL ANALYSIS

Care of Participants

Normal clinical treatment and rehabilitation will be provided to all participants as part of the standard clinical practice. All participants will be monitored closely for any adverse reactions throughout the entire intervention aerobic exercise program. During assessments for baseline and outcome physical fitness levels, a specialist in Sports Medicine will be present to oversee the entire process. During the aerobic exercises, individual patients will be closely supervised by the Senior Physiotherapist. The supervision will be a one-on-one supervision. Should any signs of discomfort or adverse effects be identified, the patient will be advised to terminate the program.

Review of Progress

A study committee consisting of members of the investigation team has already been established for this specific study. The committee is responsible for the proper conduct of the study, as well as to monitor the progress of the research. All aspects of the study, particularly the safety of patients, will be reviewed once bimonthly during the study committee meeting.

Management of Adverse Events

The prescribed aerobic exercise program has been demonstrated to be a very safe intervention program in other disease groups. However, if any signs of discomfort or adverse effects are identified in any one of the patients, he/she will be advised to terminate the program. Any adverse events will be reported to the Human Ethics Committee of the hospital.

Storage and Disposal of Data

All data generated from this study will remain confidential and no report will contain any reference to individuals' name. Upon entering the data into the electronic database, the data set will be de-identified. All personal information will be kept on a separate database with access limited only to the principal investigators. All clinical data collected as hard copies will be stored in a locked filing cabinet and electronic data will be saved on file with password protection. The database and all datasets generated subsequently will be stored in a secured drive created by the Information Technology department of the hospital. The drive will only be accessible to the principal investigators. All paper records will be kept for a period of five years and will then be destroyed.

Potential Risks

There is no particular physical risk that is related to the aerobic exercise program since the program will be specifically designed by a Sports Medicine expert according to individual abilities and needs. Participating patients will be under the strict supervision of a Senior Physiotherapist who is specialised in TBI rehabilitation. Musculoskeletal injuries and delayed onset muscle soreness (DOMS) from strenuous muscle activity are possible during and after aerobic exercise, but the risk is low in a strictly supervised situation. There may be some discomfort for the patient in exerting him/herself physically according to the requirements of the prescription, however this will be closely monitored by the treating therapist and the subject is able to stop the activity at any time.

Potential Benefits

Should positive results be obtained from this study, there are direct implications on the treatments of paediatric TBI patients. If appropriately prescribed exercise enhances the physical fitness of paediatric patients with TBI, it should be incorporated as an integral part of the standard rehabilitation program for future patients. The new program should be able to improve the physical fitness, daily activities, body weight, cognitive functioning, as well as the overall quality of life of patients. There are also indirect benefits from the positive results. An enhanced recovery from any disease or injury can have a positive effect on reducing the parental physical and psychological stresses and strains that are associated with the care of patients.

REFERENCES

Bijur PE, Haslum M, Golding J. (1990) Cognitive and behavioural sequelae of mild brain injury in children. *Pediatry;* 86: 337-344.

Bouchard C, Tremblay A, Leblanc C, *et al.* A method to assess energy expenditure in children and adults. *Am J Clin Nutr* 1983;37:461–7

Gioia GA, Isquith PK, Guy SC, Kenworthy L. (2000). *BRIEF Behavior Rating Inventory of Executive Function: Professional Manual.* Odessa, FL: Psychological Assessment Resources, Inc.

Klonoff H, Clark C, Klonoff PS. (1993). Long-term outcome of head injuries: a 23 year follow up study of children with head injuries. *J Neurol, Neriosurg & Psychia;* 56: 410-415.

Levin HS, Benton AL, Grossman RG. (1982) *Neurobehavioral consequences of closed head injuries.* New York, NY: Oxford University Press.

McBurney H, Talyor NF, Dodd KJ, Graham HK. (2003). A qualitative analysis of the benefits of strength training for young people with cerebral palsy. *Dev Med Child Neurol;* 45: 658-663.

Miller YD, Dunstan DW. (2004) The effectiveness of physical activity intervention for the treatment of overweight and obesity and type 2 diabetes. *J Sci Med Sport; 7 1 Suppl:* 52-59.

Must A, Jacques PF, Dallal GE, Bajema CJ, Dietz WH. (1992) Long-term morbidity and mortality of overweight adolescents. *N Eng J Med;* 328: 1350-1355.

Must A. (1996) Morbidity and mortality associated with elevated body weight in children and adolescents. *Am J Clin Nutr;* 63 (suppl): 445S-447S.

Patradoon-Ho P, Scheinberg A, Baur LA. (2005) Obesity in children and adolescents with acquired brain injury. *Paediatr Rehab;* 8:303-308.

Pietrobelli A, Faith MS, Allison DB, Gallagher D, Chiumello G, Heymsfield, SB. (1998). Body mass index as a measure of adiposity among children and adolescents: A validation study. *J Pediatr;* 132:204–210.

Ruijs MB, Gabreels FJ, Keyser A. The relation between neurological trauma parameters and long-term outcome in children with close brain injury. *Europ J Pediatr;* 152: 844-847.

Shore S, Shepard RJ. (1999). Immune response to exercise in children treated for cancer. *J Sports Med Phys Fitness;* 39: 240-243.

Southern MS, Loftin JM, Udall JN, Suskind RM, Ewing TL, Tang SC, Blecker U. (2000) Safety, feasibility, and efficacy of a resistance training program for preadolescent obese children. *Am J Med Sci;* 319: 370-375.

Stanghelle JK, Hjeltnes N, Bangstad HJ, Michalsen H. (1988) Effects of daily short bouts of trampoline exercise during 8 weeks on the pulmonary function and the maximal oxygen uptake of children with cystic fibrosis. *Int J Sports Med;* 9 Suppl 1: 32-36.

Takken T, Van Der Net J, Kuis W, Helders PJ. (2003). Aquatic fitness training for children with juvenile idiopathic arthritis. *Rheumatol;* 42: 1408-1414.

UDS MR. (2004). *The WeeFIM II System: Functional Assessment for Children and Adolescents with Acquired and Congenital Disability.* NY: U B Foundation Activities, Inc.

Winogron HW, Knights RM, Bawden HN. (1984) Neuropsychological deficits following brain injury in children. *J Clin Neuropsychol;* 6: 269-286.

Wood E, Rosenbaum P. (2000). The Gross Motor Function Classification System for cerebral palsy: a study of reliability and stability over time. *Develop Med & Child Neurol;* 42: 292-296.

INDEX

B

D

E

F

I

J

K

N

Q

T

Y